Periodontitis: Etiopathology and Treatment

Periodontitis:
Etiopathology and Treatment

Edited by **Regina Stuart**

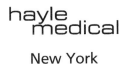

New York

Published by Hayle Medical,
30 West, 37th Street, Suite 612,
New York, NY 10018, USA
www.haylemedical.com

Periodontitis: Etiopathology and Treatment
Edited by Regina Stuart

© 2015 Hayle Medical

International Standard Book Number: 978-1-63241-319-2 (Hardback)

Contents

Preface

This book aims to highlight the current researches and provides a platform to further the scope of innovations in this area. This book is a product of the combined efforts of many researchers and scientists, after going through thorough studies and analysis from different parts of the world. The objective of this book is to provide the readers with the latest information of the field.

Pathogenesis and treatment of periodontitis consists of extensive reviews on etiopathogenic factors of periodontal tissue destruction that is associated with microbial dental plaque and the host response elements. This book discusses the modalities of adjunctive treatment. Some of the major issues presented are microbial pathogenic factors of P. gingivalis, the relationship between metabolic syndrome and periodontal disease, management of open gingival embrasures, and laser application in periodontal treatment.

I would like to express my sincere thanks to the authors for their dedicated efforts in the completion of this book. I acknowledge the efforts of the publisher for providing constant support. Lastly, I would like to thank my family for their support in all academic endeavors.

Editor

Part 1

Etiopathogenesis of Periodontal Tissue Destruction

The Role of Immuno-Inflammatory Response in the Pathogenesis of Chronic Periodontitis and Development of Chair-Side Point of Care Diagnostics

Marcela Hernández[1,2], Rolando Vernal[1], Timo Sorsa[3,4],
Taina Tervahartiala[3,4], Päivi Mäntylä[4] and Jorge Gamonal[1]
[1]Laboratory of Periodontal Biology, Faculty of Dentistry, University of Chile
[2]Department of Pathology, Faculty of Dentistry, University of Chile
[3]Department of Oral and Maxillofacial Diseases, Helsinki University Central Hospital
[4]Institute of Dentistry, University of Helsinki, Helsinki,
[1,2]Chile
[3,4]Finland

1. Introduction

Periodontitis is a chronic infection that results from the interaction of periodontopathogenic bacteria and host inflammatory and immune responses and is the most common bacterial infection worldwide. Estimates reveal that 10-15 % of adults have advanced periodontitis, and periodontal disease can contribute to widespread oral health dysfunction and enhanced susceptibility to other systemic diseases (Pussinen et al. 2007).

Bacterial biofilms are regarded to be the primary aetiological factor in the initiation of gingival inflammation and subsequent destruction of periodontal tissues (Offenbacher 1996) and three major specific pathogens have been repeatedly identified as etiologic agents, namely *Aggregatibacter (Actinobacillus) actinomycetemcomitans* (Aa), *Porphyromonas gingivalis* (Pg) and *Tannerella forsythia* (Tf) (Socransky et al. 1998). Although chronic exposure to bacteria and their products is a prerequisite for gingival inflammation and periodontal tissue destruction to occur, the major causative factor of soft- and hard- tissue breakdown associated with periodontitis is currently attributed to the host's immune-inflammatory response to bacterial challenge. Furthermore, the nature of the inflammatory response might determine the destructive character of the disease (Gemmell, Yamazaki, and Seymour 2002).

The theoretical manner in which periodontal disease progresses has long been a subject of debate. It is currently agreed that destructive periodontal disease progresses by means of asynchronous bursts of activity (Haffajee and Socransky 1986). According to this theory, periodontal tissue support is lost during short, acute episodes followed by prolonged periods of quiescence (Reddy, Palcanis, and Geurs 1997). This model implies that etiologic factors involved in periodontal tissue destruction would change according to the sequential occurrence of episodes of disease activity and quiescence or remission.

Determination of periodontal diagnosis and the extent and severity of periodontal tissue damage through standard periodontal assessment has traditionally been based on an array of clinical measurements, including probing depth (PD), clinical attachment level (CAL), bleeding on probing (BOP), plaque index (PI) and radiographic findings. Though disease activity is generally associated to the loss of soft or hard tissue attachment to the tooth, recording of clinical attachment by periodontal probing at sequential examinations is the most common method to diagnose a progressive periodontal disease (Reddy, Palcanis, and Geurs 1997). However, clinical measurements provide information about past periodontal tissue destruction and do not elucidate the current state of the disease activity nor predict the future bone resorption (Armitage 2004). Thus, despite the value of these clinical methods, such techniques often result in inconsistent diagnoses, as well as an inability to reliably predict a patient´s response to treatment (Offenbacher et al. 2007). A reason for the limited success in predicting the future course of disease in some individuals is that the clinical phenotype does not reflect the underlying biologic processes that occur at the biofilm-gingival interface (Offenbacher et al. 2007).

The biologic phenotype underlying chronic periodontitis, including the biofilm and the host response, tend to vary among individuals despite a similar clinical diagnostic category (Offenbacher et al. 2007). Consequently, disease screening should ideally be based on clinical determinations and the biologic phenotype (Page and Kornman 1997). Other associated factors include environmental exposures, as well as differences in genetic and possibly epigenetic composition (Page and Kornman 1997).

The biological changes underlying the transition process from gingival health to early inflammatory changes involve local increase in vascular permeability, edema and the recruitment and activation of polymorphonuclear neutrophils (PMN) (Delima and Van Dyke 2003). Acquired immune response becomes involved once antigen-presenting cells interact with immunocompetent cells, such as T and B lymphocytes, leading to the expansion of antibody-secreting plasma cells and the development of the chronic lesion (Gemmell and Seymour 2004). Bacterial–host interactions at the biofilm–periodontium interface trigger the synthesis of cytokines and other inflammatory mediators that promote the release of enzymes and bone-associated molecules that finally induce the alterations of the connective tissue metabolism and the destruction of the tooth supporting alveolar bone (Bhavsar, Guttman, and Finlay 2007; Graves 2008; Houri-Haddad, Wilensky, and Shapira 2007).

In addition to local periodontal tissue involvement, chronic infection of the periodontium together with continuous up-regulation of pro-inflammatory responses and immune mediators may contribute to systemic sequel including diabetes, preterm delivery of low-weight birth babies, lung inflammation, arthritis and cardiovascular diseases (CVD). In fact, numerous case-control and cohort studies have demonstrated that periodontitis patients exert increased risk for CVD, acute myocardial infarction (AMI), peripheral arterial disease and CVD, relative to patients with healthy periodontium (Mattila, Pussinen, and Paju 2005; Chen et al. 2008; Mattila et al. 2000; Alfakry et al. 2011; Persson et al. 2003). Although the associations of periodontal diseases with CVD have been investigated in several clinical studies the pathogenic mechanisms and links between both diseases are not completely clarified (Bahekar et al. 2007; Buduneli et al. 2011).

The Role of Immuno-Inflammatory Response in the Pathogenesis of Chronic Periodontitis and Development
of Chair-Side Point of Care Diagnostics

5

A major challenge in clinical periodontics is to find a reliable molecular marker of periodontal support loss with high sensitivity, specificity and utility (Buduneli & Kinane 2011). Molecules derived from inflamed host tissue and pathogenic bacteria have the potential of being used as markers of periodontitis; however, molecular markers of bone resorption have advantages as they relate to specificity for bone, easy detection, pre-analytic stability and availability of sensitive and specific assays for detection (Forde et al. 2006). Up to now, at least 90 different components in gingival crevicular fluid (GCF) and oral fluids have been evaluated as possible biomarkers for diagnosis of periodontal disease and they can be divided into three major groups: (1) host derived enzymes and their inhibitors, (2) inflammatory mediators and host response modifiers, and (3) by-products of tissue breakdown, mainly of bone resorption (Lamster and Ahlo 2007).

Recently, the use of oral fluids such as GCF, whole saliva and oral rinse as a means of evaluating host-derived products, as well as exogenous components (for instance: oral microorganisms and microbial products), has been suggested as potential sources and diagnostic markers, respectively for disease susceptibility (Sahingur and Cohen 2004; Buduneli and Kinane 2011). In fact, as whole saliva represents a pooled sample with contributions from all periodontal sites, analysis of biomarkers in saliva may provide an overall assessment of disease status as opposed to site-specific GCF analysis. This review will analyze the mechanisms involved in the breakdown of periodontal supporting tissues during chronic periodontitis, with a special focus on the role of T cells, matrix metalloproteinases (MMPs) and the development of chair side point-of-care diagnostic aids applicable to monitor both, periodontal and systemic inflammation.

2. T cells and related cytokines

Nowadays, it has been clearly demonstrated that increases in receptor activator of nuclear factor-kappa B ligand (RANKL) mRNA and protein levels in periodontal tissues stimulate the differentiation of monocyte-macrophage precursor cells into osteoclasts and the maturation and survival of the osteoclasts, leading to alveolar bone loss (Hernandez et al. 2006; Ohyama et al. 2009; Nagasawa et al. 2007; Gaffen and Hajishengallis 2008; Crotti et al. 2003; Hofbauer and Heufelder 2001; Kawai et al. 2006; Vernal et al. 2004). In this context, during inflammatory response characteristic of periodontitis, proinflammatory cytokines, such as interleukin (IL)-1β, IL-6, IL-17, and tumor necrosis factor (TNF)-α, can stimulate periodontal osteoblasts to express membrane-bound RANKL (Gaffen and Hajishengallis 2008; Acosta-Rodriguez et al. 2007; Harrington, Mangan, and Weaver 2006; Mosmann and Sad 1996; Graves 2008). In addition to osteoblasts, RANKL is expressed by a number of other cell types, mainly CD4+ T lymphocytes (Kawai et al. 2006).

CD4+ T lymphocytes represent one of the main components of the adaptive immune response and are the predominant cell type present in periodontitis gingival tissues (Hofbauer and Heufelder 2001; Kawai et al. 2006). After antigenic stimulation, naïve CD4+ T cells proliferate and may differentiate into distinct effector subsets, which have been classically divided on the basis of their cytokine production profiles into T helper (Th) 1 and Th2 cells (Mosmann et al. 1986). Th1 cells are characterized by the secretion of interferon (IFN)-γ, IL-2, IL-12, TNF-α and TNF-β, and are involved in the eradication of intracellular pathogens. Conversely, Th2 cells are characterized by secretion of IL-4, IL-5, IL-6, IL-9 and IL-13, which are potent activators of B cells, are involved in the elimination of extracellular microorganisms and parasitic infections, and are also responsible for allergic disorders (Mosmann and Sad 1996; Mosmann and Coffman 1989).

More recently, two new subsets of CD4+ T lymphocytes have been characterized, the Th17 subset, which follows different polarizing conditions and displays different functional activities than Th1 and Th2 cells, and the regulatory T (Treg) cell subset with suppressor functions (Mosmann and Sad 1996). Activated human Th17 cells are phenotypically identified as CCR2+CCR5- (Honma et al. 2007), whereas human memory CD4+ T cells producing IL-17 and expressing transcription factor related to orphan nuclear receptor C2 (RORC2) mRNA are CCR6+CCR4+ (Acosta-Rodriguez et al. 2007). Th17 cells secrete several pro-inflammatory cytokines such as IL-6, IL-17, IL-21, IL-22, IL-23, IL-26, TNF-α, and particularly RANKL (Liang et al. 2006; Harrington et al. 2005; Park et al. 2005).

The role of Th17 cells in host defence against pathogens is just emerging, particularly on their destructive potential in periodontal diseases. Increased levels of IL-17 were detected in GCF and in biopsy samples from periodontal lesions, both at the mRNA and protein levels, in patients with chronic periodontitis and these increased levels have been associated to CD4+ T cells (Takayanagi 2005; Vernal et al. 2005; Takahashi et al. 2005). Furthermore, RANKL was synthesized within periodontal lesions where IL-17 was produced by activated gingival T cells (Takahashi et al. 2005; Kramer and Gaffen 2007). These data are reinforced by the over-expression of RORC2 mRNA in active lesions from chronic periodontitis patients (Dezerega et al. 2010). Taken together, these data establish that Th17 cells represent the osteoclastogenic Th subset on CD4+ T lymphocytes, inducing osteoclastogenesis and bone resorption through synthesizing IL-17 and RANKL (Figure 1).

Diverse studies have analyzed the concentrations of RANKL and osteoprotegerin (OPG) in GCF of periodontitis patients and healthy subjects. In general, they show great variation from study to study, but the ratio of RANKL/OPG has a consistent tendency to increase from periodontal health to periodontitis and to decrease following non-surgical periodontal treatment (Bostanci et al. 2008, Buduneli et al. 2009). In a cross-sectional study, Bostanci et al. (2008) quantified the RANKL and OPG levels in GCF from 21 healthy subjects, 22 gingivitis, 28 chronic periodontitis (CP), 25 generalized aggressive periodontitis (GAgP) and 11 CP immunosuppressed patients, detecting that RANKL levels increased and OPG decreased in periodontitis patients compared with either gingivitis or healthy individuals, and concluded that RANKL/OPG ratio may predict disease occurrence (Bostanci et al. 2007). The same authors analyzed the GCF levels of TACE, an enzyme involved in the activation and secretion of RANKL from Th17 lymphocytes. They found that GCF TNF-alpha converting enzyme (TACE) levels were higher in periodontitis and TACE showed positive correlation with PD, CAL, and GCF RANKL concentration (Bostanci et al. 2008). In an intervention study (Buduneli et al. 2009), GCF levels of RANKL, OPG, and IL-17 were determined at baseline and also 4 weeks after completion of initial periodontal treatment in 10 smoker and 10 non-smoker patients with chronic periodontitis. The authors concluded that neither smoking nor periodontal inflammation seemed to influence GCF RANKL levels in systemically healthy patients with chronic periodontitis. Smoking and non-smoking patients with chronic periodontitis were affected similarly by the initial periodontal treatment with regard to GCF IL-17 and OPG concentrations.

The Role of Immuno-Inflammatory Response in the Pathogenesis of Chronic Periodontitis and Development
of Chair-Side Point of Care Diagnostics

7

On the other hand, Buduneli *et al.* (2008) selected 67 untreated CP and 44 maintenance patients and established RANKL and OPG salivary levels, demonstrating that RANKL and OPG may be affected by smoking and significant differences between treated *versus* untreated CP were found. CP patients (35 subjects) and 38 periodontally healthy subjects were analyzed by Sakellari *et al.* (2008). The GCF levels of RANKL increased in CP patients compared with healthy controls and these higher levels correlated with detection of *Treponema denticola* and *Porphyromonas gingivalis*, but not with clinical parameters (Sakellari, Menti, and Konstantinidis 2008). Arikan et al. (2011) evaluated RANKL, OPG, ICTP, and albumin levels in peri-implant sulcular fluid samples from 18 root-type implants with peri-implantitis in 12 patients and 21 clinically healthy implants in 16 other patients. The authors suggested that local levels of carboxyterminal telopeptide pyridinoline cross-links of type I collagen (ICTP) and OPG reflect an increased risk of alveolar bone loss around dental implants, and their local levels may help to distinguish diseased and healthy sites (Arikan, Buduneli, and Lappin 2011). Finally, Silva *et al.* (2008) performed a longitudinal follow-up of 56 patients affected of moderate to severe CP until determination of disease progression, detecting higher RANKL, IL-1β levels and MMP-13 activity in active sites compared with inactive sites (Silva et al. 2008). Taken together, RANKL levels are promising as discloser of periodontal disease activity. Finally, carboxyterminal telopeptide pyridinoline cross-links of type I collagen (ICTP), released into the periodontal tissues as a consequence of MMP-mediated alveolar bone resorption has been suggested to predict future bone loss, to correlate with clinical parameters and putative periodontal pathogens, and also to reduce following periodontal therapy, representing a potentially valuable diagnostic marker for periodontal disease (Giannobile, Al-Shammari, and Sarment 2003).

3. Matrix metalloproteinases (MMPs): Destructive versus regulative roles

Periodontal tissue homeostasis depends on the balanced and regulated degradation of extracellular matrix (ECM) proteins. In addition, the molecular organization of extracellular matrix is known to profoundly influence cell behavior. An unbalance in favor of collagenous matrix degradation will result in the loss of periodontal supporting tissue, the hallmark of chronic periodontitis (Reynolds and Meikle 1997). MMPs enclose a family of genetically distinct but structurally related zinc-dependent proteolytic enzymes that can synergistically degrade almost all extracellular matrix and basement membrane components and regulate several cellular processes, including inflammatory responses (McQuibban et al. 2001; McQuibban et al. 2002; Overall, McQuibban, and Clark-Lewis 2002). The 23 MMPs expressed in humans are classified based on their primary structures and substrate specificities into different groups that include collagenases (MMP-1, -8, -13), gelatinases (MMP-9, -2), membrane-type MMPs (MT-MMPs, MMP-14, -15, -16, -17, -24, -25) and other MMPs (Folgueras et al. 2004).

MMPs share a basic structure composed of three domains, namely the pro-peptide, catalytic and the hemopexin-like domain; the latter is linked to the catalytic domain via a flexible hinge region. The proteolytic activity of MMPs is subjected to a complex regulation that involves three major steps (Kessenbrock, Plaks, and Werb 2010): 1) gene expression, 2) conversion of zymogen to active enzyme and 3) specific inhibitors. MMPs are initially synthesized as pro-enzymes which are enzymatically inactive because of the interaction between the cysteine residue of the prodomain with the zinc ion of the catalytic site, known as cysteine switch. Disruption of this interaction through proteolytic removal of the prodomain or chemical modification results in enzyme activation. There are several proteinases that mediate MMP activation, including plasmin, furin and active MMPs that assemble in enzymatic amplifying loops. Once activated, the most important physiological inhibitors are tissue inhibitors of MMPs (TIMPs) -1, -2, -3 and -4 (Folgueras et al. 2004). Herein, the pathophysiological significance of increased MMP expression in periodontitis will rely ultimately on the presence of endogenous inhibitors and activating enzymes that will determine overall MMP activity (Sorsa, Mantyla et al. 2011; Buduneli and Kinane 2011).

MMPs, especially those with collagen-degrading properties, such as MMP-8, MMP-13 and MMP-9, have been recognized as the key proteases involved in destructive periodontal diseases and have widely been demonstrated in inflamed periodontal tissues and in oral fluids in association with supporting tissue loss by different analytic methods, including ELISA, immunofluorometric assays (IFMA), checkerboard method and immuno blots, (Folgueras et al. 2004; McQuibban et al. 2001; McQuibban et al. 2002; Overall, McQuibban, and Clark-Lewis 2002; Sorsa et al. 2006; Sorsa, Tjaderhane, and Salo 2004). All human MMPs are known to exist in multiple forms, i.e. latent pro-forms, active or activated forms, fragmented species, complexed species and cell-bound forms (Sorsa, Mantyla et al. 2011). The expression of different MMP isoforms in oral fluid samples can be analyzed with western immunoblotting, whereas a limitation of conventional MMP immunoassays used in periodontal research, such as ELISA, is that they do not differentiate these forms.

MMP-8 is mainly produced by neutrophils (PMN), but it can also be expressed by gingival fibroblasts, endothelial cells, epithelial cells, plasma cells, macrophages and bone cells (Heikkinen et al. 2010). MMP-8 is the major collagenolytic MMP in gingival tissue and oral fluids and elevated levels have been associated with the severity of periodontal inflammation and disease (Mantyla et al. 2006), whereas basal physiologic levels might be associated to tissue homeostasis and even to be protective against disease (Kuula et al. 2009). Among total collagenases in GCF, MMP-8 accounts for about 80%, whereas MMP-13, for up to 18% and MMP-1 is seldom detected (Golub et al. 2008).

MMP-13 has been identified in gingival sulcular epithelium, fibroblasts, macrophages, plasma cells and osteoblasts (Tervahartiala et al. 2000; Hernandez et al. 2006; Rydziel, Durant, and Canalis 2000). MMP-13 has been implicated in bone resorptive process, along with MMP-9 (Hill et al. 1995; Hill et al. 1994; Holliday et al. 1997). Total MMP-13 levels, as well as proenzyme (~60 kDa) and its active forms (~45-50 kDa), have been shown to increase in chronic periodontitis versus healthy sites in GCF in association with clinical periodontal parameters (Tervahartiala et al. 2000; Kiili et al. 2002; Ilgenli et al. 2006).

MMP-9 is the major gelatinase in oral fluids (Makela et al. 1994). As MMP-8, MMP-9 is present in granules of PMN and it is also expressed in a variety of other cell types, including resident periodontal cells, such as fibroblasts, keratinocytes and infiltrating leukocytes, like macrophages and plasma cells (Sorsa, Tjaderhane, and Salo 2004; Makela et al. 1994). Total MMP-9 levels and its active form have been demonstrated to significantly increase with periodontal inflammation in comparison to controls, composed of gingivitis and healthy subjects, and to drop along with inflammation after periodontal therapy (Makela et al. 1994; Bildt et al. 2008) (Figure 1).

Genetic variations can influence MMP transcription levels and protein synthesis. Despite the genetic background of periodontal diseases and the wide involvement of MMP-9, MMP-8 and MMP-13, MMP gene polymorphisms studied in different ethnic populations have not

The Role of Immuno-Inflammatory Response in the Pathogenesis of Chronic Periodontitis and Development
of Chair-Side Point of Care Diagnostics

9

been able to conclude specific associations with the susceptibility to develop periodontitis or disease severity. Similar allele and genotype frequencies have been demonstrated at the MMP-9 -1562 and –R+279Q polymorphic sites between periodontitis patients and healthy controls, despite the presence of significantly increased protein levels in serum and saliva of diseased subjects (Isaza-Guzman et al. ; Loo et al. 2011; de Souza et al. 2005; Chen et al. 2007; Gurkan et al. 2008). Nevertheless, the -1572T allele might be associated with a severe form of chronic periodontitis in men (Holla et al. 2006). Similarly, no differences in MMP-13- 77 A/G and -11 A /12 A polymorphic sites have been found for periodontitis patients (Pirhan et al. 2009), whereas no genetic studies are currently available for MMP-8.

Regarding, especially MMP-8, -9 and -13, it is noteworthy that clinical progression of periodontitis in active *versus* inactive sites and/or patients has been repeatedly demonstrated to be reflected as pathologically excessive elevation of either active MMP forms, i.e. conversion of latent pro-form to active form, or enzyme activity assessed by functional assays, i.e. total activated enzyme unbound to TIMPs, in GCF/peri-implant sulcular fluid (PISF), mouth-rinse and saliva samples collected from periodontitis/peri-implantitis sites and patients (Hernandez et al. 2010; Hernandez Rios et al. 2009; Sorsa, Mantyla et al. 2011). Regarding periodontitis/peri-implantitis progression in disease-active sites, pro-MMP-8, -9 and -13 have been demonstrated to be activated by independent and/or co-operative cascades involving other host proteinases (MMPs, serine proteases), reactive oxygen species and/or microbial proteases (Buduneli et al. 2011; Hernandez et al. 2010; Hernandez Rios et al. 2009). GCF collagenase activity and MMP-8 activation are also found to correlate with the levels of type I collagen breakdown fragments overcoming the protective shield provided by TIMP-1 (Reinhardt et al. 2010; Sorsa, Mantyla et al. 2011). Similarly, MMP-13 activity and ICTP have shown to increase in active sites compared with inactive sites from progressive periodontitis patients or healthy subjects (Hernandez Rios et al. 2009).

Clinical trials testing subantimicrobial dose doxycycline (SDD, synthetic FDA-approved MMP-inhibitor) medication have repeatedly reported an association between improvement of clinical parameters and reduction of GCF and serum MMP-8, -13 and -9 activation and levels (Reinhardt et al. 2010, Sorsa et al. 2011). It is possible to monitor the effect of periodontal treatment and adjunctive SDD medication by point-of-care MMP-8 immunoassays (Sorsa, Tervahartiala et al. 2011).

MMPs can also act by regulating many other MMP activation cascades. This later role could even be more significant in periodontal tissue destruction than direct collagenolytic activity, in a way that a subtle change in regulating MMPs might result in widespread MMP activation and consequent tissue destruction (Folgueras et al. 2004; Hernandez et al. 2010). MMP-14 activates the collagenases MMP-8 and MMP-13 *in vitro* (Holopainen et al. 2003; Folgueras et al. 2004; Han et al. 2007; Dreier et al. 2004; Knauper et al. 1996). Several studies using experimental models associate MMP—14, -13, -9 and -2 over expression with bone resorption, and the inhibition of bone loss by the addition of an MMP inhibitor (de Aquino et al. 2009; Rifas and Arackal 2003; Garlet et al. 2006; Cesar Neto et al. 2004; Trombone et al. 2009). *In vitro* studies have revealed that MMP-13 might initiate bone resorption by generating collagen fragments that can activate osteoclasts (Holliday et al. 1997) and proMMP-9 (Knauper et al. 1997). Active MMP-9 in turn, further digests denatured collagen derived from MMP-13 activity (Hill et al. 1995), is thought to act over preosteoclast recruitment to sites for osteoclast differentiation and bone resorption, and activates proMMP-13 and proMMP-2. On the other hand, proMMP-13 can also be activated by active MMP-14, MMP-2 and MMP-13 *in vitro* (Knauper et al. 1996). Nevertheless, whether these enzymes proteolytically interact *in vivo* is not clear, yet.

Adding of recombinant MMP-13 to gingival tissue from chronic periodontitis patients has been reported to result in elevated proMMP-9 and proMMP-2 activation rates, but only the former was significant. Furthermore, addition of MMP-13 specific synthetic inhibitor CL-82198 prevented proMMP-9 activation (Hernandez Rios et al. 2009). These results suggest an activation cascade involving MMP-13, MMP-9 and possibly MMP-2 in periodontitis progression. Higher MMP-14 levels have also been found in gingival tissue from periodontitis subjects compared to healthy gingiva (Oyarzun et al. 2010) and soluble forms of MMP-14 have been described in periodontitis GCF (Tervahartiala et al. 2000), showing a trend to be higher in active sites in comparison to inactive ones in patients with progressive periodontitis (Hernandez et al. 2010). Moreover, a positive correlation between active MMP-14 and active MMP-13 in periodontitis GCF was found, suggesting proteolytic activation to occur *in vivo* (Hernández et al. 2011). Thus, this novel proteolytic cascade could perpetuate periodontal soft and hard tissue destruction in a feed forward manner. Conversely, MMP-14 has been inversely correlated to MMP-8 in GCF from active sites in progressive periodontitis, and thus this proteolytic activation mechanism might be of minor importance in disease progression (Hernandez et al. 2010; Hernandez, Dutzan et al. 2011).

MMPs can also regulate many biological processes through limited proteolysis of matrix and non-matrix bioactive molecules, such as immune-inflammatory response and wound healing, among others, through either 1) hydrolysis of extracellular matrix to allow cell migration, 2) cleavage of binding proteins and releasing of soluble bioactive molecules from extracellular matrix reservoir or cell compartment and 3) by processing bioactive molecules, modifying their biological activity (Korpi et al. 2009; Lin et al. 2008; Tester et al. 2007; Van Den Steen et al. 2003; Van Lint et al. 2005; Gutierrez-Fernandez et al. 2007; Hernandez et al. 2011).

It has been recently reported that *Porphyromonas gingivalis*-induced experimental periodontitis in MMP-8 knock-out mouse model resulted in a more severe disease phenotype and reduced levels of mouse lipopolysaccharide (LPS)-induced CXC chemokine (LIX/CXCL5) than their wild type counterparts (Kuula et al. 2009; Hernandez et al. 2011). LIX/CXCL5 and its human homologue, granulocyte chemotactic protein-2 (GCP-2/CXCL6) have been proposed to regulate neutrophil influx to periodontal tissues at the oral interface, where they represent the first line of defense against periodontal pathogens (Kebschull et al. 2009; Hernandez et al. 2011). Accordingly, several studies support a role for MMP-8 in PMN trafficking in different inflammation models. LIX/CXCL5 levels have also shown to diminish in other MMP-8 knock-out mouse models (Gutierrez-Fernandez et al. 2007; Nilsson, Jonsson, and Dabrosin 2009), such as TNF-induced lethal hepatitis model (Van Lint et al. 2005), and reduced levels of transforming growth factor (TGF)-β1 in MMP-8-/- mice have been associated with PMN impaired infiltration and wound healing (Gutierrez-Fernandez et al. 2007). All these potential regulatory mechanisms together or alone may lead to an impaired PMN influx to the sites of inflammation in MMP-8 deficient mice and alter disease expression. Similarly, MMP-9 activity was shown to down regulate TGF-β1 protein levels in breast cancer cells exposed to tamoxifen (Nilsson, Jonsson, and Dabrosin 2009; Balbin et al. 2003). In addition, recent evidence supports that MMP-13 might also influence soluble protein levels from RANKL/OPG axis (Nannuru et al. 2010).

The Role of Immuno-Inflammatory Response in the Pathogenesis of Chronic Periodontitis and Development
of Chair-Side Point of Care Diagnostics

11

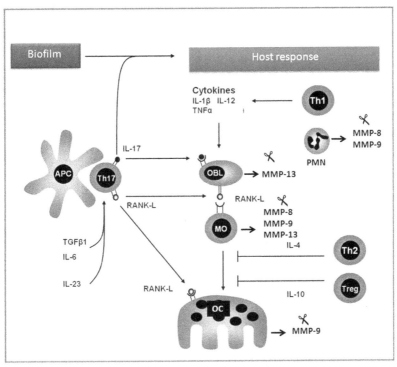

Fig. 1. The host response during periodontitis with emphasis on T cells and matrix metalloproteinases (MMPs) in periodontal tissue breakdown. As result of chronic stimuli from periodontopathogenic biofilm an immune-inflammatory response is established in periodontal tissues. The major features are the synthesis of inflammatory cytokines, such as IL-1β, IL-12, TNF-α and pathologically elevated matrix metalloproteinases (MMPs) synthesis and activation, specially MMP-8, MMP-9, and MMP-13. These MMPs degrade extracellular matrix, particularly collagen I, and they also influence periodontal immune-inflammatory response through limited proteolysis. Th17 cells may be activated as consequence of antigen presentation and contribute to bone destruction by secreting IL-17 and RANKL. IL-17 increases the inflammatory response and induces RANKL expression by osteoblastic cells. RANKL induces an increment in the osteoclast differentiation/maturation and alveolar bone resorption. MMP-13 produced by osteoblasts and MMP-9 from osteoclasts participate in the degradation of organic bone matrix. IL: interleukin; MMP: matrix metalloproteinase; TNF: tumor necrosis factor; TGF: transforming growth factor; OC: Osteoclast; APC: Antigen presenting cell; PMN: neutrophil; MO: macrophage; OBL: osteoblast.

4. Oral fluid chair-side point-of-care technologies and their systemic applications

Oral fluids [GCF, saliva, mouth-rinse, PISF] contain various molecular mediators often called biomarkers that reflect several physiological and pathological conditions. Qualitative and quantitative changes in the oral fluid biomarkers have been found to exert significance in the adjunctive diagnostics and treatment of various oral and systemic disorders.

Periodontal diseases are reflected in oral fluids as elevated levels of host cell-derived tissue destructive proteolytic enzymes, i.e. MMP-8, -9 and -13 , neutrophil elastase , α_2-macroglobulin, oxygen radical producer myeloperoxidase (MPO), pro-inflammatory mediators, (C Reactive Protein (CRP), IL-1β, TNF-α, macrophage inflammatory protein -1) and bone remodeling markers (alkaline phosphatase, ICTP, RANKL, osteoprotegrin and osteocalcin). Among these periodontitis-related oral fluid biomarkers, especially MMP-8, -9 and -13, as well as MPO are potential candidates for chair-side point-of-care oral fluid assays (Hernandez et al. 2010; Leppilahti et al. 2011; Sorsa, Tervahartiala et al. 2011). Low GCF volume and low biomarker levels in all oral fluids are characteristic during periodontal health, but the biomarker contents increase along with the severity of periodontal inflammation (Pussinen et al. 2007).

GCF, salivary and mouth-rinse biomarker analysis can provide adjunctive information for health care professionals alongside traditional oral clinical examination whether periodontal disease is present, whether treatment or medication is required or if the treatment or medication has been effective. GCF represents site specific analysis of studied biomarkers and volume. However, molecular analysis of GCF elution can be time consuming while most of the GCF analytic assays are laboratory based and usually cannot be performed in a chair-side manner. These procedures, as well as GCF sampling, are technically demanding and the GCF volume can be very small (1-5 µl). Despite these apparent diagnostic and technical disadvantages, GCF is still considered as a candidate potential oral fluid for the development of adjunctive non-invasive chair-side point of-care diagnostic technology (Sorsa et al. 1999; Sorsa et al. 2006; Sorsa, Tjaderhane, and Salo 2004; Mantyla et al. 2006; Mantyla et al. 2003; Munjal et al. 2007), especially because tissue destructive MMPs and their bioactive regulators can conveniently be measured by distinct catalytic and non-catalytic immunoassays from GCF (Sorsa et al. 2010).

In relation to GCF, collection of salivary and mouth-rinse samples is more convenient, practical, rapid and non-invasive and requires neither professional stuff nor specific materials. It could even be carried out by patients themselves. Saliva and mouth-rinse represent a pooled sample from all periodontal sites providing an overall assessment of periodontal disease and health at subject level. Whole saliva can be affected by molecular constituents and cellular remnants from other oral niches, as well as systemic conditions (Buduneli et al. 2011; Buduneli and Kinane 2011) which should be considered when it is used for diagnostics.

MMP-8 or collagenase-2/neutrophil-collagenase is the major type of interstitial collagenase present in human periodontitis-affected gingival tissue, GCF, PISF, saliva and mouth-rinse samples (Sorsa et al. 2006). Antibodies applied in the immunoassays for the detection of MMPs and their regulators affect the measurement outcome (Leppilahti et al. 2011; Gursoy et al. 2010; Sorsa et al. 2010; Sorsa, Mantyla et al. 2011). Nevertheless, especially MMP-8 immunoassays and activity assays targeting PMN-type MMP-8 isoenzyme species in oral fluids have been found to be useful to differentiate periodontitis/peri-implantitis and gingivitis sites/patients as well as healthy sites/subjects (Mantyla et al. 2006; Mantyla et al. 2003; Hernandez et al. 2010; Sorsa et al. 2010; Sorsa, Mantyla et al. 2011). Although periodontal clinical examination is necessary and cannot be substituted by any other means in periodontal diagnostics, biomarker testing could give relevant clinical adjunctive information about the individual's host response levels, although there is no known normal range at present.

The Role of Immuno-Inflammatory Response in the Pathogenesis of Chronic Periodontitis and Development
of Chair-Side Point of Care Diagnostics

13

Selective antibodies for detection of active MMP-8 in oral fluids have been utilized as adjunctive diagnostic point-of-care/chair-side tests identifying sites susceptible for periodontitis progression and periodontitis affected patients (Leppilahti et al. 2011; Mantyla et al. 2006; Sorsa, Mantyla et al. 2011; Sorsa, Tervahartiala et al. 2011). We have recently investigated levels of GCF MMP-8 with two different chair-side (dentoAnalyzer by dentognostics GmbH and MMP-8 specific chair-side dip-stick test) and two laboratory methods (immunofluorometric assay, IFMA, and commercial ELISA) (Sorsa et al. 2010). IFMA, dentoAnalyzer and MMP-8 specific chair-side dip-stick test results were well in line. Results obtained with MMP-8 commercial ELISA kit were not in line with recordings by other methods. Both IFMA and dentoAnalyzer device detected the GCF samples' MMP-8 levels with equal reliability. The chair-side dip stick test results were in line with results with these two other methods but the capability of the dip-stick test to differentiate the sample levels were rougher. The chair-side dip-stick test detected especially the sites with high MMP-8 levels.

The differences between dentoAnalyzer, IFMA, dipstick and commercial ELISA MMP-8 analysis of GCF levels can be, at least in part, explained by the evidently different specificities and sensitivities between antibodies used in these assays. DentoAnalyzer, IFMA and dipstick assays use same antibody (Hanemaaijer et al. 1997). Regarding serum and plasma MMP-8 determinations by using both IFMA and commercial ELISA, significantly higher serum MMP-8 values were recorded relative to plasma, and the differences were most notable with high serum MMP-8 concentrations as measured using IFMA (Tuomainen et al. 2008; Emingil et al. 2008). The antibody used in dentoAnalyzer, IFMA and dip-stick exerts high sensitivity to both PMN- and fibroblast-type MMP-8 isotypes and especially their active forms (Hanemaaijer et al. 1997; Sorsa et al. 1999).

Although several studies have demonstrated the central role of MMP-8 in periodontitis, it has not been shown that it is predictive of disease progression, i.e. that the increased MMP-8 concentration in GCF would precede the occurrence of attachment loss (AL). This problem arises from the nature of periodontitis and from the accuracy of diagnosing a site as progressing with clinical or radiological methods. Disease progression is regarded to be mostly episodic, occurs only infrequently and is slow in most chronic periodontitis patients. During a study period, it is likely that only a small number of sites with AL can be confirmed. Additionally, only a small group of periodontitis patients manifest multiple progressing sites (Chambers et al. 1991; Mantyla et al. 2006). In our previous study, we could not make a conclusion about the predictive value of MMP-8 testing (Mantyla et al. 2006). However, we concluded that repeatedly elevated GCF MMP-8 levels indicate the sites at risk of periodontal AL and that testing of MMP-8 site specifically from GCF is a valuable diagnostic aid which supplements the traditional methods especially from selected sites in the maintenance phase of periodontitis patients who are at continuous risk for periodontitis recurrence. Periodontitis patients' GCF MMP-8 levels decrease after conventional periodontitis hygiene phase treatment. However, the levels remain higher than in gingivitis patients' or in periodontally healthy subjects' GCF (Mantyla et al. 2003). This is valid also in periodontitis patients' shallow sites, as well as sites with no attachment loss, and tells about the elevated basic host response of periodontitis subjects (Mantyla et al. 2006; Mantyla et al. 2003) (Figure 2).

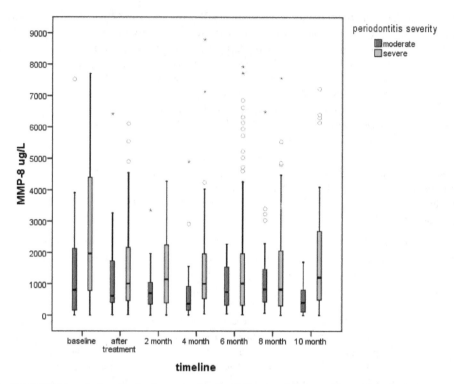

Fig. 2. MMP-8 levels in gingival crevicular fluid from subjects with moderate and severe chronic periodontitis. The box plot shows MMP-8 IFMA levels (μg/l) from patients suffering of moderate chronic periodontitis (4 patients, 34 sites) and severe chronic periodontitis (10 patients, 81 sites). Same sites from each patient were analyzed before any periodontitis treatment (baseline), one month after treatment (scaling and root planing), and with two-month interval during the maintenance phase (2-10 month). From each patient both shallow and deep sites at baseline were included into analyzed sites. The figure shows that GCF MMP-8 levels decrease in both groups after treatment but remain at comparatively high levels in severe periodontitis at each point in time indicating the higher level of host response. Box plots also show the wide ranges of MMP-8 levels, which are typical for biomarkers, and ranges become wider with the severity of the disease.

Based on other recent findings the salivary and oral rinse chair-side sample analysis of MMP-8 can be clinically useful in rough screening to identify individuals with periodontitis or to analyze the individual level of host response. Simultaneous analysis of MMP-8 and TIMP-1 could be beneficial (Leppilahti et al. 2011). The oral fluid testing could give valuable additional information about the control of inflammation which today is based on the clinical findings, that is shallower or eliminated periodontal pockets and less bleeding on probing. Salivary and oral rinse sample analysis may be useful in defining the optimal period between periodontal maintenance visits after active periodontal treatment. During the active treatment phase it could be possible to monitor the decrease of salivary and oral rinse MMP-8 levels; at the end of the active treatment phase it would show the individual optimal biomarker level to keep the host

The Role of Immuno-Inflammatory Response in the Pathogenesis of Chronic Periodontitis and Development
of Chair-Side Point of Care Diagnostics

15

response in control. At best the biomarker level could be monitored by screening home self-test to indicate when the cut-off for possibly unsafe biomarker level is reached. Also the effect of MMP-8 inhibiting SDD medication could be monitored by analyzing the salivary and oral rinse MMP-8 levels to find out when a possible break in medication would be possible or when the medication should be taken again (Golub et al. 2008; Reinhardt et al. 2010). Screening type testing from saliva or oral rinse would also be applicable for differentiation of the borderline between gingivitis and peridontitis, because gingivitis patients' MMP-8 levels are shown to be significantly lower than periodontitis patients' levels (Mantyla et al. 2003). Thus, the levels repeatedly approaching to those of periodontitis could be used to indicate patients at risk.

The point-of-care MMP-8 immuno-technologies from oral fluids and serum/plasma can be well adapted for monitoring of systemic inflammation (Tuomainen et al. 2007; Buduneli and Kinane 2011). In this regard, the elevation of serum and plasma MMP-8 has been associated with AMI, CVD and sepsis (Buduneli et al. 2011; Lauhio et al. 2011; Sorsa, Tervahartiala et al. 2011). Furthermore, a recent study on salivary MMP-8 assessed by Western immunoblot analysis in patients with or without acute myocardial infarction revealed that elevated salivary MMP-8 activation is associated with AMI (Buduneli et al. 2011). Moreover, elevated serum MMP-8 levels have recently been demonstrated to be associated with total outcome in a multicentre and prospective cohort study in sepsis; serum MMP-8 levels were significantly higher among non-survivors that among survivors. Thus elevated oral fluid and serum MMP-8 can be considered as a potential risk factor for systemic diseases such as, but not limited to, CVD, sepsis, diabetes, stroke, arthritis and pulmonary diseases (Kardesler et al. 2010; Biyikoglu et al. 2009; Buduneli et al. 2011; Ozcaka et al. 2011). In addition, oral MMP-8 activation as a consequence of AMI may contribute to progression of periodontitis and/or oral discomfort. However, oral fluid point-of-care diagnostics contains many potential confounders. The various medications together with systemic diseases (mental disorders / psychiatric diseases, nephritic syndrome) can affect the levels of potential periodontitis and CVD biomarkers in saliva and serum/plasma (Alfakry et al. 2011; Sorsa, Tervahartiala et al. 2011; Buduneli et al. 2011). Accordingly, the beneficial and reducing effects of lymecycline (a tetracycline-derivate) on serum MMP-8 levels could be monitored by MMP-8 immunoassay in reactive arthritis (Lauhio et al. 2011). In fact, serum MMP-8 levels may reflect defensive molecular processes in certain malignancies (Korpi et al. 2008) and also HIV-infection has been found to affect the level of MMPs and their regulators in oral fluid and serum/plasma (Mellanen et al. 2006).

5. Concluding remarks

Periodontal tissue destruction derived from chronic periodontitis occurs as consequence to the activation of immune-inflammatory response of the host to bacterial challenge. Major events comprise pro-inflammatory cytokine production and collagenolytic MMPs, such as MMP-8, MMP-13 and MMP-9 leading to soft periodontal tissue breakdown. Activation of Th17 subset of T lymphocytes will induce the synthesis of IL-17 and RANKL. These cytokines along with bone MMPs, will lead ultimately to octeoclastogenesis and alveolar bone resorption. Qualitative and/or quantitative changes in oral fluid biomarkers might be useful as adjunctive diagnostics and treatment of periodontitis. Among them, it appears that MMP-8 point-of-care diagnostics exert a huge potential in oral diagnostics and forms a diagnostic link from oral cavity to systemic inflammatory conditions.

6. Acknowledgment

This study was supported by project grants 1090046 and 1090461 from Scientific and Technologic Investigation Resource (FONDECYT), Santiago, Chile, and grants from The Academy of Finland (TS) and the Research Foundation of Helsinki University Central Hospital (TS). The authors are grateful to Dr. Andrea Dezerega for her artwork contribution. Timo Sorsa is an inventor of US-patents 5652227, 5736341, 5866432 and 6143476.

7. References

Acosta-Rodriguez, E. V., G. Napolitani, A. Lanzavecchia, and F. Sallusto. 2007. Interleukins 1beta and 6 but not transforming growth factor-beta are essential for the differentiation of interleukin 17-producing human T helper cells. Nat Immunol 8 (9):942-9.

Alfakry, H., S. Paju, J. Sinisalo, M. S. Nieminen, V. Valtonen, P. Saikku, M. Leinonen, and P. J. Pussinen. 2011. Periodontopathogen- and host-derived immune response in acute coronary syndrome. Scand J Immunol.

Arikan, F., N. Buduneli, and D. F. Lappin. 2011. C-telopeptide pyridinoline crosslinks of type I collagen, soluble RANKL, and osteoprotegerin levels in crevicular fluid of dental implants with peri-implantitis: a case-control study. Int J Oral Maxillofac Implants 26 (2):282-9.

Armitage, G. C. 2004. The complete periodontal examination. Periodontol 2000 34:22-33.

Bahekar, A. A., S. Singh, S. Saha, J. Molnar, and R. Arora. 2007. The prevalence and incidence of coronary heart disease is significantly increased in periodontitis: a meta-analysis. Am Heart J 154 (5):830-7.

Balbin, M., A. Fueyo, A. M. Tester, A. M. Pendas, A. S. Pitiot, A. Astudillo, C. M. Overall, S. D. Shapiro, and C. Lopez-Otin. 2003. Loss of collagenase-2 confers increased skin tumor susceptibility to male mice. Nat Genet 35 (3):252-7.

Bhavsar, A. P., J. A. Guttman, and B. B. Finlay. 2007. Manipulation of host-cell pathways by bacterial pathogens. Nature 449 (7164):827-34.

Bildt, M. M., M. Bloemen, A. M. Kuijpers-Jagtman, and J. W. Von den Hoff. 2008. Collagenolytic fragments and active gelatinase complexes in periodontitis. J Periodontol 79 (9):1704-11.

Biyikoglu, B., N. Buduneli, L. Kardesler, K. Aksu, M. Pitkala, and T. Sorsa. 2009. Gingival crevicular fluid MMP-8 and -13 and TIMP-1 levels in patients with rheumatoid arthritis and inflammatory periodontal disease. J Periodontol 80 (8):1307-14.

Bostanci, N., G. Emingil, B. Afacan, B. Han, T. Ilgenli, G. Atilla, F. J. Hughes, and G. N. Belibasakis. 2008. Tumor necrosis factor-alpha-converting enzyme (TACE) levels in periodontal diseases. J Dent Res 87 (3):273-7.

Bostanci, N., T. Ilgenli, G. Emingil, B. Afacan, B. Han, H. Toz, G. Atilla, F. J. Hughes, and G. N. Belibasakis. 2007. Gingival crevicular fluid levels of RANKL and OPG in periodontal diseases: implications of their relative ratio. J Clin Periodontol 34 (5):370-6.

Buduneli, E., P. Mantyla, G. Emingil, T. Tervahartiala, P. Pussinen, N. Baris, A. Akilli, G. Atilla, and T. Sorsa. 2011. Acute myocardial infarction is reflected in salivary matrix metalloproteinase-8 activation level. J Periodontol 82 (5):716-25.

The Role of Immuno-Inflammatory Response in the Pathogenesis of Chronic Periodontitis and Development
of Chair-Side Point of Care Diagnostics

17

Buduneli, N., B. Biyikoglu, S. Sherrabeh, and D. F. Lappin. 2008. Saliva concentrations of RANKL and osteoprotegerin in smoker versus non-smoker chronic periodontitis patients. J Clin Periodontol 35 (10):846-52.

Buduneli, N., and D. F. Kinane. 2011. Host-derived diagnostic markers related to soft tissue destruction and bone degradation in periodontitis. J Clin Periodontol 38 Suppl 11:85-105.

Cesar Neto, J. B., A. P. de Souza, D. Barbieri, H. Moreno, Jr., E. A. Sallum, and F. H. Nociti, Jr. 2004. Matrix metalloproteinase-2 may be involved with increased bone loss associated with experimental periodontitis and smoking: a study in rats. J Periodontol 75 (7):995-1000.

Crotti, T., M. D. Smith, R. Hirsch, S. Soukoulis, H. Weedon, M. Capone, M. J. Ahern, and D. Haynes. 2003. Receptor activator NF kappaB ligand (RANKL) and osteoprotegerin (OPG) protein expression in periodontitis. J Periodontal Res 38 (4):380-7.

Chambers, D. A., P. B. Imrey, R. L. Cohen, J. M. Crawford, M. E. Alves, and T. A. McSwiggin. 1991. A longitudinal study of aspartate aminotransferase in human gingival crevicular fluid. J Periodontal Res 26 (2):65-74.

Chen, C., B. Nan, P. Lin, and Q. Yao. 2008. C-reactive protein increases plasminogen activator inhibitor-1 expression in human endothelial cells. Thromb Res 122 (1):125-33.

Chen, D., Q. Wang, Z. W. Ma, F. M. Chen, Y. Chen, G. Y. Xie, Q. T. Wang, and Z. F. Wu. 2007. MMP-2, MMP-9 and TIMP-2 gene polymorphisms in Chinese patients with generalized aggressive periodontitis. J Clin Periodontol 34 (5):384-9.

de Aquino, S. G., M. R. Guimaraes, D. R. Stach-Machado, J. A. da Silva, L. C. Spolidorio, and C. Rossa, Jr. 2009. Differential regulation of MMP-13 expression in two models of experimentally induced periodontal disease in rats. Arch Oral Biol 54 (7):609-17.

de Souza, A. P., P. C. Trevilatto, R. M. Scarel-Caminaga, R. B. de Brito, Jr., S. P. Barros, and S. R. Line. 2005. Analysis of the MMP-9 (C-1562 T) and TIMP-2 (G-418C) gene promoter polymorphisms in patients with chronic periodontitis. J Clin Periodontol 32 (2):207-11.

Delima, A. J., and T. E. Van Dyke. 2003. Origin and function of the cellular components in gingival crevice fluid. Periodontol 2000 31:55-76.

Dezerega, A., P. Pozo, M. Hernandez, A. Oyarzun, O. Rivera, N. Dutzan, A. Gutierrez-Fernandez, C. M. Overall, M. Garrido, M. Alcota, E. Ortiz, and J. Gamonal. 2010. Chemokine monocyte chemoattractant protein-3 in progressive periodontal lesions in patients with chronic periodontitis. J Periodontol 81 (2):267-76.

Dreier, R., S. Grassel, S. Fuchs, J. Schaumburger, and P. Bruckner. 2004. Pro-MMP-9 is a specific macrophage product and is activated by osteoarthritic chondrocytes via MMP-3 or a MT1-MMP/MMP-13 cascade. Exp Cell Res 297 (2):303-12.

Emingil, G., B. Afacan, T. Tervahartiala, H. Toz, G. Atilla, and T. Sorsa. 2008. By mistakes we learn: determination of matrix metalloproteinase-8 and tissue inhibitor of matrix metalloproteinase-1 in serum yields doubtful results. J Clin Periodontol 35 (12):1087-8.

Folgueras, A. R., A. M. Pendas, L. M. Sanchez, and C. Lopez-Otin. 2004. Matrix metalloproteinases in cancer: from new functions to improved inhibition strategies. Int J Dev Biol 48 (5-6):411-24.

Forde, M. D., S. Koka, S. E. Eckert, A. B. Carr, and D. T. Wong. 2006. Systemic assessments utilizing saliva: part 1 general considerations and current assessments. Int J Prosthodont 19 (1):43-52.

Gaffen, S. L., and G. Hajishengallis. 2008. A new inflammatory cytokine on the block: rethinking periodontal disease and the Th1/Th2 paradigm in the context of Th17 cells and IL-17. J Dent Res 87 (9):817-28.

Garlet, G. P., C. R. Cardoso, T. A. Silva, B. R. Ferreira, M. J. Avila-Campos, F. Q. Cunha, and J. S. Silva. 2006. Cytokine pattern determines the progression of experimental periodontal disease induced by Actinobacillus actinomycetemcomitans through the modulation of MMPs, RANKL, and their physiological inhibitors. Oral Microbiol Immunol 21 (1):12-20.

Gemmell, E., and G. J. Seymour. 2004. Immunoregulatory control of Th1/Th2 cytokine profiles in periodontal disease. Periodontol 2000 35:21-41.

Gemmell, E., K. Yamazaki, and G. J. Seymour. 2002. Destructive periodontitis lesions are determined by the nature of the lymphocytic response. Crit Rev Oral Biol Med 13 (1):17-34.

Giannobile, W. V., K. F. Al-Shammari, and D. P. Sarment. 2003. Matrix molecules and growth factors as indicators of periodontal disease activity. Periodontol 2000 31:125-34.

Golub, L. M., H. M. Lee, J. A. Stoner, T. Sorsa, R. A. Reinhardt, M. S. Wolff, M. E. Ryan, P. V. Nummikoski, and J. B. Payne. 2008. Subantimicrobial-dose doxycycline modulates gingival crevicular fluid biomarkers of periodontitis in postmenopausal osteopenic women. J Periodontol 79 (8):1409-18.

Graves, D. 2008. Cytokines that promote periodontal tissue destruction. J Periodontol 79 (8 Suppl):1585-91.

Gurkan, A., G. Emingil, B. H. Saygan, G. Atilla, S. Cinarcik, T. Kose, and A. Berdeli. 2008. Gene polymorphisms of matrix metalloproteinase-2, -9 and -12 in periodontal health and severe chronic periodontitis. Arch Oral Biol 53 (4):337-45.

Gursoy, M., E. Kononen, U. K. Gursoy, T. Tervahartiala, R. Pajukanta, and T. Sorsa. 2010. Periodontal status and neutrophilic enzyme levels in gingival crevicular fluid during pregnancy and postpartum. J Periodontol 81 (12):1790-6.

Gutierrez-Fernandez, A., M. Inada, M. Balbin, A. Fueyo, A. S. Pitiot, A. Astudillo, K. Hirose, M. Hirata, S. D. Shapiro, A. Noel, Z. Werb, S. M. Krane, C. Lopez-Otin, and X. S. Puente. 2007. Increased inflammation delays wound healing in mice deficient in collagenase-2 (MMP-8). FASEB J 21 (10):2580-91.

Haffajee, A. D., and S. S. Socransky. 1986. Attachment level changes in destructive periodontal diseases. J Clin Periodontol 13 (5):461-75.

Han, Y. P., C. Yan, L. Zhou, L. Qin, and H. Tsukamoto. 2007. A matrix metalloproteinase-9 activation cascade by hepatic stellate cells in trans-differentiation in the three-dimensional extracellular matrix. J Biol Chem 282 (17):12928-39.

Hanemaaijer, R., T. Sorsa, Y. T. Konttinen, Y. Ding, M. Sutinen, H. Visser, V. W. van Hinsbergh, T. Helaakoski, T. Kainulainen, H. Ronka, H. Tschesche, and T. Salo. 1997. Matrix metalloproteinase-8 is expressed in rheumatoid synovial fibroblasts and endothelial cells. Regulation by tumor necrosis factor-alpha and doxycycline. J Biol Chem 272 (50):31504-9.

Harrington, L. E., R. D. Hatton, P. R. Mangan, H. Turner, T. L. Murphy, K. M. Murphy, and C. T. Weaver. 2005. Interleukin 17-producing CD4+ effector T cells develop via a lineage distinct from the T helper type 1 and 2 lineages. Nat Immunol 6 (11):1123-32.

The Role of Immuno-Inflammatory Response in the Pathogenesis of Chronic Periodontitis and Development
of Chair-Side Point of Care Diagnostics

19

Harrington, L. E., P. R. Mangan, and C. T. Weaver. 2006. Expanding the effector CD4 T-cell repertoire: the Th17 lineage. Curr Opin Immunol 18 (3):349-56.

Heikkinen, A. M., T. Sorsa, J. Pitkaniemi, T. Tervahartiala, K. Kari, U. Broms, M. Koskenvuo, and J. H. Meurman. 2010. Smoking affects diagnostic salivary periodontal disease biomarker levels in adolescents. J Periodontol 81 (9):1299-307.

Hernandez, M., N. Dutzan, J. Garcia-Sesnich, L. Abusleme, A. Dezerega, N. Silva, F. E. Gonzalez, R. Vernal, T. Sorsa, and J. Gamonal. 2011. Host-pathogen interactions in progressive chronic periodontitis. *J Dent Res* 90 (10):1164-70.

Hernandez, M., J. Gamonal, T. Salo, T. Tervahartiala, M. Hukkanen, L. Tjaderhane, and T. Sorsa. 2011. Reduced expression of lipopolysaccharide-induced CXC chemokine in Porphyromonas gingivalis-induced experimental periodontitis in matrix metalloproteinase-8 null mice. J Periodontal Res.

Hernandez, M., J. Gamonal, T. Tervahartiala, P. Mantyla, O. Rivera, A. Dezerega, N. Dutzan, and T. Sorsa. 2010. Associations between matrix metalloproteinase-8 and -14 and myeloperoxidase in gingival crevicular fluid from subjects with progressive chronic periodontitis: a longitudinal study. J Periodontol 81 (11):1644-52.

Hernandez, M., M. A. Valenzuela, C. Lopez-Otin, J. Alvarez, J. M. Lopez, R. Vernal, and J. Gamonal. 2006. Matrix metalloproteinase-13 is highly expressed in destructive periodontal disease activity. J Periodontol 77 (11):1863-70.

Hernandez Rios, M., T. Sorsa, F. Obregon, T. Tervahartiala, M. A. Valenzuela, P. Pozo, N. Dutzan, E. Lesaffre, M. Molas, and J. Gamonal. 2009. Proteolytic roles of matrix metalloproteinase (MMP)-13 during progression of chronic periodontitis: initial evidence for MMP-13/MMP-9 activation cascade. J Clin Periodontol 36 (12):1011-7.

Hill, P. A., A. J. Docherty, K. M. Bottomley, J. P. O'Connell, J. R. Morphy, J. J. Reynolds, and M. C. Meikle. 1995. Inhibition of bone resorption in vitro by selective inhibitors of gelatinase and collagenase. Biochem J 308 (Pt 1):167-75.

Hill, P. A., G. Murphy, A. J. Docherty, R. M. Hembry, T. A. Millican, J. J. Reynolds, and M. C. Meikle. 1994. The effects of selective inhibitors of matrix metalloproteinases (MMPs) on bone resorption and the identification of MMPs and TIMP-1 in isolated osteoclasts. J Cell Sci 107 (Pt 11):3055-64.

Hofbauer, L. C., and A. E. Heufelder. 2001. Role of receptor activator of nuclear factor-kappaB ligand and osteoprotegerin in bone cell biology. J Mol Med 79 (5-6):243-53.

Holopainen, J. M., J. A. Moilanen, T. Sorsa, M. Kivela-Rajamaki, T. Tervahartiala, M. H. Vesaluoma, and T. M. Tervo. 2003. Activation of matrix metalloproteinase-8 by membrane type 1-MMP and their expression in human tears after photorefractive keratectomy. Invest Ophthalmol Vis Sci 44 (6):2550-6.

Holla, L. I., A. Fassmann, J. Muzik, J. Vanek, and A. Vasku. 2006. Functional polymorphisms in the matrix metalloproteinase-9 gene in relation to severity of chronic periodontitis. J Periodontol 77 (11):1850-5.

Holliday, L. S., H. G. Welgus, C. J. Fliszar, G. M. Veith, J. J. Jeffrey, and S. L. Gluck. 1997. Initiation of osteoclast bone resorption by interstitial collagenase. J Biol Chem 272 (35):22053-8.

Honma, K., S. Inagaki, K. Okuda, H. K. Kuramitsu, and A. Sharma. 2007. Role of a Tannerella forsythia exopolysaccharide synthesis operon in biofilm development. Microb Pathog 42 (4):156-66.

Houri-Haddad, Y., A. Wilensky, and L. Shapira. 2007. T-cell phenotype as a risk factor for periodontal disease. Periodontol 2000 45:67-75.

Ilgenli, T., S. Vardar-Sengul, A. Gurkan, T. Sorsa, S. Stackelberg, T. Kose, and G. Atilla. 2006. Gingival crevicular fluid matrix metalloproteinase-13 levels and molecular forms in various types of periodontal diseases. Oral Dis 12 (6):573-9.

Isaza-Guzman, D. M., C. Arias-Osorio, M. C. Martinez-Pabon, and S. I. Tobon-Arroyave. Salivary levels of matrix metalloproteinase (MMP)-9 and tissue inhibitor of matrix metalloproteinase (TIMP)-1: a pilot study about the relationship with periodontal status and MMP-9(-1562C/T) gene promoter polymorphism. Arch Oral Biol 56 (4):401-11.

Kardesler, L., B. Biyikoglu, S. Cetinkalp, M. Pitkala, T. Sorsa, and N. Buduneli. 2010. Crevicular fluid matrix metalloproteinase-8, -13, and TIMP-1 levels in type 2 diabetics. Oral Dis 16 (5):476-81.

Kawai, T., T. Matsuyama, Y. Hosokawa, S. Makihira, M. Seki, N. Y. Karimbux, R. B. Goncalves, P. Valverde, S. Dibart, Y. P. Li, L. A. Miranda, C. W. Ernst, Y. Izumi, and M. A. Taubman. 2006. B and T lymphocytes are the primary sources of RANKL in the bone resorptive lesion of periodontal disease. Am J Pathol 169 (3):987-98.

Kebschull, M., R. Demmer, J. H. Behle, A. Pollreisz, J. Heidemann, P. B. Belusko, R. Celenti, P. Pavlidis, and P. N. Papapanou. 2009. Granulocyte chemotactic protein 2 (gcp-2/cxcl6) complements interleukin-8 in periodontal disease. J Periodontal Res 44 (4):465-71.

Kessenbrock, K., V. Plaks, and Z. Werb. 2010. Matrix metalloproteinases: regulators of the tumor microenvironment. Cell 141 (1):52-67.

Kiili, M., S. W. Cox, H. Y. Chen, J. Wahlgren, P. Maisi, B. M. Eley, T. Salo, and T. Sorsa. 2002. Collagenase-2 (MMP-8) and collagenase-3 (MMP-13) in adult periodontitis: molecular forms and levels in gingival crevicular fluid and immunolocalisation in gingival tissue. J Clin Periodontol 29 (3):224-32.

Knauper, V., B. Smith, C. Lopez-Otin, and G. Murphy. 1997. Activation of progelatinase B (proMMP-9) by active collagenase-3 (MMP-13). Eur J Biochem 248 (2):369-73.

Knauper, V., H. Will, C. Lopez-Otin, B. Smith, S. J. Atkinson, H. Stanton, R. M. Hembry, and G. Murphy. 1996. Cellular mechanisms for human procollagenase-3 (MMP-13) activation. Evidence that MT1-MMP (MMP-14) and gelatinase a (MMP-2) are able to generate active enzyme. J Biol Chem 271 (29):17124-31.

Korpi, J. T., P. Astrom, N. Lehtonen, L. Tjaderhane, S. Kallio-Pulkkinen, M. Siponen, T. Sorsa, E. Pirila, and T. Salo. 2009. Healing of extraction sockets in collagenase-2 (matrix metalloproteinase-8)-deficient mice. Eur J Oral Sci 117 (3):248-54.

Korpi, J. T., V. Kervinen, H. Maklin, A. Vaananen, M. Lahtinen, E. Laara, A. Ristimaki, G. Thomas, M. Ylipalosaari, P. Astrom, C. Lopez-Otin, T. Sorsa, S. Kantola, E. Pirila, and T. Salo. 2008. Collagenase-2 (matrix metalloproteinase-8) plays a protective role in tongue cancer. Br J Cancer 98 (4):766-75.

Kramer, J. M., and S. L. Gaffen. 2007. Interleukin-17: a new paradigm in inflammation, autoimmunity, and therapy. J Periodontol 78 (6):1083-93.

Kuula, H., T. Salo, E. Pirila, A. M. Tuomainen, M. Jauhiainen, V. J. Uitto, L. Tjaderhane, P. J. Pussinen, and T. Sorsa. 2009. Local and systemic responses in matrix metalloproteinase 8-deficient mice during Porphyromonas gingivalis-induced periodontitis. Infect Immun 77 (2):850-9.

The Role of Immuno-Inflammatory Response in the Pathogenesis of Chronic Periodontitis and Development
of Chair-Side Point of Care Diagnostics

21

Lamster, I. B., and J. K. Ahlo. 2007. Analysis of gingival crevicular fluid as applied to the diagnosis of oral and systemic diseases. Ann N Y Acad Sci 1098:216-29.

Lauhio, A., J. Hastbacka, V. Pettila, T. Tervahartiala, S. Karlsson, T. Varpula, M. Varpula, E. Ruokonen, T. Sorsa, and E. Kolho. 2011. Serum MMP-8, -9 and TIMP-1 in sepsis: High serum levels of MMP-8 and TIMP-1 are associated with fatal outcome in a multicentre, prospective cohort study. Hypothetical impact of tetracyclines. Pharmacol Res.

Leppilahti, J., M. M. Ahonen, M. Hernandez, S. Munjal, L. Netuschil, V. J. Uitto, T. Sorsa, and P. Mantyla. 2011. Oral rinse MMP-8 point-of-care immuno test identifies patients with strong periodontal inflammatory burden. Oral Dis. 17(1):115-22

Liang, S. C., X. Y. Tan, D. P. Luxenberg, R. Karim, K. Dunussi-Joannopoulos, M. Collins, and L. A. Fouser. 2006. Interleukin (IL)-22 and IL-17 are coexpressed by Th17 cells and cooperatively enhance expression of antimicrobial peptides. J Exp Med 203 (10):2271-9.

Lin, M., P. Jackson, A. M. Tester, E. Diaconu, C. M. Overall, J. E. Blalock, and E. Pearlman. 2008. Matrix metalloproteinase-8 facilitates neutrophil migration through the corneal stromal matrix by collagen degradation and production of the chemotactic peptide Pro-Gly-Pro. Am J Pathol 173 (1):144-53.

Loo, W. T., M. Wang, L. J. Jin, M. N. Cheung, and G. R. Li. 2011. Association of matrix metalloproteinase (MMP-1, MMP-3 and MMP-9) and cyclooxygenase-2 gene polymorphisms and their proteins with chronic periodontitis. Arch Oral Biol.

Makela, M., T. Salo, V. J. Uitto, and H. Larjava. 1994. Matrix metalloproteinases (MMP-2 and MMP-9) of the oral cavity: cellular origin and relationship to periodontal status. J Dent Res 73 (8):1397-406.

Mantyla, P., M. Stenman, D. F. Kinane, S. Tikanoja, H. Luoto, T. Salo, and T. Sorsa. 2003. Gingival crevicular fluid collagenase-2 (MMP-8) test stick for chair-side monitoring of periodontitis. J Periodontal Res 38 (4):436-9.

Mantyla, P., M. Stenman, D. Kinane, T. Salo, K. Suomalainen, S. Tikanoja, and T. Sorsa. 2006. Monitoring periodontal disease status in smokers and nonsmokers using a gingival crevicular fluid matrix metalloproteinase-8-specific chair-side test. J Periodontal Res 41 (6):503-12.

Mattila, K. J., S. Asikainen, J. Wolf, H. Jousimies-Somer, V. Valtonen, and M. Nieminen. 2000. Age, dental infections, and coronary heart disease. J Dent Res 79 (2):756-60.

Mattila, K. J., P. J. Pussinen, and S. Paju. 2005. Dental infections and cardiovascular diseases: a review. J Periodontol 76 (11 Suppl):2085-8.

McQuibban, G. A., G. S. Butler, J. H. Gong, L. Bendall, C. Power, I. Clark-Lewis, and C. M. Overall. 2001. Matrix metalloproteinase activity inactivates the CXC chemokine stromal cell-derived factor-1. J Biol Chem 276 (47):43503-8.

McQuibban, G. A., J. H. Gong, J. P. Wong, J. L. Wallace, I. Clark-Lewis, and C. M. Overall. 2002. Matrix metalloproteinase processing of monocyte chemoattractant proteins generates CC chemokine receptor antagonists with anti-inflammatory properties in vivo. Blood 100 (4):1160-7.

Mellanen, L., J. Lahdevirta, T. Tervahartiala, J. H. Meurman, and T. Sorsa. 2006. Matrix metalloproteinase-7, -8, -9, -25, and -26 and CD43, -45, and -68 cell-markers in HIV-infected patients' saliva and gingival tissue. J Oral Pathol Med 35 (9):530-9.

Mosmann, T. R., and R. L. Coffman. 1989. TH1 and TH2 cells: different patterns of lymphokine secretion lead to different functional properties. Annu Rev Immunol 7:145-73.

Mosmann, T. R., H. Cherwinski, M. W. Bond, M. A. Giedlin, and R. L. Coffman. 1986. Two types of murine helper T cell clone. I. Definition according to profiles of lymphokine activities and secreted proteins. J Immunol 136 (7):2348-57.

Mosmann, T. R., and S. Sad. 1996. The expanding universe of T-cell subsets: Th1, Th2 and more. Immunol Today 17 (3):138-46.

Munjal, S. K., N. Prescher, F. Struck, T. Sorsa, K. Maier, and L. Netuschil. 2007. Evaluation of immunoassay-based MMP-8 detection in gingival crevicular fluid on a point-of-care platform. Ann N Y Acad Sci 1098:490-2.

Nagasawa, T., M. Kiji, R. Yashiro, D. Hormdee, H. Lu, M. Kunze, T. Suda, G. Koshy, H. Kobayashi, S. Oda, H. Nitta, and I. Ishikawa. 2007. Roles of receptor activator of nuclear factor-kappaB ligand (RANKL) and osteoprotegerin in periodontal health and disease. Periodontol 2000 43:65-84.

Nannuru, K. C., M. Futakuchi, M. L. Varney, T. M. Vincent, E. G. Marcusson, and R. K. Singh. 2010. Matrix metalloproteinase (MMP)-13 regulates mammary tumor-induced osteolysis by activating MMP9 and transforming growth factor-beta signaling at the tumor-bone interface. Cancer Res 70 (9):3494-504.

Nilsson, U. W., J. A. Jonsson, and C. Dabrosin. 2009. Tamoxifen decreases extracellular TGF-beta1 secreted from breast cancer cells--a post-translational regulation involving matrix metalloproteinase activity. Exp Cell Res 315 (1):1-9.

Offenbacher, S. 1996. Periodontal diseases: pathogenesis. Ann Periodontol 1 (1):821-78.

Offenbacher, S., S. P. Barros, R. E. Singer, K. Moss, R. C. Williams, and J. D. Beck. 2007. Periodontal disease at the biofilm-gingival interface. J Periodontol 78 (10):1911-25.

Ohyama, H., N. Kato-Kogoe, A. Kuhara, F. Nishimura, K. Nakasho, K. Yamanegi, N. Yamada, M. Hata, J. Yamane, and N. Terada. 2009. The involvement of IL-23 and the Th17 pathway in periodontitis. J Dent Res 88 (7):633-8.

Overall, C. M., G. A. McQuibban, and I. Clark-Lewis. 2002. Discovery of chemokine substrates for matrix metalloproteinases by exosite scanning: a new tool for degradomics. Biol Chem 383 (7-8):1059-66.

Oyarzun, A., R. Arancibia, R. Hidalgo, C. Penafiel, M. Caceres, M. J. Gonzalez, J. Martinez, and P. C. Smith. 2010. Involvement of MT1-MMP and TIMP-2 in human periodontal disease. Oral Dis 16 (4):388-95.

Ozcaka, O., N. Bicakci, P. Pussinen, T. Sorsa, T. Kose, and N. Buduneli. 2011. Smoking and matrix metalloproteinases, neutrophil elastase and myeloperoxidase in chronic periodontitis. Oral Dis 17 (1):68-76.

Page, R. C., and K. S. Kornman. 1997. The pathogenesis of human periodontitis: an introduction. Periodontol 2000 14:9-11.

Park, H., Z. Li, X. O. Yang, S. H. Chang, R. Nurieva, Y. H. Wang, Y. Wang, L. Hood, Z. Zhu, Q. Tian, and C. Dong. 2005. A distinct lineage of CD4 T cells regulates tissue inflammation by producing interleukin 17. Nat Immunol 6 (11):1133-41.

Persson, R. E., L. G. Hollender, M. I. MacEntee, C. C. Wyatt, H. A. Kiyak, and G. R. Persson. 2003. Assessment of periodontal conditions and systemic disease in older subjects. J Clin Periodontol 30 (3):207-13.

The Role of Immuno-Inflammatory Response in the Pathogenesis of Chronic Periodontitis and Development of Chair-Side Point of Care Diagnostics

23

Pirhan, D., G. Atilla, G. Emingil, T. Tervahartiala, T. Sorsa, and A. Berdeli. 2009. MMP-13 promoter polymorphisms in patients with chronic periodontitis: effects on GCF MMP-13 levels and outcome of periodontal therapy. J Clin Periodontol 36 (6):474-81.

Pussinen, P. J., S. Paju, P. Mantyla, and T. Sorsa. 2007. Serum microbial- and host-derived markers of periodontal diseases: a review. Curr Med Chem 14 (22):2402-12.

Reddy, M. S., K. G. Palcanis, and N. C. Geurs. 1997. A comparison of manual and controlled-force attachment-level measurements. J Clin Periodontol 24 (12):920-6.

Reinhardt, R. A., J. A. Stoner, L. M. Golub, H. M. Lee, P. V. Nummikoski, T. Sorsa, and J. B. Payne. 2010. Association of gingival crevicular fluid biomarkers during periodontal maintenance with subsequent progressive periodontitis. J Periodontol 81 (2):251-9.

Reynolds, J. J., and M. C. Meikle. 1997. Mechanisms of connective tissue matrix destruction in periodontitis. Periodontol 2000 14:144-57.

Rifas, L., and S. Arackal. 2003. T cells regulate the expression of matrix metalloproteinase in human osteoblasts via a dual mitogen-activated protein kinase mechanism. Arthritis Rheum 48 (4):993-1001.

Rydziel, S., D. Durant, and E. Canalis. 2000. Platelet-derived growth factor induces collagenase 3 transcription in osteoblasts through the activator protein 1 complex. J Cell Physiol 184 (3):326-33.

Sahingur, S. E., and R. E. Cohen. 2004. Analysis of host responses and risk for disease progression. Periodontol 2000 34:57-83.

Sakellari, D., S. Menti, and A. Konstantinidis. 2008. Free soluble receptor activator of nuclear factor-kappab ligand in gingival crevicular fluid correlates with distinct pathogens in periodontitis patients. J Clin Periodontol 35 (11):938-43.

Silva, N., N. Dutzan, M. Hernandez, A. Dezerega, O. Rivera, J. C. Aguillon, O. Aravena, P. Lastres, P. Pozo, R. Vernal, and J. Gamonal. 2008. Characterization of progressive periodontal lesions in chronic periodontitis patients: levels of chemokines, cytokines, matrix metalloproteinase-13, periodontal pathogens and inflammatory cells. J Clin Periodontol 35 (3):206-14.

Socransky, S. S., A. D. Haffajee, M. A. Cugini, C. Smith, and R. L. Kent, Jr. 1998. Microbial complexes in subgingival plaque. J Clin Periodontol 25 (2):134-44.

Sorsa, T., M. Hernandez, J. Leppilahti, S. Munjal, L. Netuschil, and P. Mantyla. 2010. Detection of gingival crevicular fluid MMP-8 levels with different laboratory and chair-side methods. Oral Dis 16 (1):39-45.

Sorsa, T., P. Mantyla, H. Ronka, P. Kallio, G. B. Kallis, C. Lundqvist, D. F. Kinane, T. Salo, L. M. Golub, O. Teronen, and S. Tikanoja. 1999. Scientific basis of a matrix metalloproteinase-8 specific chair-side test for monitoring periodontal and peri-implant health and disease. Ann N Y Acad Sci 878:130-40.

Sorsa, T., P. Mantyla, T. Tervahartiala, P. J. Pussinen, J. Gamonal, and M. Hernandez. 2011. MMP activation in diagnostics of periodontitis and systemic inflammation. J Clin Periodontol 38 (9):817-9.

Sorsa, T., T. Tervahartiala, J. Leppilahti, M. Hernandez, J. Gamonal, A. M. Tuomainen, A. Lauhio, P. J. Pussinen, and P. Mantyla. 2011. Collagenase-2 (MMP-8) as a point-of-care biomarker in periodontitis and cardiovascular diseases. Therapeutic response to non-antimicrobial properties of tetracyclines. Pharmacol Res 63 (2):108-13.

Sorsa, T., L. Tjaderhane, Y. T. Konttinen, A. Lauhio, T. Salo, H. M. Lee, L. M. Golub, D. L. Brown, and P. Mantyla. 2006. Matrix metalloproteinases: contribution to pathogenesis, diagnosis and treatment of periodontal inflammation. Ann Med 38 (5):306-21.

Sorsa, T., L. Tjaderhane, and T. Salo. 2004. Matrix metalloproteinases (MMPs) in oral diseases. Oral Dis 10 (6):311-8.

Takahashi, K., T. Azuma, H. Motohira, D. F. Kinane, and S. Kitetsu. 2005. The potential role of interleukin-17 in the immunopathology of periodontal disease. J Clin Periodontol 32 (4):369-74.

Takayanagi, H. 2005. Inflammatory bone destruction and osteoimmunology. J Periodontal Res 40 (4):287-93.

Tervahartiala, T., E. Pirila, A. Ceponis, P. Maisi, T. Salo, G. Tuter, P. Kallio, J. Tornwall, R. Srinivas, Y. T. Konttinen, and T. Sorsa. 2000. The in vivo expression of the collagenolytic matrix metalloproteinases (MMP-2, -8, -13, and -14) and matrilysin (MMP-7) in adult and localized juvenile periodontitis. J Dent Res 79 (12):1969-77.

Tester, A. M., J. H. Cox, A. R. Connor, A. E. Starr, R. A. Dean, X. S. Puente, C. Lopez-Otin, and C. M. Overall. 2007. LPS responsiveness and neutrophil chemotaxis in vivo require PMN MMP-8 activity. PLoS One 2 (3):e312.

Trombone, A. P., S. B. Ferreira, Jr., F. M. Raimundo, K. C. de Moura, M. J. Avila-Campos, J. S. Silva, A. P. Campanelli, M. De Franco, and G. P. Garlet. 2009. Experimental periodontitis in mice selected for maximal or minimal inflammatory reactions: increased inflammatory immune responsiveness drives increased alveolar bone loss without enhancing the control of periodontal infection. J Periodontal Res 44 (4):443-51.

Tuomainen, A. M., M. Jauhiainen, P. T. Kovanen, J. Metso, S. Paju, and P. J. Pussinen. 2008. Aggregatibacter actinomycetemcomitans induces MMP-9 expression and proatherogenic lipoprotein profile in apoE-deficient mice. Microb Pathog 44 (2):111-7.

Tuomainen, A. M., K. Nyyssonen, J. A. Laukkanen, T. Tervahartiala, T. P. Tuomainen, J. T. Salonen, T. Sorsa, and P. J. Pussinen. 2007. Serum matrix metalloproteinase-8 concentrations are associated with cardiovascular outcome in men. Arterioscler Thromb Vasc Biol 27 (12):2722-8.

Van Den Steen, P. E., A. Wuyts, S. J. Husson, P. Proost, J. Van Damme, and G. Opdenakker. 2003. Gelatinase B/MMP-9 and neutrophil collagenase/MMP-8 process the chemokines human GCP-2/CXCL6, ENA-78/CXCL5 and mouse GCP-2/LIX and modulate their physiological activities. Eur J Biochem 270 (18):3739-49.

Van Lint, P., B. Wielockx, L. Puimege, A. Noel, C. Lopez-Otin, and C. Libert. 2005. Resistance of collagenase-2 (matrix metalloproteinase-8)-deficient mice to TNF-induced lethal hepatitis. J Immunol 175 (11):7642-9.

Vernal, R., A. Chaparro, R. Graumann, J. Puente, M. A. Valenzuela, and J. Gamonal. 2004. Levels of cytokine receptor activator of nuclear factor kappaB ligand in gingival crevicular fluid in untreated chronic periodontitis patients. J Periodontol 75 (12):1586-91.

Vernal, R., N. Dutzan, A. Chaparro, J. Puente, M. Antonieta Valenzuela, and J. Gamonal. 2005. Levels of interleukin-17 in gingival crevicular fluid and in supernatants of cellular cultures of gingival tissue from patients with chronic periodontitis. J Clin Periodontol 32 (4):383-9.

Pathogenic Factors of
P. gingivalis and the Host Defense Mechanisms

Shigenobu Kimura[1], Yuko Ohara-Nemoto[2],
Yu Shimoyama[1], Taichi Ishikawa[1] and Minoru Sasaki[1]
[1]Iwate Medical University,
[2]Nagasaki University Graduate School of Biomedical Sciences,
Japan

1. Introduction

Periodontal diseases are the inflammatory diseases triggered specifically by some selected microorganisms, *i.e.*, periodontopathic bacteria, accumulated in and around the gingival crevice. Among periodontopathic bacteria, *Porphyromonas gingivalis*, a black-pigmented gram-negative anaerobic rod, has been implicated as a major pathogen of chronic periodontitis (Hamada et al., 1991; Lamont & Jenkinson, 1998). Recent studies using DNA-DNA hybridization that permits the examination of large numbers of species in large numbers of plaque samples also indicated the increased prevalence of *P. gingivalis* as well as other 'red complex species' (*P. gingivalis*, *Treponema denticola* and *Tannerella forsythensis*) in the subjects with chronic periodontitis (Socransky & Haffajee, 2002). However, it is also evident that the colonization of the putative pathogenic bacteria in subgingival plaque is not sufficient for the initiation/onset of periodontitis, since most periodontopathic bacteria including *P. gingivalis* may also be present at sound sites (Haffajee et al., 2009). Thus, the onset and progress of chronic periodontitis is based on the balance between the pathogenesis of the periodontopathic microorganisms and the host-defense against them (host-parasite relationship).

The pathogenic factors of *P. gingivalis* including fimbriae, hemagglutinin, capsule, lipopolysaccharide (LPS), outer membrane vesicles, organic metabolites such as butyric acid, and various enzymes such as Arg- and Lys-gingipains, collagenase, gelatinase and hyaluronidase, could contribute to the induction of chronic periodontitis in diverse ways; *P. gingivalis* could colonize to gingival crevices by the fimbriae-mediated adherence to gingival epithelial cells, the proteases may have the abilities to destroy periodontal tissues directly or indirectly, and the LPS could elicit a wide variety of inflammatory responses of periodontal tissues and alveolar bone losses. Although the complex interaction to the host response fundamentally responsible for chronic periodontitis cannot be reproduced in vitro, the studies with animal models that *P. gingivalis* can induce experimental periodontitis with alveolar bone losses (Kimura et al., 2000a; Oz & Puleo, 2011) clearly indicate that *P. gingivalis* is a major causative pathogen of chronic periodontitis, and its pathogenic factors could be potentially involved solely or cooperatively in every step of the onset and progression of the disease. A recent study that the DNA vaccine expressing the adhesion/hemagglutinin domain of Arg-gingipain prevented the *P. gingivalis*–induced alveolar bone loss in mice (Muramatsu et al., 2011) may support in part the hypothesis.

In this chapter, we will address not the every pathogenic factor of *P. gingivalis* in tern, but the roles of the factors and their relationship in the pathogenic events of this microorganism, such as the colonization in gingival crevices, the invasion into gingival tissues, and the induction of inflammatory responses and alveolar bone losses.

2. Colonization in gingival crevices

The colonization of *P. gingivalis* in gingival crevices is the first step in the development of chronic periodontitis. However, it does not necessarily induce the periodontal destruction, but a prerequisite for onset of chronic periodontitis. In adults, *P. gingivalis* can be detected from periodontally healthy sites as well as diseased sites, although the number of the microorganisms is generally lower than that in diseased sites (Dzink et al., 1988; Hamada et al., 1991). In contrast, *P. gingivalis* is scarcely detected in the samples from oral cavities of children (Kimura et al., 2002; Kimura & Ohara-Nemoto, 2007). Our 2-year longitudinal study revealed that *P. gingivalis* as well as *Prevotella intermedia* and *T. denticola* appear to be transient organisms in the plaques of healthy children (Ooshima et al., 2003). From the point of view on host-parasite relationship in chronic periodontitis, the children's host-defense of antibiotic components in saliva and gingival crevicular fluid (GCF) could efficiently prevent the initial colonization and/or proliferation of these periodontal pathogens, resulting in the arrest of periodontal diseases in healthy children.

Nevertheless, it was also demonstrated that children whose parents were colonized by the BANA-positive periodontpathic species including *P. gingivalis, T. denticola,* and *T. forsythensis* were 9.8 times more likely to be colonized by these species, and children whose parents had clinical evidence of periodontitis were 12 times more likely to be colonized the species (Watson et al., 1994). The vertical transmission of *P. gingivalis,* however, has been still controversial; vertical as well as horizontal transmission was speculated in the research on 564-members of American families (Tuite-McDonnell et al., 1997), whereas vertical (parents-to-children) transmission has rarely been observed in the Netherlands (Van Winkelhoff & Boutaga, 2005), in Finland (Asikainen & Chen, 1999), and in the research of 78 American subjects (Asikainen et al., 1996). In the latter reports, since horizontal transmission of *P. gingivalis* between adult family members was considerable, it was suggested that *P. gingivalis* commonly colonizes in an established oral microbiota. According to these observations, it was also suggested that the vertical and horizontal transmission of *P. gingivalis* could be controlled by periodontal treatment involving elimination of the pathogen in diseased individuals and by oral hygiene instructions.

The major habitat of *P. gingivalis* is subgingival plaques in gingival crevices. However, *P. gingivalis* can be detected in the tongue coat samples from periodontally healthy and diseased subjects (Dahlén et al., 1992; Kishi et al., 2002). Clinical studies suggested that tongue coat could be a dominant reservoir of *P. gingivalis* (Kishi et al., 2002; Faveri et al., 2006). Furthermore, our recent study with 165 subjects aged 85 years old indicated that *P. gingivalis* as well as *P. intermedia, T. denticola* and *T. forsythensis* was found more frequently in tongue coat samples from dentate than edentulous subjects, and the prevalence of *P. gingivalis* was significantly related to the number of teeth with a periodontal pocket depth ≥ 4 mm (Kishi et al., 2010). Thus, it can be speculated that an adequately stable circulation of *P. gingivalis* between subgingival plaque and tongue coat occurs over time in dentate individuals. In addition, tooth loss, which is synonymous with loss of the gingival crevice, may affect the oral microflora population, resulting in a significant decrease in *P. gingivalis*.

Despite the host defense mechanisms in saliva and GCF, *P. gingivalis* can adhere and then colonize in gingival crevices to a variety of surface components lining the gingival crevicular cells and the tooth surface. The adhesive ability of *P. gingivalis* is mainly mediated by the fimbriae, although other bacterial components such as vesicles, hemagglutinin, and proteases may play an adjunctive role (Naito et al, 1993). Fimbriae are the thin, filamentous, and proteinaceous surface appendages found in many bacterial species, and these fimbriae are claimed to play an important role in the virulence of a number of oral and non-oral pathogens such as uropathogenic *Escherichia coli* and *Neisseria gonorrehoeae*. Fimbriae of *P. gingivalis* were first recognized on the outer surface by electron microscopic observation (Slots & Gibbons, 1978; Okuda et al., 1981), and were isolated and purified to a homogeneity from strain 381 by a simple and reproducible method using DEAE Sepharose chromatography (Yoshimura et al., 1984). Fimbriae of *P. gingivalis* 381 are composed of constituent (subunit) protein, fimbrillin, with a molecular weight of 40-42 kDa by sodium dodecyl sulfate-polyacrylamide gel electrophoresis (Ogawa et al., 1991; Hamada et al., 1994). Lee et al. (1991) compared fimbriae diversities of size and amino terminal sequence of fimbrillins from various *P. gingivalis* strains; they differed in molecular weights ranging from 40.5 to 49 kDa and were classified into four types (types I to IV) based on the amino terminal sequences of fimbrillins. Further molecular and epidemiological studies using PCR method to differentiate possibly varied bacterial pathogenicity revealed that *P. gingivalis* fimbriae are classified into six genotypes based on the diversity of the *fimA* genes encoding each fimbrillin (types I to V, and type Ib), and that *P. gingivalis* with type II *fimA* is most closely associated with the progression of chronic periodontitis (Amano et al., 1999a; Nakagawa et al., 2000 & 2002b) (Table 1). A recent study with the mutants in which *fimA* of ATCC 33277 (type I strain) was substituted with type II *fimA* and that of OMZ314 (type II strain) with type I *fimA* indicated that type II fimbriae is a critical determinant of *P. gingivalis* adhesion to epithelial cells (Kato et al., 2007).

fimA type	Odds ratio	95% confidence interval	*P* value
I	0.20	0.1 – 0.4	0.0000
Ib	6.51	2.9 – 14.6	0.0000
II	77.80	31.1 – 195.4	0.0000
III	2.51	1.1 – 5.8	0.0246
IV	7.54	3.5 – 16.0	0.0000
V	1.05	0.6 – 1.8	0.8525

Table 1. Relationship of *fimA* types in chronic periodontitis

P. gingivalis fimbriae possess a strong ability to interact with host proteins such as salivary proteins, extracellular matrix proteins, epithelial cells, and fibroblast, which promote the colonization of *P. gingivalis* to the oral cavity (Naito & Gibbons, 1988; Hamada et al., 1998). These bindings are specific and occur via protein-protein interactions through definitive domains of fimbriae and host proteins. The real-time observation by biomolecular interaction analysis (BIAcore) showed specific and intensive interaction to salivary proteins and extracellular matrix proteins (Table 2). The binding components in saliva are acidic proline-rich protein (PRP), proline-rich glycoprotein (PRG), and statherin (Amano et al., 1996a, 1996b & 1998). *P. gingivalis* fimbriae also show significant interactions with extracellular matrix proteins including fibronectin and laminin (Kontani et al., 1996; Amano et al., 1999b). Therefore, *P. gingivalis* cells can bind to tooth surface and upper gingival crevice that is covered with saliva. Although a deeper portion of the gingival crevice could not be contaminated with saliva, *P. gingivalis* can bind directly to sulcular epithelial cells via interaction with extracellular matrix proteins.

In addition, Arg-gingipains produced by *P. gingivalis* can enhance the adherence of purified fimbriae to fibroblasts and matrix proteins; Arg-gingipains can expose a cryptitope in the matrix protein molecule, i.e. the C-terminal Arg residue of the host matrix proteins, so that the organism can adhere to the surface layer in gingival crevices through fimbrial-Arg interaction (Kontani et al., 1996 & 1997).

Host protein	k_a (1/M/s)	K_{dis} (1/s)	K_a (1/M)
PRP	2.61×10^3	1.60×10^{-3}	1.63×10^6
PRG	3.38×10^3	2.08×10^{-3}	1.62×10^6
Statherin	2.49×10^3	1.68×10^{-3}	1.48×10^6
Laminin	3.62×10^3	1.68×10^{-3}	2.15×10^6
Fibronectin	3.46×10^3	1.60×10^{-3}	2.16×10^6
Thrombospondin	3.01×10^3	1.33×10^{-3}	2.26×10^6
Type I collagen	3.04×10^3	1.10×10^{-3}	2.76×10^6
Vitronectin	4.16×10^3	1.10×10^{-3}	3.79×10^6
Elastin	3.72×10^3	1.21×10^{-3}	3.08×10^6
Anti-fimbriae IgG	6.11×10^3	5.00×10^{-3}	1.22×10^7

Table 2. Binding constants of *P. gingivalis* fimbriae to host proteins

In gingival crevices, serum antimicrobial components consecutively exude through the junctional epithelium, termed GCF. GCF originates from plasma exudates, thus contains IgG, IgA, complements and cellular elements. It is noted that 95% of the cellular elements are polymorphonuclear leukocytes (PMNL) and the remainder being lymphocytes and monocytes, even in the GCF from clinically healthy gingival crevices, indicating that PMNL are the principal cell of GCF (Genco & Mergenhagen, 1982). PMNL come into direct contact with plaque bacteria in the gingival crevice and actively phagocytose them. The protective function of PMNL in human periodontal diseases is demonstrated by the fact that patients with PMNL disorders, e.g. Chédiak-Higashi syndrome, lazy leukocyte syndrome, cyclic neutropeni, chronic granulomatous disease and diabetes mellitus, have usually rapid and severe periodontitis (Genco, 1996; da Fonseca & Fontes, 2000; Delcourt-Debruyne et al., 2000; Meyle & Gonzáles, 2001; Lalla et al., 2007). Furthermore, quantitative analyses using flow cytometer revealed that about 50% of the patients with localized and generalized aggressive periodontitis exhibited depression of phagocytic function of peripheral blood PMNL (Kimura et al., 1992 & 1993), suggesting that the functional abnormalities of PMNL are implicated in the pathogenesis of both forms of aggressive periodontitis. Thus, PMNL could play an important role in gingival crevices as innate immunity to prevent the colonization and/or proliferation of *P. gingivalis*, resulting in the arrest of periodontal diseases in healthy subjects.

The gingival crevice is bathed in saliva that contains a lot of antibiotic agents, such as lysozyme, lactoferrin, peroxydase and secretary IgA. In addition, the sulcular epithelium acts as a physical barrier against intruders (Cimasoni, 1983). Furthermore, our recent study indicated that the sulcular epithelial cells could be a substantial producer of secretory leukocyte protease inhibitor (SLPI) that functions inhibitory to the pathogenic *P. gingivalis* infection (Ishikawa et al., 2010). SLPI has been recognized as not only a protease inhibitor but also an important defense component in innate immunity in mucosal secretory fluids. To elucidate the functional role in innate immunity in gingival crevices, we investigated the SLPI production from a gingival epithelial cell line, GE1, with or without the stimulation of the lyophilized whole cells of *P. gingivalis* (Pg-WC) and the LPS (Pg-LPS), and the inhibitory effect of SLPI on *P. gingivalis* proteases. The real-time RT-PCR analyses indicated that the unstimulated GE1 cells showed low, but significant levels of SLPI mRNA expression, which was augmented by the stimulation with Pg-LPS as well as Pg-WC (Fig. 1). The augmentation of SLPI mRNA expression in GE1 cells was accompanied by the inductions of IL-6, TNF-α and IL-1β mRNA expressions. Although it was reported that IL-6 could induce macrophages to produce SLPI, the kinetics analyses suggested that the augmentation of SLPI production in GE1 cells could not be a second response to the IL-6 induced by the stimulant, but a direct response by the *P. gingivalis* antigens. Further experiments using rSLPI indicated that SLPI showed a direct inhibitory effect on the *P. gingivalis* protease of Lys-gingipain (Fig. 2). Thus the results suggested that the SLPI production by gingival epithelial cells could increase in response to *P. gingivalis* through the stimulation with its pathogenic constituents.

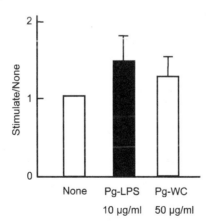

Fig. 1. SLPI mRNA expression of GE1 cells and the augmentation with *P. gingivalis* LPS. GE1 cells were incubated without or with Pg-LPS or Pg-WC. The mRNA levels of SLPI were measured by real-time RT-PCR. Mean ± S.D.

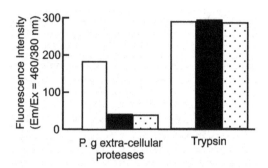

Fig. 2. Inhibitory effect of SLPI on the Lys-gingipain activity. Proteolytic activity toward His-Glu-Lys-MCA was measured with *P. gingivalis* extracellular proteases or trypsin without SLPI (open bar) or with 50 μg/ml (closed bar) and 100 μg/ml (dotted bar) of rSLPI.

3. Invasion into gingival tissues

Ultrastructural study demonstrated bacterial invasion in the apical gingiva of patients suffering from advanced chronic periodontitis (Frank, 1980; Saglie et al., 1986; Kim et al., 2010). In disease legions, the barrier of PMNL present in the gingival crevice (periodontal pocket) is insufficient to prevent plaque bacterial invasion of the pocket walls, and subgingival plaque bacteria including *P. gingivalis* penetrate gingival epithelium. The bacterial penetration and access to the connective tissue is augmented by enlargement of the intercellular spaces of the junctional epithelium caused by destruction of intercellular junctions. *P. gingivalis* Arg- and Lys-gingipains are involved in degradation of several types of intercellular junctions and extracellular matrix proteins in host tissues. Intercellular presence of subgingival plaque bacteria was specifically demonstrated in the regions. However, intracellular bacteria have not been inevitably noticed in the cases of advanced chronic periodontitis except bacteria in phagocytic vacuoles of PMNL by ultrastructural studies.

On the other hand, invasion or internalization of *P. gingivalis* is observed in the cultures of gingival epithelial cells (Lamont et al., 1992 & 1995), oral epithelial KB cells (Duncan et al., 1993), and aortic and heart endothelial cells (Deshpande et al., 1998). Invasion of bacteria is quantitated by the standard antibiotic protection assay using gentamicin and metronidazole. Under optimal inoculation conditions at a multiplicity of infection of 1:100, approximately 10% of *P. gingivalis* are recovered intracellularly from epithelial cells at 90 to 300 min after incubation. The invasion efficiency for KB cells and endothelial cells is reported to be much lower, around 0.1%. With these cells, adherence of *P. gingivalis* to the cell surface commonly induces microvilli protruding and the attached bacterial cells are surrounded by microbilli on the cell surface (Fig. 3A). Adherence of *P. gingivalis* to eukaryotic cell surface is relevantly mediated with fimbriae, and it was reported that a fimbriae-deficient mutant exhibited a greater reduction in invasion compared with adherence (Weinberg et al., 1997). Therefore, it is speculated that fimbrillin interacts with cell surface receptor, permitting *P. gingivalis* invasion. Among the six *fimA* types, the adhesion to a human epithelial cell line was more significant in *P. gingivalis* harboring the type II *fimA* than those with other *fimA* types. Accordingly, invasion of the type II *fimA* bacteria was most efficiently demonstrated (Nakagawa et al., 2002b). Host receptor candidates including β2 and α5β1-integrin have been reported to interact with *P. gingivalis* fimbrillin.

Following the attachment of *P. gingivalis* to cells, the invasion process requires the involvement of both microfilament (actin polymerization) and microtubule activities. This property is similar to those of *N. gonorrhoeae* and enteropathogenic *E. coli*. In addition, proteolytic activity is involved in *P. gingivalis* invasion, whereas *de novo* protein synthesis both in *P. gingivalis* and eukaryotic cells are not inevitably needed (Lamont et al., 1995; Deshpande et al., 1998).

Although effects of staurosporine, a broad-spectrum inhibitor of protein kinases, on invasion are varied among targeted cells, protein phosphorylation is surely involved in *P. gingivalis* invasion. A recent report by Tribble et al. (2006) demonstrated that a haloacid dehalogenase family serine phosphatase, SerB653, secreted from *P. gingivalis* regulates microtubule dynamics in human immortalized gingival keratinocytes. The dephosphorylation activity of SerB653 is closely related to the optimal invasion and intracellular survival of the microorganism. The pull-down assay revealed Hsp90 and GAPDH as interactive candidates for SerB653. Both proteins are known to be phosphorylated and may play a role in modulation of microtubules for initiation of the bacterial invasion into epithelial cells.

We have recently succeeded in monitoring the *P. gingivalis* invasion process into porcine carotid endothelial cells in culture by time-laps movie (a part of the results is shown as Fig. 3B) (Hayashi M., Ohara-Nemoto, Y. & Kawamura, T., unpublished data of Cine-Science Lab. Co., Tokyo, Japan). Our movie clearly showed swift entering of the bacteria inside the cell through cell membrane. Intracellular movement of *P. gingivalis* was also observed, suggesting an interaction of the bacteria with microtubules. After 3-h invasion, *P. gingivalis* was located around the nuclei (Fig. 3B). This observation is in good accord with previous data, which showed accumulation of internalized recombinant FimA-microspheres around the epithelial cell nuclei (Nakagawa et al., 2002a).

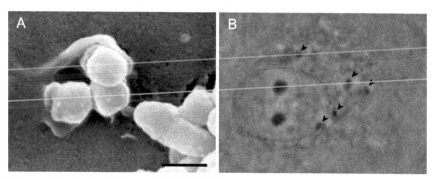

Fig. 3. Entry of *P. gingivalis* into endothelial cells. *P. gingivalis* ATCC 33277 was co-cultured with porcine carotid endothelial cells. (A) Scanning electron micrograph. *P. gingivalis* (observed in white) was surrounded by microvilli protruding from endothelial cell. Bar = 0.5 μm. (B) *P. gingivalis* inside the cell. A representative scene at 3 h after internalization from time-laps microscopic imaging with phase contrast microscopy. Arrowheads indicate *P. gingivalis* observed near the nucleus.

Molecular events of intracellular signal transduction that occur after invasion of *P. gingivalis* have been poorly defined. *P. gingivalis* invasion induces transient increase in cytosolic Ca^{2+}

concentration in gingival epithelial cells, suggesting an involvement of a Ca^{2+}-dependent signaling pathway (Izutsu et al., 1996). *P. gingivalis* internalization inhibits secretion of IL-8 by gingival epithelial cells (Darveau et al., 1998; Nassar et al., 2002), whilst interaction via integrin induced expression of IL-1β and TNF-α genes in mouse peritoneal macrophages (Takeshita et al., 1998). Since challenge of oral bacterial substances or purified *P. gingivalis* LPS to an immortal mouse gingival epithelial cell line GE1 induced gene expression of IL-1α, IL-1β, IL-6, TNF-α and SLPI (Hatakeyama et al., 2001; Ishikawa et al., 2010), the cytokine production may be induced not only by bacterial invasion but also via a Toll-like receptor pathway activated by pathogen-associated molecular patterns in host cells. These findings raise a possibility that signal transduction caused by *P. gingivalis* invasion modulates cell promotion, resulting in gingival tissue destruction.

We monitored the dysfunction of endothelial cells for the first time on co-culture with *P. gingivalis* ATCC 33277 by time-laps microscopic imaging. Endothelial cell attachment became loose at 3 h after bacterial inoculation. Furthermore, cell atrophy was evident at 22 h (Fig. 4) (Hayashi M., Ohara-Nemoto, Y. & Kawamura, T., unpublished data). Therefore, it is of interest whether cellular dysfunction is caused by *P. gingivalis* invasion into host cells or mediated by intercellular signaling through host cell surface.

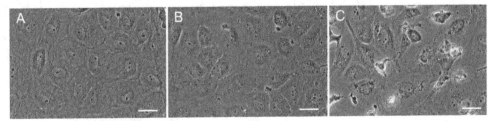

Fig. 4. Dysfunction of endothelial cells caused by co-culture with *P. gingivalis*. Porcine carotid endothelial cells were cultured with *P. gingivalis* ATCC 33277 at 37°C. Time-laps microscopic imaging was taken for 22 h. (A) Normal endothelial cells. Images at 3 h (B) and 22 h (C) after addition of *P. gingivalis*. Bar = 30 μm.

4. Induction of inflammatory responses

Chronic periodontitis is recognized as a B-cell-rich lesion that includes immunoglobulin G-producing plasma cells. However, the immunohistopathological studies revealed that B cell activation in periodontitis lesions by substances from plaque bacteria is, at least in major part, polyclonal, since the immunoglobulin showed a broad spectrum of antibody specificities, as is expected of polyclonal activation (Page, 1982). LPS from the outer membrane of gram-negative bacteria elicits a wide variety of responses that may contribute to inflammation and host defense. LPS stimulates various cell types including pre-B cells and B cells, and LPS activates most B cells (polyclonal B cell activation) without regard to its antigen specificity (Snow, 1994). Although *P. gingivalis* LPS is composed of unique constituents and exhibits characteristic immunological activities (Fujiwara et al., 1990 & 1994; Kimura et al., 1995 & 2000b), *P. gingivalis* LPS can be a potent polyclonal activator of B cells (Mihara et al., 1994), thus, it appears that *P. gingivalis* LPS could play a central role in the B cell activation in periodontitis lesions.

P. gingivalis LPS in gingival tissues could not only elicit a wide variety of responses of gingival fibroblasts and periodontal ligament fibroblasts to produce inflammatory cytokines (Agarwal et al., 1995; Yamaji et al., 1995), but also modulate immunocompetent cell responses, especially B cell activation, that may deteriorate the inflammatory condition. The immunoregulatory disorder is demonstrated in chronic periodontitis patients (Kimura et al., 1991).

It is also possible that the proteolytic enzymes of gingipains and collagenase produced by *P. gingivalis* could destroy periodontal tissue directly or indirectly, leading the progression of the disease (Holt et al., 1999; Potempa et al., 2000). Moreover, the organic metabolites such as ammonia, propionate and butyrate could exhibit the ability of disruption of the host immune system and the toxicity against the gingival epithelium (Tsuda et al., 2010). Thus, in chronic periodontitis, the pathogenic factors of *P. gingivalis* could contribute to the gingival inflammation in diverse ways, which results in the alveolar bone losses.

5. Induction of alveolar bone losses

In order to investigate the host-parasite relationship in periodontal diseases, animal models are critically important, since they provide the information about the complex pathogenic mechanism in periodontal diseases. To date, various models including rodents, rabbits, pigs, dogs, and nonhuman primates, have been used to model human periodontitis, and there are clear evidences from the literatures demonstrating alveolar bone losses in the animals infected with *P. gingivalis* (Holt et al., 1988; Kimura et al., 2000a, Wang et al., 2007; Oz & Puleo, 2011). In rodent models, however, a relatively large number of bacteria have often been used for a successful establishment (Klausen, 1991), since some periodontopathic bacteria including *P. gingivalis* are reported to be not easily established in the murine mouth (Wray & Grahame, 1992). In many instances, 10^8-10^9 bacteria in the suspension were applied into the oral cavity two or three times, with or without ligation (Oz & Puleo, 2011). In these studies, therefore, the precise inoculum size of the bacteria into the gingival crevice was unknown. Furthermore, it is possible that the pathogenicity of the bacteria with higher activity in the initial colonization in the oral cavity may have been overestimated, regardless of their bone resorbing potential. Then, we developed *P. gingivalis*-adhered ligatures on which 4.29 ± 0.23 logCFU/mm of *P. gingivalis* 381 cells were pre-adhered, and had applied it (1×10^5 *P. gingivalis* cells per mouse) on the first molar in the right maxillary quadrant of a mouse with sterile instruments (Kimura et al., 2000a). *P. gingivalis* was recovered in 95% of the infected mice on 1 week, and 58% on 15 weeks after the single infection with a *P. gingivalis*-adhered ligature in mouse gingival sulcus, indicating that, by means of this method, the establishment of *P. gingivalis* in murine mouths is not transient. The long-lasting infection of *P. gingivalis* in mice resulted in the site-specific alveolar bone breakdown on weeks 13 to 15, although sham-infected mice showed some alveolar bone breakdown in the ligation sites. These findings are supported by the linear regression analysis showing a significant positive correlation between the number of recovered *P. gingivalis* and alveolar bone loss. Furthermore, the *P. gingivalis*-induced alveolar bone loss seemed to be localized around the infected site. Thus, it is strongly suggested that the colonization of a critical amount of *P. gingivalis* for a certain period in gingival crevices may cause the periodontal breakdown at the site of colonization.

P. gingivalis could induce alveolar bone loss in diverse ways; *P. gingivalis* could influence both bone metabolism by Toll-like receptor signaling and bone remodeling by the receptor activator of NF-κB (RANK) signaling (Zhang et al., 2011). Among the pathogenic factors of *P. gingivalis*, a major causative factor in alveolar bone losses may be ascribed to the LPS. *P. gingivalis* LPS can induce in vitro the osteoclast formation directly, and also indirectly by the cytokine production from gingival fibroblasts (Slots and Genco, 1984; Zubery, 1998; Scheres et al., 2011). Moreover, an in vivo study indicated that *P. gingivalis* LPS injection resulted in significantly more bone loss versus PBS injections in both the rats with and without diabetes on normal diets (Kador et al., 2011).

In addition, an alternative hypothesis of etiology of development/onset of chronic periodontitis, 'polymicrobial pathogenicity', has been proposed, although a number of findings supporting the pathogenicity of *P. gingivalis* in periodontal diseases. The hypothesis is based on the observation in periodontitis patients that the colonization of 'red complex species' (*P. gingivalis*, *T. denticola* and *T. forsythensis*) strongly related to pocket depth and bleeding on probing (Socransky et al., 1998), and in a rat model that the rats infected with the polymicrobial consortium of the 'red complex species' exhibited significantly increased alveolar bone loss compared to those in the rats infected with one of the microbes (Kesavalu et al., 2007). However, the synergistic pathogenicity is still controversial; Orth et al. (2011) reported that co-inoculation with *P. gingivalis* and *T. denticola* induced alveolar bone losses synergistically in a murine model, whereas no synergistic virulence of the mixed infection with *P. gingivalis* and *T. denticola* was showed in a rat experimental periodontitis model (Verma et al., 2010).

The hypothesis of the synergistic polymicrobial pathogenicity does not exclude the pathogenicity of *P. gingivalis*, but acknowledges also the significant role of the local environmental conditions in subgingival plaques that could govern the periodontopathic potential of *P. gingivalis*. Further studies are obviously required to elucidate the mechanism of the polymicrobial pathogenicity in periodontal breakdown and what kinds of putative periodontopathic bacteria could participate in the synergistic pathogenicity with *P. gingivalis*.

6. References

Agarwal, S., Baran, C., Piesco, N. P., Quintero, J. C., Langkamp, H. H., Johns, L. P. & Chandra, C. S. (1995) Synthesis of proinflammatory cytokines by human gingival fibroblasts in response to lipopolysaccharides and interleukin-1β. *J. Periodont. Res.* vol. 30, pp. 382-389, 0022-3484

Amano, A., Sharma, A., Lee, J. Y., Sojar, H. T., Raj, P. A. & Genco, R. J. (1996a) Structural domains of *Porphyromonas gingivalis* recombinant fimbrillin that mediate binding to salivary proline-rich protein and statherin. *Infect. Immun.* vol. 64, pp. 1631-1637, 0019-9567

Amano, A., Kataoka, K., Raj, P. A., Genco, R. J. & Shizukuishi, S. (1996b) Binding sites of salivary statherin for *Porphyromonas gingivalis* recombinant fimbrillin. *Infect. Immun.* vol. 64, pp. 4249-4254, 0019-9567

Amano, A., Shizukuishi, S., Horie, H., Kimura, S., Morisaki, I. & Hamada, S. (1998) Binding of *Porphyromonas gingivalis* fimbriae to proline-rich glycoproteins in parotid saliva via a domain shared by major salivary components. *Infect. Immun.* vol. 66, pp. 2072-2077, 0019-9567

Amano, A., Nakagawa, I., Kataoka, K., Morisaki, I. & Hamada, S. (1999a) Distribution of *Porphyromonas gingivalis* strains with *fimA* genotypes in periodontitis patients. *J. Clin. Microbiol.* vol. 37, pp. 1426-1430, 0095-1137

Amano, A., Nakamura, T., Kimura, S., Morisaki, I., Nakagawa, I., Kawabata, S. & Hamada, S. (1999b) Molecular interactions of *Porphyromonas gingivalis* fimbriae with host proteins: kinetic analyses based on surface plasmon resonance. *Infect. Immun.* vol. 67, pp. 2399-2405, 0019-9567

Asikainen, S., Chen, C. & Slots, J. (1996) Likelihood of transmitting *Actinobacillus actinomycetemcomitans* and *Porphyromona gingivalis* in families with periodontitis. *Oral Microbiol. Immunol.* vol. 11, pp. 387-394, 0902-0055

Asikainen, S. & Chen, C. (1999) Oral ecology and person-to-person transmission of *Actinobacillus actinomycetemcomitans* and *Porphyromona gingivalis*. *Periodontology 2000* vol. 20, pp. 65-81, 0906-6713

Cimasoni, G. (1983) Crevicular fluid updated. Monogr. Oral Sci. vol. 12:III-VII, pp. 1-152, 0077-0892

da Fonseca, M. A. & Fontes, F. (2000) Early tooth loss due to cyclic neutropenia: long-term follow-up of one patient. *Spec. Care Dentist.* Vol. 20, pp. 187-190, 0275-1879

Dahlén, G., Manji, F., Baelum, V. & Fejerskov, O. (1992) Putative periodontopathogens in "diseased" and "non-diseased" persons exhibiting poor oral hygiene. *J. Clin. Periodontol.* vol. 19, pp. 35-42, 0303-6979

Darveau, R. P., Belton, C. M., Reife, R. A. & Lamont, R. J. (1998) Local chemokine paralysis, a novel pathogenic mechanism of *Porphyromonas gingivalis*. *Infect. Immun.* vol. 66, pp. 1660-1665, 0019-9567

Delcourt-Debruyne, E. M., Boutigny, H. R. & Hildebrand, H. F. (2000) Features of severe periodontal disease in a teenager with Chédiak-Higashi syndrome. *J. Periodontol.* vol. 71, pp. 816-824, 0022-3492

Deshpande, R. G., Khan, M. B. & Genco, C. A.(1998) Invasion of aortic and heart endothelial cells by *Porphyromonas gingivalis*. *Infect. Immun.* vol. 66, pp. 5337-5343, 0019-9567

Duncan, M. J., Nakao, S., Skobe, Z. & Xie, H. (1993) Interactions of *Porphyromonas gingivalis* with epithelial cells. *Infect. Immun.* vol. 61, pp. 2260-2265, 0019-9567

Dzink, J. L., Socransky, S. S. & Haffajee, A. D .(1988) The predominant cultivable microbiota of active and inactive lesions of destructive periodontal diseases. *J. Clin. Periodontol.* vol. 15, pp. 316-323, 0303-6979

Faveri, M., Feres, M., Shibli, J. A., Hayacibara, R. F., Hayacibara, M. M. & de Figueiredo, L. C. (2006) Microbiota of the dorsum of the tongue after plaque accumulation: an experimental study in humans. *J. Periodontol.* vol. 77, pp. 1539-1546, 0022-3492

Frank, R. M. (1980) Bacterial penetration in the apical pocket wall of advanced human periodontitis. *J. Periodont. Res.* vol. 15, pp. 563-573, 0022-3484

Fujiwara, T., Ogawa, T., Sobue, S. & Hamada, S. (1990) Chemical, immunobiological and antigenic characterizations of lipopolysaccharides from *Bacteroides gingivalis* strains. *J. Gen. Microbiol.* vol. 136, pp. 319-326, 0022-1287

Fujiwara, T., Nakagawa, I., Morishima, S., Takahashi, I. & Hamada, S. (1994) Inconsistency between the fimbrilin gene and the antigenicity of lipopolysaccharides in selected strains of *Porphyromonas gingivalis*. *FEMS Microbiol. Lett.* vol. 124, pp. 333-341, 0378-1097

Genco, R. J. & Mergenhagen, S. E. eds. (1982) *Host-parasite interaction in periodontal diseases,* American Society for Microbiology, 0-914826-37-9, Washington, D.C.

Genco, R. J. (1996) Current view of risk factors for periodontal diseases. *J. Periodontol.* vol. 67, pp. 1041-1049, 0022-3492

Haffajee, A. D., Teles, R. P., Patel, M. R., Song, X., Veiga, N. & Socransky, S. S. (2009) Factors affecting human supragingival biofilm composition. I. Plaque mass. *J. Periodont. Res.* vol. 44, pp. 511-519, 0022-3484

Hamada, S., Holt, S. C. & McGhee, J. R. eds. (1991) *Periodontal disease: Pathogens and host immune responses,* Quintessence Publishing Co., 4-87417-342-X C3047, Tokyo, Japan

Hamada, S., Fujiwara, T., Morishima, T., Takahashi, I., Nakagawa, I., Kimura, S. & Ogawa, T. (1994) Molecular and immunological characterization of the fimbriae of *Porphyromonas gingivalis. Microbiol. Immunol.* vol. 38, pp. 921-930, 0385-5600

Hamada, S., Amano, A., Kimura, S., Nakagawa, I., Kawabata, S. & Morisaki, I. (1998) The importance of fimbriae in the virulence and ecology of some oral bacteria. *Oral Microbiol. Immunol.* vol. 13, pp. 129-138, 0902-0055

Hatakeyama, S., Ohara-Nemoto, Y., Yanai, N., Obinata, M., Hayashi, S. & Satoh, M. (2001) Establishment of gingival epithelial cell lines from transgenic mice harboring temperature sensitive simian virus 40 large T-antigen gene. *J. Oral Pathol. Med.* vol. 30. pp. 296-304, 0904-2512

Holt, S. C., Ebersole, J., Felton, J., Brunsvold, M. & Kornman, K. S. (1988) Implantation of *Bacteroides gingivalis* in nonhuman primates initiates progression of periodontitis. *Science* vol. 239(4835), pp. 55-57, 0036-8075

Holt, S. C., Kesavalu, L., Walker, S. & Genco, C. A. (1999) Virulence factors of *Porphyromonas gingivalis. Periodontology 2000* vol. 20, pp. 168-238, 0906-6713

Ishikawa, T., Ohara-Nemoto, Y., Tajika, S., Sasaki, M. & Kimura, S. (2010) The production of secretory leukocyte protease inhibitor from gingival epithelial cells in response to *Porphyromonas gingivalis* lipopolysaccharides. *Interface Oral Health Sci. 2009,* pp. 275-276, 978-4-431-99643-9

Izutsu, K. T., Belton, C. M., Chan, A., Fatherazi, S., Kanter, J. P., Park, Y. & Lamont, R. J. (1996) Involvement of calcium in interactions between gingival epithelial cells and *Porphyromonas gingivalis. FEMS Microbiol. Lett.* vol. 144, pp. 145-150, 0378-1097

Kador, P. F., O'Meara, J. D., Blessing, K., Marx, D. B. & Reinhardt, R. A. (2011) Efficacy of structurally diverse aldose reductase inhibitors on experimental periodontitis in rats. *J. Periodontol.* vol. 82, pp. 926-933, 0022-3492

Kato, T., Kawai, S., Nakano, K., Inaba, H., Kuboniwa, M., Nakagawa, I., Tsuda, K., Omori, H., Ooshima, T., Yoshimori, T. & Amano, A. (2007) Virulence of *Porphyromonas gingivalis* is altered by substitution of fimbria gene with different genotype. *Cell. Microbiol.* vol. 9, pp. 753-765, 1462-5814

Kesavalu, L., Sathishkumar, S., Bakthavatchalu, V., Matthews, C., Dawson, D., Steffen, M. & Ebersole, J. L. (2007) Rat model of polymicrobial infection, immunity, and alveolar bone resorption in periodontal disease. *Infect. Immun.* vol. 75, pp. 1704-1712, 0019-9567

Kim, Y. C., Ko, Y., Hong, S. D., Kim, K. Y., Lee, Y. H., Chae, C. & Choi, Y. (2010) Presence of *Porphyromonas gingivalis* and plasma cell dominance in gingival tissues with periodontitis. *Oral Dis.* vol. 16, pp. 375-381, 1354-523X

Kimura, S., Fujimoto, N. & Okada, H. (1991) Impaired autologous mixed-lymphocyte reaction of peripheral blood lymphocytes in adult periodontitis. *Infect. Immun.* vol. 59, pp. 4418-4424, 0019-9567

Kimura, S., Yonemura, T., Hiraga, T. & Okada, H. (1992) Flow cytometric evaluation of phagocytosis by peripheral blood polymorphonuclear leukocytes in human periodontal diseases. *Arch. Oral Biol.* vol. 37, pp. 495-501, 0003-9969

Kimura, S., Yonemura, T. & Kaya, H. (1993) Increased oxidative product formation by peripheral blood polymorphonuclear leukocytes in human periodontal diseases. *J. Periodont. Res.* vol. 28, pp. 197-203, 0022-3484

Kimura, S., Koga, T., Fujiwara, T., Kontani, M., Shintoku, K., Kaya, H. & Hamada, S. (1995) Tyrosine protein phosphorylation in murine B lymphocytes by stimulation with lipopolysaccharide from *Porphyromonas gingivalis*. *FEMS Microbiol. Lett.* vol. 130, pp. 1-6, 0378-1097

Kimura, S., Nagai, A., Onitsuka, T., Koga, T., Fujiwara, T., Kaya, H. & Hamada, S. (2000a) Induction of experimental periodontitis in mice with *Porphyromonas gingivalis*-adhered ligatures. *J. Periodontol.* vol. 71, pp. 1167-1173, 0022-3492

Kimura, S., Tamamura, T., Nakagawa, I., Koga, T., Fujiwara, T. & Hamada, S. (2000b) CD14-dependent and independent pathways in lipopolysaccharide-induced activation of a murine B-cell line, CH12. LX. *Scand. J. Immunol.* vol. 51, pp. 392-399, 0300-9475

Kimura, S., Ooshima, T., Takiguchi, M., Sasaki, Y., Amano, A., Morisaki, I. & Hamada, S. (2002) Periodontopathic bacterial infection in childhood. *J. Periodontol.* vol. 73, pp. 20-26, 0022-3492

Kimura, S. & Ohara-Nemoto, Y. (2007) Early childhood caries and childhood periodontal diseases, In: *Pediatric Infectious Diseases Revisited*, H. Schroten & S. Wirth (Eds.), 177-197, Birkhäuser-Verlag AG, 978-37643-7997, Basel, Switzerland

Kishi, M., Kimura, S., Ohara-Nemoto, Y., Kishi, K., Aizawa, F., Moriya, T. & Yonemitsu, M. (2002) Oral malodor and periodontopathic microorganisms in tongue coat of periodontally healthy subjects. *Dent. Japan*, vol. 38, pp. 24-28, 0070-3737

Kishi, M., Ohara-Nemoto, Y., Takahashi, M., Kishi, K., Kimura, S. & Yonemitsu, M. (2010) Relationship between oral status and prevalence of periodontopathic bacteria on the tongues of elderly individuals. *J. Med. Microbiol.* vol. 59, pp. 1354-1359, 0022-2615

Klausen, B. (1991) Microbiological and immunological aspects of experimental periodontal disease in rats: a review article. *J. Periodontol.* vol. 62, pp. 59-73, 0022-3492

Kontani, M., Ono, H., Shibata, H., Okamura, Y., Tanaka, T., Fujiwara, T., Kimura, S. & Hamada, S. (1996) Cysteine protease of *Porphyromonas gingivalis* 381 enhances binding of fimbriae to cultured human fibroblasts and matrix proteins. *Infect. Immun.* vol. 64, pp. 756-762, 0019-9567

Kontani, M., Kimura, S., Nakagawa, I. & Hamada, S. (1997) Adherence of *Porphyromonas gingivalis* to matrix proteins via a fimbrial cryptic receptor exposed by its own arginine-specific protease. *Mol. Microbiol.* vol. 24, pp. 1179-1187, 0950-382X

Lalla, E., Cheng, B., Lal, S., Kaplan, S., Softness, B., Greenberg, E., Goland, R. S. & Lamster, I. B. (2007) Diabetes mellitus promotes periodontal destruction in children. *J. Clin. Periodontol.* vol. 34, pp. 294-298, 0303-6979

Lamont, R. J., Oda, D., Persson, R. E. & Persson, G. R. (1992) Interaction of *Porphyromonas gingivalis* with gingival epithelial cells maintained in culture. *Oral Microbiol. Immunol.* vol. 7, pp. 364–367, 0902-0055

Lamont, R. J., Chan, A., Belton, C. M., Izutsu, K. T., Vasel, D. & Weinberg, A. (1995) *Porphyromonas gingivalis* invasion of gingival epithelial cells. *Infect. Immun.* vol. 63, pp. 3878–3885, 0019-9567

Lamont, R. J. & Jenkinson, H. F. (1998) Life below the gum line: Pathogenic mechanisms of *Porphyromonas gingivalis. Microbiol. Mol. Biol. Rev.* vol. 62, pp. 1244-1263, 1092-2172.

Lee, J. Y., Sojar, H. T., Bedi, G. S. & Genco, R. J. (1991) *Porphyromonas (Bacteroides) gingivalis* fimbrillin: size, amino-terminal sequence, and antigenic heterogeneity. *Infect. Immun.* vol. 59, pp. 383-389, 0019-9567.

Meyle, J. & Gonzáles, J. R. (2001) Influences of systemic diseases on periodontitis in children and adolescents. *Periodontology 2000* vol. 26, pp. 92-112, 0906-6713

Mihara, J., Fukai, T., Morisaki, I., Fujiwara, T. & Hamada, S. (1994) Decrease in mitogenic responses with age in senescence accelerated mouse spleen cells to LPS from *Porphyromonas gingivalis,* In: *The SAM model of senescence,* T. Takeda (Ed.), 219-222, Excerpta Medica, 0-444-81695-X, Amsterdam, Netherlands

Muramatsu, K., Kokubu, E., Shibahara, T., Okuda, K. & Ishihara, K. (2011) HGP44 induces protection against *Porphyromonas gingivalis*-Induced alveolar bone loss in mice. *Clin. Vaccine Immunol.* vol. 18, pp. 888-891, 1556-6811

Naito, Y & Gibbons, R. J. (1988) Attachment of *Bacteroides gingivalis* to collagenous substrata. *J. Dent. Res.* vol. 67, pp. 1075-1080, 0022-0345

Naito, Y., Tohda, H., Okuda, K. & Takazoe, I. (1993) Adherence and hydrophobicity of invasive and noninvasive strains of *Porphyromonas gingivalis. Oral Microbiol. Immunol.* vol. 8, pp. 195-202, 0902-0055

Nakagawa, I., Amano, A., Kimura, R. K., Nakamura, T., Kawabata, S. & Hamada, S. (2000) Distribution and molecular characterization of *Porphyromonas gingivalis* carrying a new type of *fimA* gene. *J. Clin. Microbiol.* vol. 38, pp. 1909-1914, 0095-1137

Nakagawa, I., Amano, A., Kuboniwa, M., Nakamura, T., Kawabata, S. & Hamada, S. (2002a) Functional differences among FimA variants of *Porphyromonas gingivalis* and their effects on adhesion to and invasion of human epithelial cells. *Infect. Immun.* vol. 70, pp. 277-285, 0019-9567

Nakagawa, I., Amano, A., Ohara-Nemoto, Y., Endoh, N., Morisaki, I., Kimura, S., Kawabata, S. & Hamada, S. (2002b) Identification of a new variant of *fimA* gene of *Porphyromonas gingivalis* and its distribution in adults and disabled populations with periodontitis. *J. Periodont. Res.* vol. 37, pp. 425-432, 0022-3484

Nassar, H., Chou, H. H., Khlgatian, M., Gibson, F. C. 3rd, Van Dyke, T. E. & Genco, C. A. (2002) Role for fimbriae and lysine-specific cysteine proteinase gingipain K in expression of interleukin-8 and monocyte chemoattractant protein in *Porphyromonas gingivalis*-infected endothelial cells. *Infect. Immun.* vol. 70, pp. 268-276, 0019-9567

Ogawa, T., Kusumoto, Y., Uchida, H., Nagashima, S., Ogo, H. & Hamada, S. (1991) Immunobiological activities of synthetic peptide segments of fimbrial protein from *Porphyromonas gingivalis. Biochem. Biophys. Res. Commun.* vol. 180, pp. 1335-1341, 0006-291X

Okuda, K., Slots, J. & Genco, R. J. (1981) *Bacteroides gingivalis, Bacteroides asaccharolyticus* and *Bacteroides melaninogenicus* subspecies: cell surface morphology and adherence to erythrocytes and human buccal epithelial cells. *Curr. Microbiol.* vol. 6, pp. 5-12, 0343-8651

Ooshima, T., Nishiyama, N., Hou, B., Tamura, K., Amano, A., Kusumoto, A. & Kimura, S. (2003) Occurrence of periodontal bacteria in healthy children: a 2-year longitudinal study. *Community Dent. Oral Epidemiol.* vol. 31, pp. 417-425, 0301-5661

Orth, R. K., O'Brien-Simpson, N. M., Dashper, S. G. & Reynolds, E. C. (2011) Synergistic virulence of *Porphyromonas gingivalis* and *Treponema denticola* in a murine periodontitis model. *Mol. Oral Microbiol.* vol. 26, pp. 229-240, 2041-1006

Oz, H. S. & Puleo, D. A. (2011) Animal models of periodontal disease. *J. Biomed. Biotechnol.* vol. 2011, Article ID 754867, pp. 1-8, 1110-7243

Page, R. C. (1982) Lymphoid cell responsiveness and human periodontitis, In: *Host-parasite interaction in periodontal diseases*, R. J. Genco & S, E. Mergenhagen (Eds.), 217-224, American Society for Microbiology, 0-914826-37-9, Washington D.C., USA

Potempa, J., Banbula, A. & Travis, J. (2000) Role of bacterial proteinases in matrix destruction and modulation of host responses. *Periodontology 2000* vol. 24, pp. 153-192, 0906-6713

Saglie, F. R., Smith, C. T., Newman, M. G., Carranza, F. A. Jr., Pertuiset, J. H., Cheng, L., Auil, E & Nisengard, R. J. (1986) The presence of bacteria in the oral epithelium in periodontal disease. II. Immunohistochemical identification of bacteria. *J. Periodontol.* vol. 57, pp. 492-500, 0022-3492

Scheres, N., de Vries, T. J., Brunner, J., Crielaard, W., Laine, M. L. & Everts, V. (2011) Diverse effects of *Porphyromonas gingivalis* on human osteoclast formation. *Microb. Pathog.* vol. 51, pp. 149-155, 0882-4010

Slots, J. & Gibbons, R. J. (1978) Attachment of *Bacteroides melaninogenicus* subsp. *asaccharolyticus* to oral surfaces and its possible role in colonization of the mouth and of periodontal pockets. *Infect. Immun.* vol. 19, pp. 254-264, 0019-9567

Slots, J. & Genco, R. J. (1984) Black-pigmented *Bacteroides* species, *Capnocytophaga* species, and *Actinobacillus actinomycetemcomitans* in human periodontal disease: virulence factors in colonization, survival, and tissue destruction. *J. Dent. Res.* vol. 63, pp. 412-421, 0022-0345

Snow, E. C. ed. (1994) *Handbook of B and T lymphocytes*, Academic Press, 0-12-653955-3, San Diego, USA

Socransky, S. S., Haffajee, A. D., Cugini, M. A., Smith, C. & Kent, R. L. Jr. (1998) Microbial complexes in subgingival plaque. *J. Clin. Periodontol.* vol. 25, pp. 134-144, 0303-6979

Socransky, S. S. & Haffajee, A. D. (2002) Dental biofilms: difficult therapeutic targets. *Periodontology 2000.* vol. 28, pp. 12-55, 0906-6713

Takeshita, A., Murakami, Y., Yamashita, Y., Ishida, M., Fujisawa, S., Kitano, S. & Hanazawa, S. (1998) *Porphyromonas gingivalis* fimbriae use β2 integrin (CD11/CD18) on mouse peritoneal macrophages as a cellular receptor, and the CD18 β chain plays a functional role in fimbrial signaling. *Infect. Immun.* vol. 66, pp. 4056–4060, 0019-9567

Tribble, G. D., Mao, S., James, C. E. & Lamont, R. J. (2006) A *Porphyromonas gingivalis* haloacid dehalogenase family phosphatase interacts with human phosphoproteins and is important for invasion. *Proc. Natl. Acad. Sci. USA* vol. 103, pp. 11027-11032, 0027-8424

Tsuda, H., Ochiai, K., Suzuki, N. & Otsuka, K. (2010) Butyrate, a bacterial metabolite, induces apoptosis and autophagic cell death in gingival epithelial cells. *J. Periodont. Res.* vol. 45, pp. 626-634, 0022-3484

Tuite-McDonnell, M., Griffen, A. L., Moeschberger, M. L., Dalton, R. E., Fuerst, P. A. & Leys, E. J. (1997) Concordance of *Porphyromona gingivalis* colonization in families. *J. Clin. Microbiol.* vol. 35, pp. 455-461, 0095-1137

Van Winkelhoff, A. J. & Boutaga, K. (2005) Transmission of periodontal bacteria and models of infection. *J. Clin. Periodontol.* vol. 32 Suppl 6, pp. 16-27, 0303-6979

Verma, R. K., Rajapakse, S., Meka, A., Hamrick, C., Pola, S., Bhattacharyya, I., Nair, M., Wallet, S. M., Aukhil, I. & Kesavalu, L. (2010) *Porphyromonas gingivalis* and *Treponema denticola* mixed microbial infection in a rat model of periodontal disease. *Interdiscip. Perspect. Infect. Dis.* vol. 2010, article ID 605125, 10 pages, 1687-708X

Wang, S., Liu, Y., Fang, D. & Shi, S. (2007) The miniature pig: a useful large animal model for dental and orofacial research. *Oral Dis.* vol. 13, pp. 530-537, 1354-523X

Watson, M. R., Bret, W. A. & Loesche, W. J. (1994) Presence of *Treponema denticola* and *Porphyromonas gingivalis* in children correlated with periodontal disease of their parents. *J. Dent. Res.* vol. 73, pp. 1636-1640, 0022-0345

Weinberg, A., Belton, C. M., Park, Y. & Lamont, R. J. (1997) Role of fimbriae in *Porphyromonas gingivalis* invasion of gingival epithelial cells. *Infect. Immun.* vol. 65, pp. 313–316, 0019-9567

Wray, D. & Grahame, L. (1992) Periodontal bone loss in mice induced by different periodontopathic organisms. *Arch. Oral Biol.* vol. 37, pp. 435-438, 0003-9969

Yamaji, Y., Kubota, T., Sasaguri, K., Sato, S., Suzuki, Y., Kumada, H. & Umemoto, T. (1995) Inflammatory cytokine gene expression in human periodontal ligament fibroblasts stimulated with bacterial lipopolysaccharides. *Infect. Immun.* vol. 63, pp. 3576-3581, 0019-9567

Yoshimura, F., Takahashi, K., Nodasaka, Y. & Suzuki, T. (1984) Purification and characterization of a novel type of fimbriae from the oral anaerobe *Bacteroides gingivalis*. *J. Bacteriol.* vol. 160, pp. 949-957, 0021-9193

Zhang, P., Liu, J., Xu, Q., Harber, G., Feng, X., Michalek, S. M. & Katz, J. (2011) TLR2-dependent modulation of osteoclastogenesis by *Porphyromonas gingivalis* through differential induction of NFATc1 and NF-κB. *J. Biol. Chem.* vol. 286, pp. 24159-24169, 0021-9258

Zubery, Y., Dunstan, C. R., Story, B. M., Kesavalu, L., Ebersole, J. L., Holt, S. C. & Boyce, B. F. (1998) Bone resorption caused by three periodontal pathogens in vivo in mice is mediated in part by prostaglandin. *Infect. Immun.* vol. 66, pp. 4158-4162, 0019-9567

Exopolysaccharide Productivity and Biofilm Phenotype on Oral Commensal Bacteria as Pathogenesis of Chronic Periodontitis

Takeshi Yamanaka[1], Kazuyoshi Yamane[1],
Chiho Mashimo[1], Takayuki Nambu[1], Hugo Maruyama[1],
Kai-Poon Leung[2] and Hisanori Fukushima[1]
[1]*Osaka Dental University,*
[2]*US Army Dental and Trauma Research Detachment, Institute of Surgical Research,*
[1]*Japan*
[2]*USA*

1. Introduction

Exopolysaccharide (EPS) productivities in many bacteria have been associated with pathogenicity in mammalian hosts as providing extracellular matrices to form biofilm (Costerton et al., 1995). Bacteria assuming biofilm-forming capacity have enormous advantages in establishing persistent infections (Costerton et al., 1999). Chronic periodontitis is caused by dental plaque known as a complex biofilm which consists of several hundred different species of bacteria (Chen, 2001; Socransky and Haffajee, 2002; Lovegrove, 2004). While sucrose-derived homopolysaccharides are well known substrates which mediate adhesion of bacteria to the tooth surface and co-aggregation interactions between species of oral bacteria in the dental plaque (Russell, 2009), recent studies suggest that each bacterium produces distinctive EPS components in a sucrose-independent manner and can form so called single species biofilm (Branda et al., 2005). In the oral cavity, several species of oral bacteria are known to produce their own EPS with this manner (Okuda et al., 1987; Dyer and Bolton, 1985; Kaplan et al., 2004; Yamane et al., 2005; Yamanaka et al., 2009; Yamanaka et al., 2010). In this chapter, we will describe a possibility that a single species biofilm in the oral cavity can cause persistent chronic periodontitis along with the importance of dental plaque formation and maturation with sucrose-derived polysaccharides.

2. Dental plaque formation with sucrose-derived polysaccharides

Dental plaque is defined as a community of oral bacteria on a tooth surface in which microorganisms are found embedded in EPS and intimately communicate each other via several different communication pathways such as auto-/co-aggregation, metabolic communication, quorum sensing and competent stimulation peptides (Rickard et al., 2008). A recent study using pyrosequencing technique showed that dental plaque harbors nearly 7000 species-level phylotypes (Keijser et al., 2008). Therefore, dental plaque is described as mix-/multi-species biofilm as well. A widely accepted theory of dental plaque formation is an organized sequence of events (Marsh, 2004). 1) The enamel surface of tooth is covered by acquired pellicle which consists of salivary proteins. 2) Initial colonizers of oral bacteria adhere on the tooth surface via physico-chemical interactions between the bacterial cell surface and the pellicle matrices, and then establish firmer adhesin-receptor mediated attachment. A study (Nyvad and Kilian, 1987) using cultivation technique showed that the initial colonizers are predominated by streptococci such as *Streptococcus sanguinis*, *Streptococcus oralis* and *Streptococcus mitis*. Gram-positive rod *Actinomyces* spp, veillonellae, and *Rothia mucilaginosa* were frequently found in the early stage of plaque formation (Nyvad and Kilian, 1987). After the colonization of these pioneers, bacteria that have glucosyltransferase (GTF) or fructosyltransferase (FTF) start to provide sucrose-derived EPS as plaque substrates (Russell, 2009). The EPS can be soluble or insoluble and the latter make a major contribution to the structural integrity of dental plaque and can consolidate the attachment of bacteria in dental plaque. Among previously known initial colonizers, *S. sanguinis* can provide water-soluble/insoluble EPSs because this organism possesses both GTF and FTF. In this environmental niche, co-adhesion between initial colonizers and secondary colonizers occurs. 4) Then, more secondary species adhere to the developing dental plaque resulting in the increased number of bacteria through the continued integration and cell divisions (Rickard et al., 2008). 5) When dental plaque as multi-species biofilm has developed and become matured, the flora gradually changes from Gram-positive cocci and *Actinomyces* to the one containing certain amount of Gram-negative organisms (Chen, 2001; Herrera et al., 2008; Paster et al., 2001; Socransky et al., 1998). The change in dental plaque flora is also associated with the extension of the plaque subgingivally, and it is evidently shown that this phenomenon causes the plaque-associated complex symptoms in periodontal tissues (Darby and Curtis, 2001; Dahlen, 1993). This theory well explains the dental plaque formation, maturation and the plaque-associated complex in modern day since the production and consumption of sucrose increased dramatically in nineteenth century. However, considering the facts that ancient specimens showed carious lesions localized on the root surfaces and simultaneous absence of coronal lesions, oral microorganisms might have a strategy in sucrose-independent manner to form dental plaque on the tooth surface around the gingival crevice. The periodontal bone loss is also found on the ancient specimens (Meller et al., 2009; Gerloni et al., 2009). Therefore, it is conceivable that the dental plaque developed in sucrose-independent manner could be pathogenic for periodontal tissues and can cause chronic periodontitis lesions.

2.1 Initial colonizers on the tooth surface and their capacity to form biofilm

More recent studies using molecular methods and a retrievable enamel chip model have revealed a new line-up of initial colonizers though the early dental plaque microflora varies at subject-specific basis (Diaz et al., 2006; Kolenbrander et al., 2005). In initial plaque on the chip at four to eight hours, *Streptococcus* spp. was dominant while *Veillonella*, *Gemella*, *Prevotella*, *Niesseria*, *Actinomyces* and *Rothia* were also frequently found. Among streptococci, *S. oralis*, *S. mitis*, *S. infantis*, *S. sanguinis*, *S. parasanguinis*, *S. gordonii*, *S. cristatus* and *S. bovis* were found in the early dental plaque. Although this bacterial community can be given substrates by bacteria which synthesize EPS in sucrose-dependent manner, we recently found that several bacteria newly nominated as initial colonizers have the ability to produce their own EPS in sucrose-independent manner and to form biofilms.

Exopolysaccharide Productivity and Biofilm Phenotype on Oral Commensal Bacteria as Pathogenesis of
Chronic Periodontitis

43

The presence of dense meshwork structures under scanning electron microscopy (SEM) is a typical feature for biofilm forming organisms. The appearances of *Escherichia hermannii* (Yamanaka et al., 2010) with or without EPS production in SEM observation are shown in Figure 1. *E. hermannii* YS-11 isolated from persistent apical periodontitis lesions produced EPS and exhibited cell surface meshwork structures (Fig. 1A). The meshwork structures of *E. hermannii* YS-11 disappeared when *wzt*, one of the ABC-transporter genes, was disrupted by transposon random insertion mutagenesis (Fig. 1B). Complementation of this gene to the transposant restored and dramatically augmented the formation of meshwork structures (Fig. 1, C and D). Such phenotypes are similar to those of *Pseudomonas aeruginosa*, a prototype of biofilm-forming bacteria (Kobayashi, 1995; Yasuda et al., 1999), *Escherichia coli* (Prigent-Combaret et al., 2000; Uhlich et al., 2006), *Salmonella* (Anriany et al., 2001; Jain and Chen, 2006), and *Vibrio cholerae* (Wai et al., 1998).

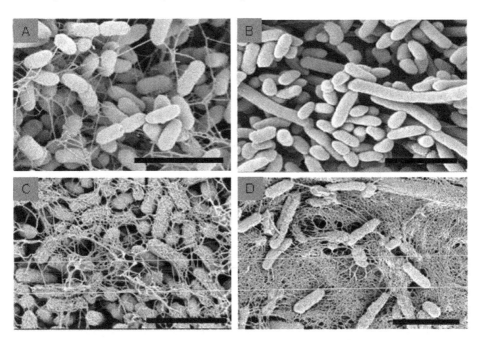

Fig. 1. Scanning electron micrographs showing surface structures of *Escherichia hermannii* strain YS-11 (A; wild type), strain 455 (B; *wzt* transposant) and strain 455-LM (strain 455 with pWZT; C: without IPTG induction; D: with IPTG induction). Bars = 3 μ m

When we observed the surface structures of isolates from saliva of healthy volunteers or from chronic peripheral periodontitis lesions by SEM, similar cell surface-associated meshwork-like structures were observed on *Neisseria, S. parasanguinis, S. mitis, Rothia dentocariosa, Rothia mucilaginosa* (Yamane et al., 2010), *Prevotella intermedia* (Yamanaka et al., 2009), *Prevotella nigrescens* (Yamane et al., 2005) and *Actinomyces oris* (Fig. 2). We have investigated the clinical isolates of *P. intermedia* and *P. nigrescens* with meshwork structures and found that the organisms can produce their own unique EPS in sucrose-independent manner (see below). However, it is still unclear whether other initial colonizers posses the meshwork structures with the same manner. It is important to note that similar tubule-like structures are formed by bacterial nanotubes (Dubey and Ben-Yehuda, 2011) or amyloids (Dueholm et al., 2010).

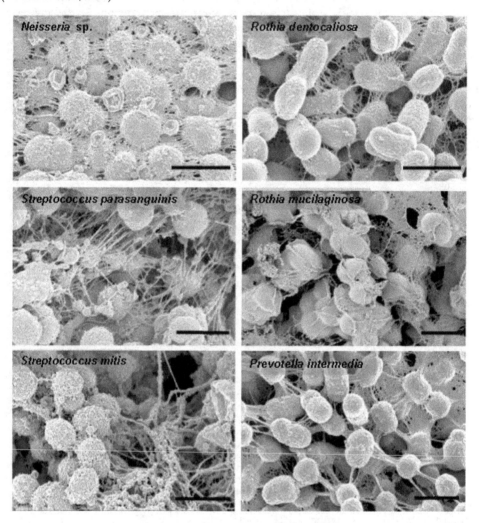

Fig. 2. Scanning electron micrographs showing cell surface structures of oral bacteria known as initial colonizers. A colony of each clinical isolate was used for SEM observation and identification by 16S rRNA gene sequencing. Bars = 2 μm.

2.1.1 Single species biofilm with unique EPS production on the outside of oral cavity

Practically all bacteria living in their own environmental niche have the capacity to form biofilm by a self-synthesized matrix that holds the cells together and tightly attaches the bacterial cells to the underlying surface. Polysaccharide is a major component of the matrix in most bacterial biofilms although recent studies have shown that constituents of biofilm matrix vary and that extracellular nucleic acids (Wu and Xi, 2009) or secreted proteins (Latasa et al., 2006) are also used as the matrix. Recent investigations have revealed that each biofilm-forming bacterium produces distinctive EPS components *e.g.* alginate and/or Psl found in *P. aeruginosa* (Ryder et al., 2007), acidic polysaccharide of *Burkholderia cepacia* (Cerantola et al., 1999), collanic acid, poly-β-1,6-GlcNAc (PGA) or cellulose found in *E. coli* (Junkins and Doyle, 1992) (Wang et al., 2004; Danese et al., 2000), cellulose of *Salmonella* (Solano et al., 2002; Zogaj et al., 2001), amorphous EPS containing *N*-acetylglucosamine (GlcNAc), D-mannose, 6-deoxy-D-galactose and D-galactose of *V. cholerae* (Wai et al., 1998; Yildiz and Visick, 2009), polysaccharide intercellular adhesin (PIA) of *Staphylococcus* (Rupp et al., 1999), and glucose and mannose rich components found in *Bacillus subtilis* biofilm (Hamon and Lazazzera, 2001; Ren et al., 2004; Yamane et al., 2009). An enteric pathogen *Campylobacter jejuni* produces EPS that reacts with calcofulor white, indicating the polysaccharide harbors β1-3 and/or β1-4 linkages. The production of this EPS is considered to be involved in the stress response of this organism together with its surface-associated lipooligosaccharide and capsular polysaccharides (McLennan et al., 2008). Persistent infections caused by biofilm-forming bacteria have been abundantly reported, however, understanding the molecular basis for the synthesis of biofilm matrices is still limited. The bacteria assuming the ability to produce their own polysaccharides and causing infectious diseases (biofilm infections) are listed in Table 1.

EPS-producing bacteria	Constituents of EPS	Biofilm infection
Pseudomonas aeruginosa	Alginate, Psl (mannose- and galactose-rich polysaccharide) or Pel (glucose rich polysaccharide)	Cystic fibrosis pneumonia, contact lenses infection, central venous catheter infections
Burkholderia cepacia	Acidic branched heptasaccharide	Cystic fibrosis pneumonia (cepacia syndrome)
Escherichia coli	Cellulose, colonic acid or poly-β-1,6-GlcNAc (PGA)	Intestinal disorders, urinary tract infections, urinary catheter infections
Vibrio cholerae	Glucose- and galactose-rich polysaccharide	Cholera, diarrheal diseases (the EPS protects this organism from environmental stress)
Salmonella enterica serovar Typhimurium	Cellulose	Gastroenteritis
Staphylococcus aureus *Staphylococcus epidermidis*	Staphylococcal polysaccharide intercellular adhesion (PIA)	Endocarditis, central venous catheter infections, urinary catheter infections
Bacillus subtilis	Glucose- and mannose-rich polysaccharide	Opportunistic infections, apical periodontitis
Campylobacter jejuni	EPS contains β1-3 and/or β1-3 linkages	Bacterial gastroenteritis

Table 1. EPS-producing bacteria on the outside of oral cavity, constituents of EPS and related diseases.

Oral streptococci such as anginosus group, mitis-group and salivarius-group and *Rothia* are known to cause biofilm infections on prosthetic heart valves and artificial voice prosthesis (Donlan, 2001). Interestingly, some clinical isolates of *Streptococcus intermedius* and *Streptococcus salivarius* exhibit dense meshwork structures around their cells suggesting these organisms can form single species biofilm on medical devices though we still do not know the constituents of the matrices (Matsumoto-Mashimo et al., 2008) (Fig. 3).

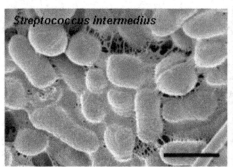 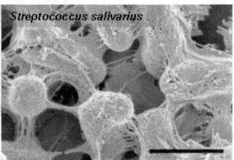

Fig. 3. Scanning electron micrographs showing cell surface structures of clinically isolated *S. intermedius* and *S. salivarius*. Bars = 2 μ m.

2.1.2 Biofilm-forming bacteria from chronic periodontitis lesions and the chemical composition of their EPS

As described above, several periodontopathic bacteria are known to produce EPS or capsular polysaccharides. The production of mannose-rich polysaccharide by *Capnocytophaga ochracea* has been reported (Dyer and Bolton, 1985). The mannose-rich EPS provides this organism with a protection from attack by the human innate immune system (Bolton et al., 1983). Kaplan et al. (2004) reported that *Aggregatibacter actinomycetemcomitans* has a gene cluster which is homologous to *E. coli pgaABCD* and encodes the production of poly-ß-1,6-GlcNAc (PGA) (Wang et al., 2004). We found that *P. intermedia* strain 17 produced a large amount of EPS, with mannose constituting more than 80% of the polysaccharides (Yamanaka et al., 2009). The growth of strain 17 was slower than that of *P. intermedia* ATCC 25611 (a reference strain for *P. intermedia*). Viscosity of spent culture media of strain 17 was higher than that of ATCC 25611. Transmission electron microscopy of negatively stained purified EPS showed fine fibrous structures that are formed in bundles. Meshwork structures were represented on latex beads coated with the purified EPS (Fig. 4).

We have also reported that a clinical isolate of *P. nigrescens* can produce a copious amount of EPS consisting of mannose (88%), glucose (4.3%), fructose (2.7%), galactose (2.1%), arabinose (1%) and small amounts of xylose, rhamnose and ribose. Methylation analysis suggested that the EPS is composed of highly branched (1-2)-linked mannose residues (Yamane et al., 2005). Okuda et al. (1987) reported that *P. intermedia* 25611, *Porphyromonas gingivalis* 381 and *P. gingivalis* ATCC 33277 had capsular structures around the cells and that the capsular polysaccharides extracted from *P. gingivalis* 381 contained galactose and glucose as their major constituents. *P. gingivalis* W83 is known to produce capsular polysaccharides, and the

genetic locus for capsule biosynthesis has been identified (Aduse-Opoku et al., 2006).
However, these reference strains in our laboratory do not produce capsular polysaccharide
or EPS. One possibility is that the tested strains had lost their ability to produce capsular
polysaccharides or EPS because of multiple *in vitro* passages of the organisms in the
laboratory. Although the molecular basis for biofilm formation in *Rothia* still needs to be
elucidated, Yamane et al. (2010) determined the whole genome sequence of *R.mucilaginosa*
DY-18, a clinical isolate from persistent apical periodontitis lesions with an ability to
produce EPS and exhibit cell surface meshwork structures.

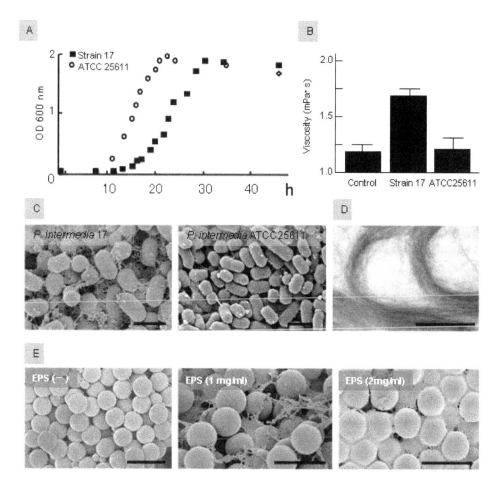

Fig. 4. Comparison of growth (A), viscosity of spent culture media (B) and phenotype
between *P. intermedia* strain 17 and ATCC 25611. Bars in C = 1 μ m. Transmission electron
micrograph of negatively stained purified EPS from *P. intermedia* 17 cultures (D).
Bar = 500 nm. Meshwork structures represented on EPS-coated latex beads
(2 μ m in diameter)(E). Bars = 5 μ m.

2.1.3 EPS productivity and biofilm phenotype as virulence factors

It is evidently shown that the slime/EPS production is critical for bacteria to exhibit the resistance to the neutrophil phagocytosis, though some EPS are not essential to bacterial adherence to host cells or for systemic virulence. Jesaitis et al. (2003) demonstrated that human neutrophils that settled on *P. aeruginosa* biofilms became phagocytically engorged, partially degranulated, and engulfed planktonic bacteria released from the biofilms. Deighton et al. (1996) compared the virulence of slime-positive *Staphylococcus epidermidis* with that of slime-negative strain in a mouse model of subcutaneous infection and showed that biofilm-positive strains produced significantly more abscesses that persisted longer than biofilm-negative strains. Our previous studies showed that *P. nigrescens* as well as *P. intermedia* with mannose-rich EPS showed stronger ability to induce abscesses in mice than those of a naturally occurring variant or chemically-induced mutant that lack the ability to produce EPS. TEM observations revealed that test strains with mannose-rich EPS appeared to be recognized by human neutrophils but not internalized (Yamane et al., 2005; Yamanaka et al., 2009). Leid et al. (2002) have shown that human neutrophils can easily penetrate *S. aureus* biofilms but fail to phagocytose the bacteria. Similarly, in the murine model of systemic infection, the deletion of *ica* locus necessary for the biosynthesis of surface polysaccharide of *S. aureus* significantly reduces its virulence. A study in the early 1970s clearly showed that addition of the slime from *P. aeruginosa* cultures to *E. coli* or *S. aureus* dramatically inhibited phagocytosis by neutrophils (Schwarzmann and Boring III, 1971). In our previous study, we observed the restoration of the induction of abscess formation in mice when the purified EPS from the biofilm-forming strain of *P. nigrescens* was added to the cultures of a biofilm-non-forming mutant and injected into mice (Yamane et al., 2005). Though we have to carefully investigate the possibility that multiple mutations exist in EPS negative variants and lead to the observed incapability to induce abscesses in mice, it is conceivable that biofilm bacteria being held together by EPS might present a huge physical challenge for phagocytosing neutrophils. As a consequence of these neutrophils being frustrated by their inability to phagocytose this bacterial mass, this might trigger the unregulated release of bactericidal compounds that could cause tissue injury as shown in the inflammatory pathway associated with lung injury or chronic wounds (Moraes et al., 2006; Bjarnsholt et al., 2008). The cellular components from neutrophils themselves are known to exert a stimulatory effect on the developing *P. aeruginosa* biofilm when the host fails to eradicate the infection. We recently compared the level of pathogenicity on the clinical strains of *P. intermedia* with EPS productivity to those of several laboratory reference strains of periodontopathic bacteria (*P.intermedia* ATCC 25611, *P. gingivalis* ATCC 33277, *P. gingivalis* 381 and *P. gingivalis* W83; strains without producing polysaccharides as described above) in terms of the abscess formation in mice. EPS-producing *P. intermedia* strains 17 and OD1-16 induced abscess lesions in mice at 10^7 CFU, but other periodontopathic bacteria did not when tested at this cell concentration (Yamanaka et al. 2011). Resistance of *P. intermedia* with EPS productivity against the phagocytic activity of human neutrophils was stronger than those of *P. intermedia* ATCC 25611 and *P. gingivalis* ATCC 33277 that lack the capacity to produce polysaccharides (Fig. 5). Therefore, it is plausible that the antiphagocytic effect of EPS confers the ability to *P. intermedia* to induce abscess in mice at a small inoculation size.

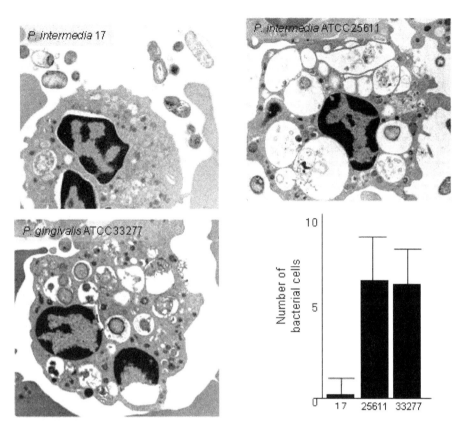

Fig. 5. Resistance of EPS-producing *P. intermedia* strain 17 against the phagocytic activity of
human neutrophils. Test strains were co-cultured with human neutrophils for 90 min.
Under transmission electron microscopy (TEM), 30 neutrophils were arbitrarily selected,
and the number of bacterial cells engulfed in each cell was counted. Strain 17 cells were not
engulfed by neutrophils. In contrast, *P. intermedia* ATCC 25611 and *P. gingivalis* ATCC 33277
cells were internalized and found within cytoplasmic vacuoles.

3. Conclusion

The matured dental plaque via the ordered sequence of events is undoubtedly a very
important reservoir of periodontopathic pathogens. However, combined recent evidences
together, it is plausible that initial colonizers including Gram-negative anaerobes can form
biofilm by a self-synthesized matrix. If the initial colonizers assume an ability to produce
EPS, this could contribute to the pathogenicity of the organisms by conferring their ability to
evade the host's innate defense response. Some of the initial colonizers who have formed
their own biofilm might be recognized by neutrophils in the gingival crevice but the
neutrophils can not eradicate the bacterial cells due to the existence of EPS as the matrix of
biofilm. This could be one of many etiologies of tissue injury found in chronic periodontitis
lesions. Our hypothetical idea is described in Figure 6.

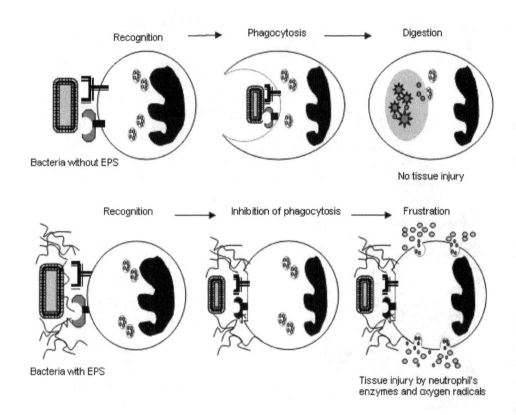

Fig. 6. Schematic depiction of tissue injury by neutrophils frustrated with unsuccessful phagocytosis of EPS-producing bacterial cells.

Finally, it is important to point out that many virulence phenotypes, especially the EPS productivity, expressed in natural environmental niches could be immediately lost through laboratory passages (Fux et al., 2005). Therefore, freshly isolated clinical strains are needed to re-evaluate the pathogenicity of periodontopathic bacteria isolated from the dental plaque or periodontal lesions.

4. Acknowledgment

We are grateful to Mr. Hideaki Hori (the Institute of Dental Research, Osaka Dental University) for his excellent assistance with electron microscopy. A part of this research was performed at the Institute of Dental Research, Osaka Dental University. This study was supported in part by Osaka Dental University Joint Research Funds (B08-01), Grant-in-Aid for Young Scientists (B) (23792118, to T. Nambu) and Grant-in-Aid for Scientific Research (C) (23592724, to H. Fukushima) from the Ministry of Education, Culture, Sports, Science and Technology.

5. References

Aduse-Opoku J, Slaney JM, Hashim A, Gallagher A, Gallagher RP, Rangarajan M, Boutaga K, Laine ML, Van Winkelhoff AJ, Curtis MA (2006). Identification and characterization of the capsular polysaccharide (K-Antigen) locus of *Porphyromonas gingivalis*. *Infect Immun* 74(1):449-460.

Anriany YA, Weiner RM, Johnson JA, De Rezende CE, Joseph SW (2001). *Salmonella enterica* serovar Typhimurium DT104 displays a rugose phenotype. *Appl Environ Microbiol* 67(9):4048-4056.

Bjarnsholt T, Kirketerp-Moller K, Jensen PO, Madsen KG, Phipps R, Krogfelt K, Hoiby N, Givskov M (2008). Why chronic wounds will not heal: a novel hypothesis. *Wound Rep Reg* 16(1):2-10.

Bolton RW, Dyer JK, Reinhardt RA, Okano DK (1983). Modulation of in vitro human lymphocyte responses by an exopolysaccharide from *Capnocytophaga ochracea*. *J Dent Res* 62(12):1186-9.

Branda SS, Vik S, Friedman L, Kolter R (2005). Biofilms: the matrix revisited. *Trends Microbiol* 13(1):20-6.

Cerantola S, Lemassu-Jacquier A, Montrozier H (1999). Structural elucidation of a novel exopolysaccharide produced by a mucoid clinical isolate of *Burkholderia cepacia*. Characterization of a trisubstituted glucuronic acid residue in a heptasaccharide repeating unit. *Eur J Biochem* 260(2):373-83.

Chen C (2001). Periodontitis as a biofilm infection. *J Calif Dent Assoc* 29(5):362-9.

Costerton JW, Lewandowski Z, Caldwell DE, Korber DR, Lappin-Scott HM (1995). Microbial biofilms. *Annu Rev Microbiol* 49, 711-745.

Costerton JW, Stewart PS, Greenberg EP (1999). Bacterial biofilms: a common cause of persistent infections. *Science* 284(5418):1318-22.

Dahlen GG (1993). Black-pigmented gram-negative anaerobes in periodontitis. *FEMS Immunol Med Microbiol* 6(2-3):181-92.

Danese PN, Pratt LA, Kolter R (2000). Exopolysaccharide production is required for development of *Escherichia coli* K-12 biofilm architecture. *J Bacteriol* 182(12):3593-6.

Darby I, Curtis M (2001). Microbiology of periodontal disease in children and young adults. *Periodontol 2000* 26(1):33-53.

Deighton MA, Borland R, Capstick JA (1996). Virulence of *Staphylococcus epidermidis* in a mouse model: significance of extracellular slime. *Epidemiol Infect* 117(2):267-80.

Diaz PI, Chalmers NI, Rickard AH, Kong C, Milburn CL, Palmer RJ, Jr., Kolenbrander PE (2006). Molecular characterization of subject-specific oral microflora during initial colonization of enamel. *Appl Environ Microbiol* 72(4):2837-2848.

Donlan RM (2001). Biofilm formation: A clinically relevant microbiological process. *Clin Infect Dis* 33(8):1387-1392.

Dubey GP, Ben-Yehuda S (2011). Intercellular nanotubes mediate bacterial communication. *Cell* 144(4):590-600.

Dueholm MS, Petersen SV, Sonderkaer M, Larsen P, Christiansen G, Hein KL, Enghild JJ, Nielsen JL, Nielsen KL, Nielsen PH, Otzen DE (2010). Functional amyloid in *Pseudomonas*. *Mol Microbiol* 77(4):1009-1020.

Dyer JK, Bolton RW (1985). Purification and chemical characterization of an exopolysaccharide isolated from *Capnocytophaga ochracea*. *Can J Microbiol* 31(1):1-5.

Fux CA, Shirtliff M, Stoodley P, Costerton JW (2005). Can laboratory reference strains mirror 'real-world' pathogenesis? *Trends Microbiol* 13(2):58-63.

Gerloni A, Cavalli F, Costantinides F, Bonetti S, Paganelli C (2009). Dental status of three Egyptian mummies: radiological investigation by multislice computerized tomography. *Oral Surg Oral Med Oral Pathol Oral Radiol Endod* 107(6):e58-64.

Hamon MA, Lazazzera BA (2001). The sporulation transcription factor Spo0A is required for biofilm development in *Bacillus subtilis*. *Mol Microbiol* 42(5):1199-209.

Herrera D, Contreras A, Gamonal J, Oteo A, Jaramillo A, Silva N, Sanz M, Botero JE, Leon R (2008). Subgingival microbial profiles in chronic periodontitis patients from Chile, Colombia and Spain. *J Clin Periodontol* 35(2):106-13.

Jain S, Chen J (2006). Antibiotic resistance profiles and cell surface components of Salmonellae. *J Food Prot* 69(5):1017-23.

Jesaitis AJ, Franklin MJ, Berglund D, Sasaki M, Lord CI, Bleazard JB, Duffy JE, Beyenal H, Lewandowski Z (2003). Compromised host defense on *Pseudomonas aeruginosa* biofilms: characterization of neutrophil and biofilm interactions. *J Immunol* 171(8):4329-4339.

Junkins AD, Doyle MP (1992). Demonstration of exopolysaccharide production by enterohemorrhagic *Escherichia coli*. *Curr Microbiol* 25(1):9-17.

Kaplan JB, Velliyagounder K, Ragunath C, Rohde H, Mack D, Knobloch JK, Ramasubbu N (2004). Genes involved in the synthesis and degradation of matrix polysaccharide in *Actinobacillus actinomycetemcomitans* and *Actinobacillus pleuropneumoniae* biofilms. *J Bacteriol* 186(24):8213-20.

Keijser BJ, Zaura E, Huse SM, van der Vossen JM, Schuren FH, Montijn RC, ten Cate JM, Crielaard W (2008). Pyrosequencing analysis of the oral microflora of healthy adults. *J Dent Res* 87(11):1016-20.

Kobayashi H (1995). Airway biofilm disease: clinical manifestations and therapeutic possibilities using macrolides. *J Infect Chemother* 1:1-15.

Kolenbrander PE, Egland PG, Diaz PI, Palmer J, Robert J. (2005). Genome-genome interactions: bacterial communities in initial dental plaque. *Trends Microbiol* 13(1):11-15.

Latasa C, Solano C, Penades JR, Lasa I (2006). Biofilm-associated proteins. *C R Biol* 329(11):849-57.

Leid JG, Shirtliff ME, Costerton JW, Stoodley aP (2002). Human leukocytes adhere to, penetrate, and respond to *Staphylococcus aureus* biofilms. *Infect Immun* 70(11):6339-6345.

Lovegrove JM (2004). Dental plaque revisited: bacteria associated with periodontal disease. *J N Z Soc Periodontol* 87: 7-21.

Marsh PD (2004). Dental plaque as a microbial biofilm. *Caries Res* 38(3):204-11.

Matsumoto-Mashimo C, Kotsu Y, Furukawa T, Ishida T, Nishimura K, Motoyama H, Kato H, Ueda M, Yamanaka T, Fukushima H (2008). Biofilm-forming bacteria in periodontal pockets screened by measurement of viscosity of culture media and observation of cell surface structures. *J Osaka Dent Univ* 42:1-7.

McLennan MK, Ringoir DD, Frirdich E, Svensson SL, Wells DH, Jarrell H, Szymanski CM, Gaynor EC (2008). *Campylobacter jejuni* biofilms up-regulated in the absence of the stringent response utilize a calcofluor white-reactive polysaccharide. *J Bacteriol* 190(3):1097-1107.

Meller C, Urzua I, Moncada G, von Ohle C (2009). Prevalence of oral pathologic findings in an ancient pre-Columbian archeological site in the Atacama Desert. *Oral Dis* 15(4):287-94.

Moraes TJ, Zurawska JH, Downey GP (2006). Neutrophil granule contents in the pathogenesis of lung injury. *Curr Opin Hematol* 13(1):21-7.

Nyvad B, Kilian M (1987). Microbiology of the early colonization of human enamel and root surfaces in vivo. *Scand J Dent Res* 95(5):369-80.

Okuda K, Fukumoto Y, Takazoe I, Slots J, Genco RJ (1987). Capsular structures of black-pigmented *Bacteroides* isolated from human. *Bull Tokyo dent Coll* 28(1):1-11.

Paster BJ, Boches SK, Galvin JL, Ericson RE, Lau CN, Levanos VA, Sahasrabudhe A, Dewhirst FE (2001). Bacterial diversity in human subgingival plaque. *J Bacteriol* 183(12):3770-83.

Prigent-Combaret C, Prensier G, Le Thi TT, Vidal O, Lejeune P, Dorel C (2000). Developmental pathway for biofilm formation in curli-producing *Escherichia coli* strains: role of flagella, curli and colanic acid. *Environ Microbiol* 2(4):450-64.

Ren D, Bedzyk LA, Setlow P, Thomas SM, Ye RW, Wood TK (2004). Gene expression in *Bacillus subtilis* surface biofilms with and without sporulation and the importance of *yveR* for biofilm maintenance. *Biotechnol Bioeng* 86(3):344-64.

Rickard AH, Bachrach G, Davies D (2008). Cell-cell communication in oral microbial communities, In:. *Molecular Oral Microbiology*, Rogers AH, 87-108, Caister Academic Press, 978-1-904455-24-0, Norfolk, UK.

Rupp ME, Ulphani JS, Fey PD, Bartscht K, Mack D (1999). Characterization of the importance of polysaccharide intercellular adhesin/hemagglutinin of *Staphylococcus epidermidis* in the pathogenesis of biomaterial-based infection in a mouse foreign body infection model. *Infect Immun* 67(5):2627-2632.

Russell RRB (2009). Bacterial polysaccharides in dental plaque, In:. *Bacterial Polysaccharides*, Ullrich M, 143-156, Caister Academic Press, 978-1-904455, Nortfork, UK.

Ryder C, Byrd M, Wozniak DJ (2007). Role of polysaccharides in *Pseudomonas aeruginosa* biofilm development. *Curr Opin Microbiol* 10(6):644-8.

Schwarzmann S, Boring III JR (1971). Antiphagocytic effect of slime from a mucoid strain of *Pseudomonas aeruginosa*. *Infect Immun* 3, 762-767.

Socransky SS, Haffajee AD (2002). Dental biofilms: difficult therapeutic targets. *Periodontol 2000* 28, 12-55.

Socransky SS, Haffajee AD, Cugini MA, Smith C, Kent RL, Jr. (1998). Microbial complexes in subgingival plaque. *J Clin Periodontol* 25(2):134-44.

Solano C, Garcia B, Valle J, Berasain C, Ghigo J-M, Gamazo C, Lasa I (2002). Genetic analysis of *Salmonella enteritidis* biofilm formation: critical role of cellulose. *Mol Microbiol* 43(3):793-808.

Uhlich GA, Cooke PH, Solomon EB (2006). Analyses of the red-dry-rough phenotype of an *Escherichia coli* O157:H7 strain and its role in biofilm formation and resistance to antibacterial agents. *Appl Environ Microbiol* 72(4):2564-2572.

Wai SN, Mizunoe Y, Takade A, Kawabata S-I, Yoshida S-I (1998). *Vibrio cholerae* O1 strain TSI-4 produces the exopolysaccharide materials that determine colony morphology, stress resistance, and biofilm formation. *Appl Environ Microbiol* 64(10):3648-3655.

Wang X, Preston JF, 3rd, Romeo T (2004). The *pgaABCD* locus of *Escherichia coli* promotes the synthesis of a polysaccharide adhesin required for biofilm formation. *J Bacteriol* 186(9):2724-2734.

Wu J, Xi C (2009). Evaluation of different methods for extracting extracellular DNA from the biofilm matrix. *Appl Environ Microbiol* 75(16):5390-5.

Yamanaka T, Furukawa T, Matsumoto-Mashimo C, Yamane K, Sugimori C, Nambu T, Mori N, Nishikawa H, Walker CB, Leung K-P, Fukushima H (2009). Gene expression profile and pathogenicity of biofilm-forming *Prevotella intermedia* strain 17. *BMC Microbiol* 9(1):11.

Yamanaka T, Sumita-Sasazaki Y, Sugimori C, Matsumoto-Mashimo C, Yamane K, Mizukawa K, Yoshida M, Hayashi H, Nambu T, Leung K-P, Fukushima H (2010). Biofilm-like structures and pathogenicity of *Escherichia hermannii* YS-11, a clinical isolate from a persistent apical periodontitis lesion. *FEMS Immunol Med Microbiol* 59(3):456-65.

Yamanaka T, Yamane K, Furukawa T, Matsumoto-Mashimo C, Sugimori C, Nambu T, Obata N, Walker C, Leung K-P, Fukushima H (2011). Comparison of the virulence of exopolysaccharide-producing *Prevotella intermedia* to exopolysaccharide non-producing periodontopathic organisms. *BMC Infect Dis* 11(1):228.

Yamane K, Nambu T, Yamanaka T, Mashimo C, Sugimori C, Leung K-P, Fukushima H (2010). Complete genome sequence of *Rothia mucilaginosa* DY-18: a clinical isolate with dense meshwork-like structures from a persistent apical periodontitis lesion. *Sequencing* 2010(Article ID 457236):1-6.

Yamane K, Ogawa K, Yoshida M, Hayashi H, Nakamura T, Yamanaka T, Tamaki T, Hojoh H, Leung KP, Fukushima H (2009). Identification and characterization of clinically isolated biofilm-forming gram-positive rods from teeth associated with persistent apical periodontitis. *J Endod* 35(3):347-52.

Yamane K, Yamanaka T, Yamamoto N, Furukawa T, Fukushima H, Walker CB, Leung K-P (2005). A novel exopolysaccharide from a clinical isolate of *Prevotella nigrescens*: purification, chemical characterization and possible role in modifying human leukocyte phagocytosis. *Oral Microbiol Immunol* 20(1):1-9.

Yasuda H, Koga T, Fukuoka T (1999). In vitro and in vivo models of bacterial biofilms. *Methods Enzymol* 310(577-95.

Yildiz FH, Visick KL (2009). *Vibrio* biofilms: so much the same yet so different. *Trend Microbiol* 17(3):109-118.

Zogaj X, Nimtz M, Rohde M, Bokranz W, Romling U (2001). The multicellular morphotypes of *Salmonella typhimurium* and *Escherichia coli* produce cellulose as the second component of the extracellular matrix. *Mol Microbiol* 39(6):1452-1463.

4

Growth Factors and Connective Tissue Homeostasis in Periodontal Disease

Catalina Pisoschi, Camelia Stanciulescu and Monica Banita
University of Medicine and Pharmacy, Craiova
Romania

1. Introduction

Periodontal disease is one of the major dental pathologies that affect human populations worldwide at high prevalence rates (Petersen, 2003). Periodontal diseases represents a family of heterogeneous chronic inflammatory lesions that involve the periodontium, a connective tissue protected by the epithelium, important to attach the teeth to the bone in the jaws and to support the teeth during function (Taylor, 2003). It is well known that periodontal diseases are caused by the interaction between periodontopathogens, almost gram-negative bacteria that grows on the teeth, and the host immune response to the chronic infection which results in tissue destruction (Ratcliff & Johnson, 1999; Reynolds & Meikle, 1997).

Gingivitis and periodontitis are the two main periodontal diseases and may be present concurrently. Gingivitis is a form of periodontal disease in which gingival tissues are inflamed but their destruction is mild and reversible while periodontitis is a chronic inflammatory response to the subgingival bacteria with irreversible changes (Armitage, 1999). Periodontium destruction is characterized by loss of connective tissue attachment and bone around the teeth in conjunction with the formation of periodontal pockets due to apical migration of the junctional epithelium (Champagne et al., 2003). Periodontal disease progression is episodic in nature on a tooth site level, but more recently, it has been realized that it is principally patient-based rather than site-based (Zia et al., 2011); the host related risk factors could be the key to better understand disease evolution. The available evidence shows that important risk factors for periodontal disease relate to poor oral hygiene, tobacco use, excessive alcohol consumption, stress, and diabetes mellitus (Laurina et al., 2009; Taylor & Borgnakke, 2008). Degrees of inflammation and fibrosis depend on these risk factors but recently the genetic basis of many aspects of the periodontal host response has been discussed in reference to disorders predisposing to periodontal disease (Bartold & Narayanan, 2006; Kinane & Hart, 2003).

Clinical hallmarks of periodontal disease are represented by the redness and swelling of the gingival margin around the neck of the teeth, recession of the gums, tooth looseness, changes in tooth alignment and halitosis (Taylor, 2003). Recently, it has been accepted that during chronic periodontal disease, morphological changes in the architecture of the extracellular matrix of the gingiva could occur and lead to gingival enlargement. This refers to the overgrowth of the gingiva characterized by the expansion and accumulation of the connective tissue with occasional presence of increased cell number. These changes are unspecific, appearing in gingival enlargement associated to chronic inflammation but also when other risk factors exist (inheritance, systemic diseases, such as diabetes mellitus, and drugs administration). The most common form of gingival overgrowth is that drug-induced, by anti-seizure drugs, such as phenytoin, immunosuppressive agents, such as cyclosporine, and some calcium antagonists (verapamil, diltiazem, dihidropyridines, most notably nifedipine) (Dongari-Bagtzoglou et al., 2004; Seymour, 2006).

Histological assessment showed that independently of the etiological factor involved, changes of the mucosa refer both to the gingival epithelium and the lamina propria (Banita et al., 2008, 2011). There is now general agreement that all gingival overgrowth lesions contain fibrotic or expanded connective tissue with various levels of inflammation and an enlarged gingival epithelium. As soon as plaque accumulates adjacent to the gingival margin, inflammatory cells infiltrate in the subjacent connective tissue and initiate its destruction. Simultaneously with collagen destruction, wound repair occurs, which results in fibrosis and scarring coexisting at the foci of inflammation (Bartold & Narayanan, 2006). According to this sequence of events, the stages of inflammation, matrix destruction and repair succeed each other in the development of periodontal disease.

Important player for the regulation of gingival connective tissue homeostasis is the fibroblast, cell able to synthesize and breakdown the collagen fibers and other proteins from the ground substance. *In vitro* studies have shown that fibroblasts from human normal gingiva produce collagens type I and type III, while cells derived from gingiva of patients with chronic periodontitis failed to produce detectable amounts of type III collagen (Hammouda et al., 1980; Chavier et al., 1984, as cited in Bartold & Narayanan, 2006). Buduneli et al. (2001a) investigated total collagen content and collagen type I, III, IV, V and VI content in gingival connective tissue of chronic periodontitis as well as aggressive periodontitis patients and clinically healthy subjects. It was suggested that different collagen types present in various periodontitis categories may be related with diverse pathogenic mechanisms acting in these diseases. In our previous studies we observed the abundance of type I collagen in the extracellular matrix of the gingival tissue obtained from patients with chronic periodontitis. In accordance with reference data, we suggest two explanations for this: despite the degradation of the fibrilar collagen, cells are able to synthesize a new type of collagen, type I trimer which accumulates in the gingiva (Narayanan et al., 1985, as cited in Bartold & Narayanan, 2006) or that inflamed human gingiva contains fibroblasts with different phenotype than those from the normal tissue, the myofibroblasts, able to synthesize a large amount of collagen.

Pathogenic pathways involved in the imbalance of connective tissue homeostasis in periodontal inflammatory diseases are complex, and specific mediation is not completely understood. Activation of matrix metalloproteinases (MMPs) is one of the most important evolving under a rigorous control.

Growth factors and cytokines play an important role in regulation of the gingival extracellular matrix turnover. Tumor necrosis factor-α (TNF-α) and interleukins induce the expression of MMPs while transforming growth factor-β (TGF-β) down-regulates their synthesis and secretion and promotes the production of their natural tissue inhibitors, TIMPs (Bartold & Narayanan, 2006). Connective tissue growth factor (CTGF) is another important mediator of tissue remodelling which stimulates fibroblasts to produce extracellular matrix constituents, so its expression correlates positively with the degree of gingival fibrosis (Heng et al., 2006; Trackman & Kantarci, 2004). Local conditions favour angiogenesis in periodontal tissues being characterized by an increased expression of the vascular endothelial growth factor (VEGF), this cytokine acting also to complete the greater ability of regeneration of the gingiva (Lucarini et al. 2009).

At the beginning, specialists tried to diagnose the stage of periodontal disease depending on the relation between the clinical appearances and the presence of some specific cell populations or specific matrix components (Havemose-Poulsen & Holmstrup, 1997; Romanos et al., 1993). Traditional clinical measurements (probing pocket depth, bleeding on probing, clinical attachment loss, plaque index) used for the diagnosis of periodontium health are often of limited usefulness because they are not sufficiently accurate to discern between previous periodontal disease and present disease activity. There is a need for development of new diagnostic tools to allow earlier detection of active disease, predict disease progression and evaluate the response to periodontal therapy, thereby improving the clinical management of patients with periodontal diseases. Advances in periodontal diseases diagnostic research are moving toward methods whereby periodontal risk can be identified and quantified by objective measures such as biomarkers. Gingival crevicular fluid (GCF) and salivary levels of several growth factors, cytokines and enzymes of host origin appear to hold the greatest promise as valuable biomarkers in assessing development of periodontal disease (Buduneli & Kinane, 2011; Giannobile et al., 2003; Gurkan et al., 2008; Goncalves et al., 2009; Kaufman & Lamster, 2000; Pisoschi et al., 2010; Wright et al., 2000).

In the last decade, scientists began to use signaling molecules such as growth factors in their quest to restore destroyed tooth support (Anusaksathien & Giannobile, 2002) and this reason request a very good knowledge of the biological actions of growth factors, both summative and redundant, in the specific "milieu" of periodontal diseases.

This paper highlights a brief review of the literature on growth factors involvement in periodontal disease and our contribution in this field, in order to sustain their use as biomarkers of active periodontal disease and future therapeutic tools.

2. Changes of the gingival tissues in periodontal disease

Periodontium includes four tissues located near the teeth: i) root cementum, ii) periodontal ligament; iii) alveolar bone, and iv)the part of the gingiva facing the tooth (dentogingival junction) (Nanci & Bosshardt, 2006). Gingiva or gums represent the mucosal tissue that covers the alveolar bone. Healthy gingiva is pale pink or pigmented and wrap tightly around the neck of the teeth (Taylor, 2003). Histologically, gingiva consists of two types of tissues - the epithelium that covers a connective tissue, chorion or lamina propria. A keratinized stratified squamous epithelium protects the lamina propria of the gingiva on its masticatory surfaces and a non-keratinized epithelium protects the lamina propria on its crevicular and junctional surfaces. During normal or pathological conditions such as inflammation, the periodontal connective tissues, including the gingiva, undergo many changes. Clinically detected gingival overgrowth – term used to substitute the former "gingival hypertrophy" or "gingival hyperplasia", because the changes of this clinical condition are more complex (Dongari-Bagtzoglou et al., 2004) - is one of the alterations recently postulated to occur in chronic periodontitis. It is caused by a variety of etiological factors and is exacerbated by local bacterial biofilm accumulation, because the periodontopathogens products act on the gingival tissues activating cellular events that induce the alteration of connective tissue homeostasis and the destruction of the alveolar bone (Reynolds & Meikle, 1997). Clinical characteristics of different forms of gingival overgrowth have been previously reviewed (Marshall & Bartold, 1998, 1999; Seymour et al., 2000). Gingival overgrowth is characterized by enlarged and occasionally inflamed gums (the interdental papilla and the free gingival margins increase in size and thickness progressively covering the tooth crown). Besides the one associated with periodontal disease, gingival overgrowth can be inherited (hereditary gingival fibromatosis), sometimes associated with other systemic diseases (such as diabetes mellitus) or with idiopathic origin. The majority of cases, however, occur as a side-effect of systemic medications, including the anti-seizure drug phenytoin, the immunosuppressive agent cyclosporin A and certain anti-hypertensive calcium-channel-blockers (verapamil, diltiazem and dihidropyridines, most notably nifedipine) (Seymour, 2006; Trackman & Kantarci, 2004). There is now general agreement that all gingival overgrowth lesions contain fibrotic or expanded connective tissues with various levels of inflammation and an enlarged gingival epithelium. The degrees of inflammation, fibrosis, and cellular pattern depend on the risk factor if it is identified: the duration, dose, and identity of the drug, the quality of oral hygiene, and the individual susceptibility that stems from genetic factors and environmental influences. Histological assessment showed that independently of the etiological factor involved, changes of the mucosa are unspecific and refer both to the gingival epithelium and the lamina propria. Our previous studies of chronic periodontitis gingival samples revealed epithelial hypertrophy with a thick stratified squamous epithelium showing an alternation between keratinized and non-keratinized areas with the increase of the spinous layer (acanthosis) associated with acantholysis (Banita et al., 2008, 2011). Epithelium bended deeply into the lamina propria to form the so called "rete pegs" (Fig.1.).

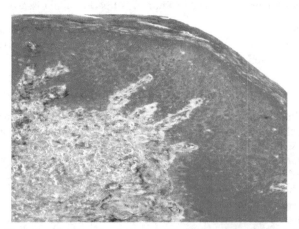

Fig. 1. Gingival enlarged epithelium in chronic periodontitis (Masson staining x 10)

Gingival tissues assessed showed also the thickness of the lamina propria due to an excessive deposition of connective tissue. It was an important accumulation of thick collagen bundles with a various number of fibroblasts and the constant presence of pro-inflammatory cells (lymphocytes and macrophages) and numerous *de novo* capillaries (Fig.2).

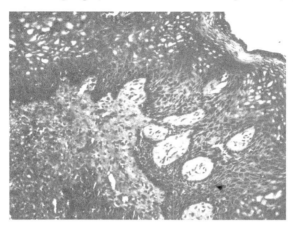

Fig. 2. Infiltration of connective tissue with inflammatory cells in periodontitis, de novo capillaries (Haematoxylin & Eosin staining x 10)

Using silver impregnation we noticed that the ratio between collagen types was changed, the extent of the yellowish coloured areas proving the presence of more type I collagen (Fig.3).

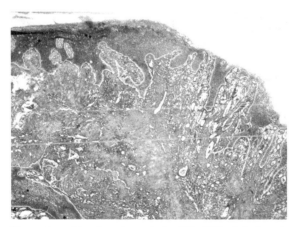

Fig. 3. Abundant collagen type I in chronic periodontitis (Gömöri silver impregnation x 4,5)

Our observations are in agreement with those of Lorencini and coworkers (2009) who, in their experimental model of ligature-induced periodontal disease noticed also this paradigm. They hypothesized that a kind of "frustrated repair" of the extracellular matrix can occur simultaneously with collagen breakdown and that the new configuration of the fibers can contribute to periodontal disease progression (Lorencini et al., 2009). Other authors postulated that with the developing of inflammatory lesion, the gingival collagens become more soluble, with increasing amount of collagen type V and the appearance of a new collagen, type I trimer (Narayanan et al., 1985, as cited by Bartold & Narayanan, 2006). Taken together these results prove without doubt that there is a permanent link between inflammatory cell populations and extracellular matrix turnover in inflammatory gingival overgrowth. Gingival tissues are recognized for their remarkable ability of regeneration and healing after wounding. The ability of regeneration of the gingival epithelium is compulsory in order to maintain the homeostasis of the gingival mucosa. Lamina propria has also the ability to heal very quickly after wounding. Some areas of interest for researchers are the biological processes that control how the periodontal tissues respond to wounding, and how cells from the different tissues of the periodontium interact when more than one periodontal tissue is affected. It is generally agreed that gingival overgrowth results from an increase of extracellular matrix macromolecules infiltrated with various numbers of inflammatory cells.

3. Extracellular matrix homeostasis in periodontal disease

Connective tissue remodelling is essential for normal growth and development and many diseases have long been associated with the imbalance of the breakdown of the collagenous matrix of different tissues. Complex pathogenic pathways control the balance synthesis/degradation of the extracellular matrix. Macromolecules of interstitial connective tissues and basement membranes may be degraded by: *i)* matrix metalloproteinase (MMP)-dependent, *ii)* plasmin-dependent, *iii)* polymorphonuclear leukocyte serine proteinase-dependent reactions, and *iv)* a phagocytic pathway based on intracellular digestion of internalized material by lysosomal cathepsins (Birkedal-Hansen et al., 1993).

Since the early 1990s, interest has focused on works showing that connective tissue cells synthesize and secrete a family of proteinases, the MMPs, which can digest extracellular matrix macromolecules and play a major role in connective tissue breakdown.

3.1 Matrix metalloproteinases

Matrix metalloproteinases (MMPs), or matrixins, are enzymes derived from many types of mesenchymal cells, monocytes, macrophages and keratinocytes and can synergistically digest most of extracellular matrix (ECM) macromolecules (Reynolds et al., 1994; Whittaker & Ayscough, 2001). The MMP gene family encodes more than 20 human metal-dependent endopeptidases (Stamenkovic, 2003) divided into major five groups (see Tabel 1).

As we already mentioned, gingival tissue remodelling involve the balance between synthesis and accumulation of matrix components and their breakdown under the catalitic action of metalloproteases. Several MMPs have been identified in the inflamed gingival tissues: MMP-1, -2, -3, -8, -9, -13, produced by the keratinocytes, macrophages, polymorphonuclear leukocytes (Banita et al., 2011; Bartold & Narayanan, 2006; Bildt et al., 2008; Kubota et al., 2008; Kumar et al., 2006). Their activity could be different depending on the severity of disease and the needs for extracellular matrix digestion.

In a previous study regarding the expression of MMPs in gingival samples of chronic periodontitis we observed an enhanced expression of MMP-1 in keratinocytes from diseased epithelial layers (Fig.4). In some cases, MMP-1 expression extended to the lamina propria as inflammation progressed. MMP-1 increased activity could explain the change of collagen quality and quantity, since its preferred substrates are the type I and type III collagens.

Type of MMPs	Substrates	Members
Collagenases	Native fibrilar collagens (I, II, III, VII, VIII, X) Gelatins (limited) Other ECM molecules	MMP-1 (Collagenase 1) MMP-8 (Neutrophil collagenase) MMP-13 (Collagenase 3)
Gelatinases	Denaturated collagens (gelatins) Type IV collagen Other ECM molecules	MMP-2 (Gelatinase A) MMP-9 (Gelatinase B)
Stromelysins	Collagens III-V Gelatins (limited) Other ECM molecules MMPs	MMP-3 (Stromelysin 1) MMP-10 (Stromelysin 2)
Matrilysins	Collagen IV and X, gelatins Other ECM molecules MMPs	MMP-7 (Matrilysin 1) MMP-26 (Matrylisin 2)
Membrane type - MMPs	Collagen (I, II, III) Pro-MMP-2 Other ECM molecules	MT1-MMP - MT6-MMP (MMP-14, MMP-15, MMP-16, MMP-17, MMP-24, MMP-25)

Table 1. Major types of matrix metalloproteinases (MMPs)

Several other researchers reported an intense MMP-1 collagenolytic activity in fibroblasts and macrophages resident in the periodontal tissue (Beklen et. al., 2007; Kubota et al., 2008) and focused on the interrelation between MMP-1 and MMP-3 in order to amplify the proteolysis in chronic periodontitis (Beklen et. al., 2007).

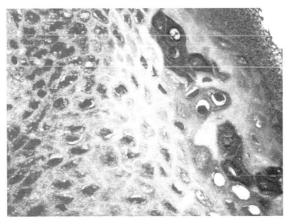

Fig. 4. Expression of MMP-1 in gingival epithelium in chronic periodontitis (IHCx40)

Regarding MMP-2, we observed an increased expression of this enzyme in many keratinocytes from the basal layer and in some cells from the basement membrane (Fig. 5); the active form of MMP-2 increased significantly as inflammation progressed.

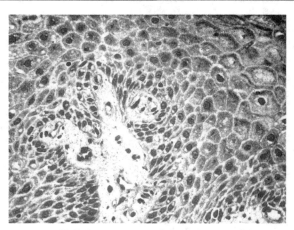

Fig. 5. Increased expression of MMP-2 in gingival epithelium and basement membrane in chronic periodontitis (IHCx20)

Its expression and distribution is justified by the fact that this gelatinase has an important role in the degradation of denatured collagen (predigested with MMP-1) and type IV collagen of the basement membrane, and these processes are increased in various stages of periodontal disease progression. MMP-2 is also able to increase matrix degradation by MMP-13 and neutrophil collagenase (De Souza & Line, 2002). The degenerative process causes the loss of attachment apparatus between tooth, epithelium, and connective tissue which accelerates inflammation and deepening of periodontal pocket. In the last decade, many research groups reported the putative role of other MMPs (MMP-7, MMP-25, MMP-26, MT1-MMP) as mediators of the alternating sequence inflammation-fibrosis during progression of periodontal disease (Emingil et al., 2006a, 2006b; Oyarzun et al., 2010).

3.2 Tissue inhibitors of matrix metalloproteinases

MMPs activity is controlled *in vivo* in three ways: *i)* these enzymes are synthesized and secreted as latent, inactive precursors and conversion to the active form require activation; *ii)* production of MMPs can be regulated by growth factors and cytokines; *iii)* their activity can be inhibited by endogenous serum and tissue inhibitors (Nagase, 1997, as cited by Bartold & Narayanan, 2006). Various tissues express one or more of the members of the most important group of inhibitors known as tissue inhibitors of MMP (TIMPs). These are specific inhibitors that bind MMPs in a 1:1 stoichiometry. All the four currently known TIMPs (TIMP-1, TIMP-2, TIMP-3, and TIMP-4) are very well conserved since they have been identified in vertebrates, including humans, insects and even in the nematode, *Caenoharbditis elegans* (Brew et al., 2000). Their expression is rigorous regulated during development and tissue remodelling under pathological conditions associated with unbalanced MMP activities, and changes of TIMP levels are considered to be important because they directly affect the level of MMP activity (Visse & Nagase, 2003). TIMP-1 and TIMP-3 expression is inducible, whereas TIMP-2 is largely constitutive (Verstappen & Van den Hoff, 2006). TIMPs are produced in many tissues, although not every tissue expresses all four inhibitors. Most mesenchymal and epidermal cells are able to produce TIMPs in various conditions (Rowe et al., 1997, as cited by Verstappen & Van den Hoff, 2006), but TIMP-4 expression is restricted to neural tissue, gonads, breast and skeletal muscle (Lambert et al., 2004).

Our studies regarding the modulation of MMP/TIMP balance in gingival overgrowth associated with periodontitis lead to the following observations related to TIMP activity. We noticed that the immune reaction for TIMP-1 was positive in few epithelial cells in periodontitis-affected gingival samples assessed (Banita et al., 2011). For TIMP-2 the immune response was quite different. We observed extended areas of TIMP-2 intense positive cells in the epithelium (Fig.6) and a lot of TIMP-2 positive pro-inflammatory cells and few fibroblasts in the lamina propria (Fig.7).

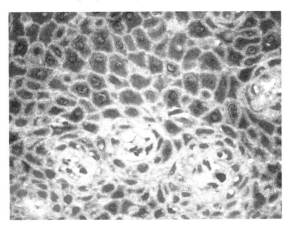

Fig. 6. TIMP-2 expression in gingival epithelium in periodontitis–affected gingiva (IHCx40)

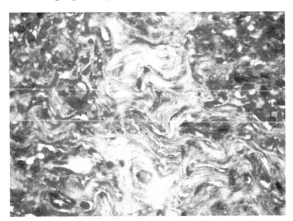

Fig. 7. TIMP-2 expression in periodontitis-affected gingival lamina propria (IHCx20)

Our results showed increased levels for both MMPs and TIMPs assessed in periodontitis-affected gingival tissue and are in accordance with other similar studies. Up-regulated MMPs and TIMPs expression with a modified MMPs/TIMPs ratio depending on the type of lesion (destruction or fibrosis) indicate that the imbalance between degradation and synthesis of the extracellular matrix components persists in periodontitis-affected gingiva and is responsible for an increased tissue breakdown in periodontitis. The reciprocal regulation of TIMPs and MMPs expression may depend on endogenous growth factors and cytokines.

4. Growth factors and cytokines in periodontal disease

The balance between MMPs and TIMPs influence on extracellular matrix homeostasis in different types of tissues is tightly controlled by growth factors, a class of polypeptide hormones. Other polypeptide mediators that affect matrix synthesis include several cytokines - interleukins (IL-1, IL-4, IL-6, IL-10) and tumour necrosis factor-α (TNF-α). By binding to specific cell-surface tyrosine kinase receptors, growth factors are able to regulate significant cellular events in tissue regeneration and repair, including cell growth, proliferation and differentiation, chemotaxis, angiogenesis, and extracellular matrix synthesis (Giannobile, 1996). Growth factors are classified as biological mediators that lack specificity sequestered in the extracellular matrix and molecules available from the circulation (Bartold & Narayanan, 2006). Growth factors demonstrate pleiotropic or multiple effects on wound repair in almost all tissues, including the periodontium.

Some of the most important growth factors exerting functions in healthy and diseased periodontium are listed below:

a.   Platelet-Derived Growth Factor (PDGF)
b.   Fibroblast Growth Factors (a-FGF and b-FGF)
c.   Transforming Growth Factors (TGF-α and -β)
d.   Connective Tissue Growth Factor (CTGF)
e.   Vascular Endothelial Growth Factor (VEGF)
f.   Insulin-like Growth Factors (IGF-I, IGF-II)
g.   Epidermal Growth Factor (EGF)
h.   Hepatocyte Growth Factor (HGF)

After an injury occurs, healing proceeds in a succession of "well orchestrated" cell-cell and cell-extracellular matrix interactions. In the process of normal wound healing, the growth factors act in conjunction to form a complex arrangement of molecules that regulate cellular activity and bordering the wound (Giannobile, 1996). Table 2 lists the sources and the main effects of some growth factors and cytokines important for extracellular matrix remodelling.

The role of growth factors is now recognized in connective tissue homeostasis during inflammation and fibrosis. Tissue repair studies conducted on animals provide evidence that soft tissue wound healing is enhanced by EGF, TGF-α and β, PDGF, acidic and basic FGF. Combinations of different growth factors yield greater repair than can be achieved by individual factors alone (Giannobile, 1996).

Growth factors mediate many events associated with turnover, repair and regeneration of periodontal tissues. Gingival epithelial cells, gingival fibroblasts, and periodontal ligament fibroblasts are the major cells involved in tissue repair. An appropriate response of these target cells to various growth factors depends on the expression of corresponding receptors.

a) Platelet-Derived Growth Factor. In vitro and *in vivo* studies suggest PDGF as the most thoroughly described growth factor associated with periodontal health. There are different isoforms of PDGF (PDGF-AA, -AB, -BB), and all have been shown to have a fibroblast proliferative activity *in vitro* (Giannobile, 1996). PDGF is present in increased levels in the human inflamed gingiva and is mainly localized to the pocket epithelium (Pinheiro et al., 2003).

Growth Factor	Source	Effect
PDGF isoforms	Platelets Macrophages Keratinocytes	Fibroblast and macrophage chemotaxis Fibroblast proliferation Extracellular matrix synthesis
FGF	Macrophages Endothelial cells	Fibroblast proliferation Angiogenesis
TGF-β1, 2	Platelets Macrophages	Fibroblast and macrophage chemotaxis Extracellular matrix synthesis Secretion of protease inhibitors
CTGF	Epithelial cells Vascular cells	Extracellular matrix synthesis
EGF TGF-α	Platelets Macrophages Keratinocytes	Reepithelization
IGF	Plasma Platelets	Endothelial and fibroblast proliferation Collagen synthesis
VEGF	Keratinocytes Macrophages	Angiogenesis
IL-1	Neutrophils	Activate growth factor expression in macrophages, keratinocytes and fibroblasts
TNF-α	Neutrophils	Activate growth factor expression in macrophages, keratinocytes and fibroblasts

Table 2. Sources and major functions of several growth factors and cytokines

It is possible that expression of PDGF contributes to the inflammatory changes that occur during periodontal diseases. PDGF supports the healing in the periodontal soft tissues in a variety of ways. Since PDGF is chemotactic for fibroblasts, it induces collagen synthesis, but also stimulates fibroblasts to synthesize the proteoglycans that supply the framework for extracellular matrix development. Lipopolysaccharide, the major constituent of the cell walls of gram-negative bacteria, inhibits the proliferation of gingival fibroblasts and PDGF decreases this inhibitory effect (Bartold & Narayanan, 1992). Reported data suggest that there may be cell specific differences in response to PDGF isoforms critical to periodontal healing that may be exploited in the development of efficient therapies (Mumford et al., 2001).

b) Transforming Growth Factor-β (TGF-β). TGF-β superfamily consists of several multifunctional structurally related growth and differentiation factors associated to the inflammatory response, known also to be involved in apoptosis, angiogenesis, wound healing and fibrosis (Frank et al., 1996; Lawrence, 1995). There are three TGF-β isoforms important for humans, TGF-β1, 2 and 3; their amino acid sequences are 70-80% homologous but they can be distinguished by the effects on cell growth, biological interactions and receptor binding abilities (Frank et al., 1996). TGF-β1 is expressed in epithelial, hematopoietic, and connective tissue cells (Massague, 1998). Because TGF-β1 exhibits both pro-inflammatory and anti-inflammatory properties besides its ability to stimulate synthesis of ECM molecules and to inhibit the breakdown of ECM, it has been intensively evaluated in relation to all types of gingival overgrowth.

Regarding TGF-β1 expression in chronic periodontitis, we noticed a positive reaction in some keratinocytes from the gingival basal epithelial layer (Fig.8), and pro-inflammatory cells infiltrating lamina propria (Fig.9).

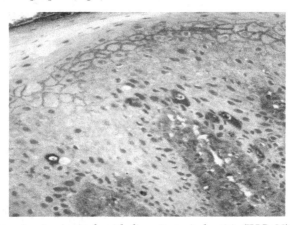

Fig. 8. TGF-β1 expression in gingival epithelium in periodontitis (IHCx20)

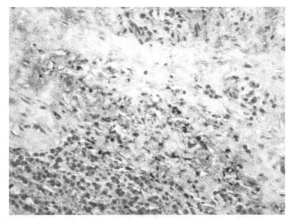

Fig. 9. TGF-β1 expression in inflammatory cells infiltrating lamina propria of periodontitis-affected gingiva (IHCx20)

Our results confirm that increased gingival inflammation is associated with high levels of TGF-β isoforms. It is well known that TGF-β is one of several cytokines able to regulate inflammation and immune responses and the fact that TGF-β mediates leukocyte recruitment, adhesion and activation suggests that it play a key role in the host response to bacterial and immunological insults (Prime et al., 2004), even there is not a clear evidence for its role in the pathogenesis of the periodontal disease. But TGF-β has also a marked effect on ECM homeostasis, being an important mediator of fibroblast proliferation and ECM synthesis. The inverse relationship between TGF-β1 and MMP-1 expression in the gingival epithelium noticed in our studies could be in accordance with TGF- β1 action as inhibitor of MMP-1 activity and proves that TGF-β mediates a tight control of the MMP/TIMPs equilibrium and synthesis of matrix macromolecules. TGF-β1 pro-fibrotic role could be explained also by the stimulation of collagen synthesis in lamina propria. There are considerable data supporting the fact that under pathological conditions, TGF-β1 orchestrates a cross talk between parenchymal, inflammatory and collagen expressing cells and have a key role in control inflammation and fibrosis (Buduneli et al., 2001b; Ellis et al., 2004; Wright et al., 2001). The role of TGF-β1 in gingival overgrowth must be considered in line with natural development of the periodontal lesion, as inflammation preceedes fibrosis, and with its stadial activity. First, it acts as a pro-inflammatory cytokine that mediate the recrutation of monocytes-macrophages, their adhesion and action at site lesion, suggesting a key role in the host-response to the presence of the bacterial products. Finally, as the inflammation progresses, TGF-β1 overexpression in epithelial and fibroblasts could be a response to paracrine stimulation by other cytokines secreted by the pro-inflammatory cells. Despite the great interest for this growth factor, the precise role of TGF-β1 in the pathogenesis of periodontitis-induced gingival overgrowth is still under debate.

c) Connective Tissue Growth Factor (CTGF). The CCN family consists of six multifunctional members including CCN1 (Cyr61), CCN2 (connective tissue growth factor, CTGF), CCN3 (Nov), CCN4 (WISP1), CCN5 (WISP2), and CCN6 (WISP3) (Brigstock, 2003). The functions of this family include embryogenesis, wound healing, and regulation of ECM production. CTGF is a matricellular cysteine-rich peptide that plays a variety of important roles in cell development and differentiation and acts to promote fibrosis in many different tissues in cooperation with other growth factors and extracellular matrix proteins (Leask & Abraham, 2003). These findings rise the hypothesis that CTGF could play a role in gingival fibrosis.

In periodontitis, we observed a different pattern of CTGF distribution in gingival structures. Many samples showed an intense positive reaction in basal and parabasal epithelial layers but also in structures from the lamina propria (Fig.10). Higher CTGF staining in overgrown gingiva was accompanied by an increased number of fibroblasts and collagen fibers, in accordance with CTGF contribution to increase fibrosis. Fibrosis, as well as physiological wound repair and inflammation, involves the same molecules and cellular events (Bartold & Narayanan, 2006). As a consequence of inflammation, fibrosis can be the result of several events: abnormal release of mediators and persistence of changes in the abnormal growth factor/cytokine profile, and proliferation of cells with an abnormal phenotype responsible for the excessive extracellular matrix synthesis that characterize fibrosis. CTGF alone does not promote fibrosis. Recent studies indicate that CTGF binds to other factors, resulting in either inhibition or stimulation activity (Kantarci et al., 2006, Trackman & Kantarci, 2004). CTGF binding to VEGF results in inhibition of VEGF while CTGF binding to TGF-β1 is reported to be stimulatory (Trackman & Kantarci, 2004). Therefore simultaneous production of both TGF-β1 and CTGF is required to sustain fibrosis in gingival overgrowth.

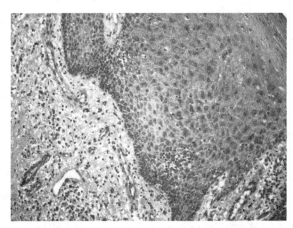

Fig. 10. Intense expression of CTGF in periodontitis-affected gingival epithelium (IHCx20)

d) Basic Fibroblast Growth Factor (bFGF or FGF-2). FGFs are a family of at least 23 structurally related polypeptides known to play a critical role in angiogenesis and mesenchymal cell mitogenesis. In periodontium, FGF-2 is present in the extracellular matrix, as well as in the cementum and can function as a local factor at the site (Gao et al., 1996). In periodontitis, the presence of bFGF was reported in the gingival epithelium, inflammatory cells and connective tissue (Laurina et al., 2009). They noted also a more increased expression of FGF receptor (FGFR) in hyperplasic gingival tissue compared to normal. One of their conclusions was that the expression of growth factors and their receptors in sulcular epithelium was lower than into the gingival epithelium and seems to be specific for periodontitis (Laurina et al., 2009).

e) Epidermal Growth Factor (EGF). EGF is a multifunctional cytokine with a variety of biological functions including epithelial growth and differentiation, and wound healing. In the periodontium, EGF seems to exert only a minor effect on the promotion of mitogenesis, chemotaxis, or matrix synthesis in periodontal ligament fibroblasts (Giannobile, 1996). He supposed that EGF receptors (EGF-R) localization in periodontal ligament fibroblasts may stabilize the periodontal ligament fibroblast phenotype or cellular physical characteristics.

Buduneli et al. (2001c) evaluated the expression of EGF-receptor (EGFR) in frozen sections of cyclosporine (CsA)-induced gingival overgrowth using immunohistochemical and semiquantitative techniques. Gingival biopsies were obtained from 12 renal transplant patients receiving CsA as well as from 9 systemically and periodontally healthy individuals. The authors suggested that CsA affects EGFR metabolism in gingival keratinocytes resulting in an increased number of cell surface receptors, which may eventually play a role in the pathogenesis of gingival tissue alterations. In chronic periodontitis, EGFR was regionally detected in gingival epithelium in some cases (Laurina et al., 2009). Other *in vivo* studies are needed to reveal the precise effects of EGF on soft periodontal tissue healing.

f) Insulin-Like Growth Factors (IGFs). IGFs are a family of mitogenic proteins that control growth, differentiation, and the maintenance of differentiated function in numerous tissues. The IGF family includes three ligands (insulin, IGF-I, and IGF-II), their corresponding cell surface receptors (IR, IGF-IR, and IGF-IIR), and at least six IGF-binding proteins (IGFBPs) able to bind circulating IGFs and modulate their biological actions. Studies have suggested that IGF-I has an important involvement in periodontal wound healing and regeneration. IGF-I is chemotactic for cells that come from the periodontal ligament and demonstrates significant effects on the mitogenesis of periodontal ligament fibroblasts (Giannobile, 1996). IGF-I is able to prevent apoptosis in fibroblasts, to regulate DNA and protein synthesis in periodontal ligament fibroblasts *in vitro* and to enhance soft tissue wound healing in *vivo* (Werner & Katz, 2004). Regarding the IGF-IR expression in chronic periodontitis, Laurina et al. (2009) reported only a weak presence in the sulcular epithelium suggesting a potential role in regeneration of periodontal tissue. The effect of IGF-II on the metabolism of gingival fibroblasts is still uncertain.

h) Hepatocyte growth factor (HGF). HGF is a multifunctional cytokine involved in the repair and regeneration of various tissues and their protection from injury (Matsumoto & Nakamura, 1997) and recently, it has been linked also to the development of periodontal disease (Ohshima et al., 2001; Ohnishi & Daikuhara, 2003). HGF may be closely involved in the pathogenesis and progression of periodontal disease because it stimulates excessive proliferation and invasion of gingival epithelial cells and impair the regeneration of deep collagenous structures in the periodontium (Ohshima et al., 2001).

g) Vascular Endothelial Growth Factor (VEGF). Over the last two decades researchers have demonstrated that VEGF is a key regulator of physiological and pathological angiogenesis, because it induces endothelial cell proliferation, stimulates angiogenesis and increases vascular permeability (Ferrara, 2009). In the last decade, many groups focused their research on the angiogenic factors that contribute to periodontal healing. In periodontitis patients, VEGF was detected within vascular endothelial cells, neutrophils, plasma cells, and junctional, pocket and gingival epithelium (Booth et al, 1998). In a previous study on biopsies obtained from patients with type 2 diabetes associated gingival overgrowth, we detected VEGF expression in keratinocytes from the basal and spinous layers and in many *de novo* capillaries (Pisoschi et al., 2009). Other authors reported increased VEGF expression in epithelial cells and endothelial cells in periodontitis-affected gingiva (Guneri et al., 2004; Keles et al., 2010; Lucarini et al., 2009). Giannobile et al. (2003) suggested that VEGF could be an important growth factor for the onset of gingivitis and its progression to periodontitis. Taken together these observations conclude that VEGF expression is related to both maintenance of periodontal health and periodontal tissue destruction but the precise mechanism of neovascularization remains in debate.

5. Gingival crevicular fluid and salivary growth factors as potential biomarkers of periodontal disease

Traditional periodontal diagnostic methods include assessment of clinical parameters (probing pocket depth, bleeding on probing, clinical attachment loss, plaque index), and radiographs but these conventional techniques are of limited usefulness because they are not sufficiently accurate to discern between previous periodontal disorders and present disease activity. For this reason, development of non-invasive diagnostic tools has presented a significant challenge to periodontology. Recently, gingival crevicular fluid (GCF) and saliva are in the middle of high-throughput techniques aimed to validate tests for the objective diagnosis of disease, monitoring, and prognostic indicators. Oral fluids contain locally and systemically derived mediators of periodontal disease, including pathogens, host-response, and bone-specific markers (Kinney et al., 2007). Most biomarkers assessed in oral fluids are inflammatory cytokines, but some collagen degradation products and bone turnover-related molecules have emerged as possible markers of periodontal disease activity, too. Most biomarkers in GCF and saliva are indicators of soft-tissue inflammatory events (pathogens infection and host inflammatory response) that precede the destruction of the alveolar bone (Buduneli & Kinane, 2011).

The detection of connective tissue-derived molecules may provide a more precise assessment of the breakdown of periodontal tissues, especially in light of the variability in the host response of different individuals (Giannobile et al. 2003).

Among those which are the potential candidates for oral fluid-based diagnostics of periodontal disease are included: alkaline phosphatase, MMP-8, MMP-9, MMP-13, osteocalcin, osteonectin, osteopontin, and pyridinoline cross-linked carboxyterminal telopeptide of type I collagen (Arikan et al., 2008, 2011; Buduneli et al., 2008; Kinney et al., 2007; Miller et al., 2006; Ozçaka et al., 2011) but the list is still open.

Extracellular matrix molecules that are derived from the periodontium have been identified in GCF and saliva. Although growth factors function as molecular mediators of periodontal tissues repair their value as diagnostic biomarkers of periodontal tissue inflammation and/or destruction has yet elucidated.

Research in this area has reported the assessment of GCF and salivary levels of several growth factors for their potential to diagnose periodontal disease, including EGF, TGF-β, PDGF, HGF, and VEGF (Buduneli et al., 2001b; Chang et al., 1996; Gurkan et al., 2006; Hormia et al., 1993; Kamimoto et al., 2002; Sakallioglu et al., 2007; Wilczynska-Borawska et al., 2006).

We were also interested to seek a relationship between salivary levels of growth factors and other molecules (MMPs, TIMPs, TNFα) related to host response and morphological and clinical changes observed in periodontitis. We compared the salivary concentration of TGF-β1 and CTGF in patients with periodontal disease and healthy control subjects. We didn't obtain any significant difference for the salivary TGF-β1 levels between healthy subjects and those with gingivitis. Only the values obtained for salivary TGF-β1 in chronic periodontitis differ significantly from those found for control subjects but even in this case we observed a great difference between the smallest and the highest values (Pisoschi et al., 2010). This variation could be explained by the duration of the candidate risk factors on TGF-β1 levels, being well known that periodontal disease is characterized by periods of active tissue destruction and quiescence. Our findings are in accordance with the results reported by other researchers for the variation of TGF-β1 levels in patients with aggressive and chronic periodontitis (Gurkan et al., 2006). We also obtained a good correlation between salivary concentration and gingival expression of TGF-β1. So far, we didn't find any significant differences between salivary CTGF levels of patients with gingivitis, chronic periodontitis and controls (unpublished data). However, CTGF concentrations were higher in samples obtained from patients with type 2 diabetes associated gingival overgrowth (Pisoschi et al., 2011). Regarding the level of circulating and oral fluids TGF-β1 and CTGF, we agree with other researchers that variation in the analytical technique used in sample assessment might influence the values.

As we mentioned before, many reports sustained the importance of VEGF in the pathogenesis of periodontal disease. Therefore researchers attempted to find a correlation between GCF or salivary VEGF levels and its tissue expression in order to link this biomarker with the degree of periodontal damage. A recent study of Pradeep et al. (2011) that included patients with gingivitis and chronic periodontitis, reported an increase of VEGF concentration in GCF and a positive correlation between GCF and serum VEGF levels. Moreover a correlation between growth factor levels and clinical periodontal parameters before and after nonsurgical periodontal treatment was observed.

Even the results of much research have confirmed the presence of several growth factors in GCF and saliva, for many of them the relation between their variation and the severity of the periodontal disease is still unclear. In the future, high-throughput proteomic and metabolomic technologies will be critical in establishing whether a biomarker could be accurate to diagnose and predict the severity of the periodontal disease.

6. Growth factors as therapeutic tools in periodontal disease

Therapeutic approaches for treatment of periodontitis are divided into two categories: *i) anti-infective treatment*, and *ii) regenerative therapy*.

Several restoring techniques have been developed to regenerate periodontal tissues including guided tissue regeneration, bone grafting, and use of enamel matrix derivatives. Principles of guided tissue regeneration dictate that one of the goals of therapy is to modulate the repopulation of the wound with cells derived from the periodontal ligament rather than from the gingival tissues (Mumford et al., 2001). However, this technique is not associated with complete periodontal regeneration and a major complication and limiting factor in the achievement of periodontal regeneration is the presence of microbial periodontopathogens that contaminate wounds and reside on tooth surfaces as plaque-associated biofilms.

For more than a decade, periodontal researchers have been studying the potential of growth factors to achieve predictable periodontal regeneration. It is accepted that many growth factors are produced as inactive propeptides and stored in the cytoplasm (Anusaksathien & Giannobile, 2002). Cleavage of these propeptides and extracellular secretion of the mature forms provide the growth factors able to bind on their specific receptors.

Growth factor therapies are directed to stimulate the specific progenitor cells which are responsible for the regeneration of mineralized and nonmineralized tissues in the periodontium but also to limit periodontal degradation. Therapeutic application of growth factors to restore damaged tissue aims the regeneration through biomimetic processes, or mimicking the processes that occur during embryonic and post-natal development (Schilephake, 2002). The complexity of these events suggests that creating an optimal regenerative environment requires the combination of different growth factors as found in natural processes. But also the use of a single recombinant growth factor may induce several molecular, biochemical and morphological cascades that will result in tissue regeneration. Almost all the growth factors are believed to be potential targets for the periodontal regenerative therapy but few strategies are subjected to various phases of clinical trials. Growth factors tested for their contribution to periodontal regeneration include PDGF, IGF-I, TGF-β1, bFGF and some bone morphogenetic proteins (Giannobile et al., 1996, 2001;

Murakami et al., 1999; Taba et al., 2005). Results from the in vivo studies have shown that all of the above mentioned bioactive molecules, with the exception of TGF-β1, exhibited ability to promote periodontal tissue regeneration and suggest that there may be cell-specific differences critical to periodontal wound healing that may be exploited in the development of new therapies.

PDGF was the first growth factor to be evaluated in preclinical periodontal regenerative studies. In vitro studies had shown that exogenous application of PDGF at different concentrations (between 0,01 and 10 ng/ml) resulted in proliferation, migration and matrix synthesis in cultures of periodontal cells, including gingival and periodontal ligament fibroblasts, cementoblasts, preosteoblasts and osteoblasts in a time and dose dependence (Kaigler et al., 2006). From all its isoforms, PDGF-BB is the most effective on periodontal ligament cell mitogenesis and extracellular matrix macromolecules biosynthesis (Bartold, 1993; Ojima et al., 2003). Even periodontal ligament fibroblasts and gingival fibroblasts have been shown to proliferate rapidly, gingival fibroblasts have been shown to fill a wound space significantly faster than periodontal ligament cells and this is an unwanted effect (Mumford et al., 2001). Studies on combination growth factor therapy involving PDGF and IGF-I have consistently promoted the periodontal regeneration (greater osseous and new attachment response) in animal models and lead to the first study in humans using growth factors for periodontal regeneration. In their human phase I/II clinical trial, PDGF/IGF-I were considered safe when applied topically to periodontal osseous lesions, resulting in a significant improvement in bone growth and fill of periodontal defects, compared with standard therapy (Howell et al., 1997, as cited by Kaigler et al., 2006).

TGF-β plays a significant role in periodontal regeneration. It is pleiotropic, and can stimulate or inhibit cell growth, an action that can interfere with its therapeutic use (Clokie & Bell, 2003). TGF-β1 has been used for this application. The results of rhTGF-β1 for periodontal regeneration have not been consistent preclinically as shown in dogs and sheeps investigations (Mohamed et al., 1998; Tatakis et al, 2000, as cited by Kraigler et al., 2006). These studies showed little advantages in new bone formation and no improvement in cementum regeneration when treated with rhTGF-β1. Other research demonstrated that TGF-β1 increased the amount of bone healing adjacent to dental implants in minipigs (Clokie & Bell, 2003). TGF-β can also modulate other growth factors, such as PDGF, EGF, and FGF, by altering their cellular response or by inducing their expression. Combined therapies, which involved PDGF and TGF-β, have demonstrated synergistic effects and enhanced regeneration. Together, PDGF and TGF-β have stimulated gingival fibroblasts and periodontal ligament cells. Some authors reported that TGF-β, both alone and in combination with PDGF, led to a greater proliferation of periodontal ligament cells compared to the gingival fibroblasts. On the contrary, PDGF stimulated a significantly greater proliferation of gingival fibroblasts compared to periodontal ligament cells. Since periodontal proliferation at the diseased site is a desired feature in periodontal regeneration and because of the limited number of studies and inconsistent results, the use of TGF-β will be further emphasized and thoroughly investigated.

Several studies reported that FGFs can stimulate mitogenesis and chemotaxis in periodontal ligament cells (Takayama et al., 1997; Terranova et al., 1989). FGFs increased osteoblast proliferation, although they do not directly increase collagen production by differentiated osteoblasts. They have shown bFGF stimulates human endothelial and periodontal ligament cell migration and proliferation on the dentin surfaces, and that the combination of bFGF with fibronectin can further enhanced periodontal ligament cell chemotaxis. Despite different concentrations of bFGF and different delivery systems used in the studies, all showed an improvement in the periodontal tissue regeneration. Studies that evaluated more than one concentration of bFGF suggested that its effects are dose dependent (Murakami et al., 2003).

The results from preclinical and initial clinical studies using growth factors are encouraging; however, some limitations exist with respect to bone volume and predictability. Trials utilizing topical growth factors have revealed difficulties in maintaining therapeutic levels of proteins and to obtain optimal outcomes *in vivo*; of great importance is to enhance the half-life of growth factors and their biological stability (Yun et al., 2010). Based on the results of studies that support *in vitro* biological functions of FGFs for tissue regeneration, the largest *in vivo* study in the field of periodontal regenerative therapy was initiated by Kitamura's team. This was a human clinical trial projected to determine the safety and efficiency of FGF-2 for clinical application. Their results support that topical application of three doses of FGF-2 during periodontal surgery could be efficient for the regeneration of periodontal tissue (Kitamura et al., 2008).

Future clinical application of growth factors in the regeneration of periodontal tissues will be achieved when their biological functions are maximized by the appropriate use of biomaterials and stem cells.

7. Conclusions

The biology of periodontal connective tissues is important to be understood in terms of development, pathology, regeneration and interrelationship between periodontitis interactions and various systemic diseases. Although growth factors function as molecular mediators of periodontal tissues, their value as diagnostic biomarkers for periodontal tissue inflammation and/or fibrosis is yet to be elucidated. High-throughput technologies applied for assessment of gingival crevicular fluid and saliva will give new promises for the use of growth factors as objective biomarkers in periodontal disease.

In earlier studies, the application of growth factors provided different degrees of success in stimulating wound healing in the periodontal areas. There is an imperious need to further evaluate the biologic mechanisms that may be responsible for the promotion of tissue regeneration by growth factors. Finally, studies on growth factors delivery and improved stability seek evidence to conclusively support the addition of growth factors strategy to the therapeutic protocol for regeneration of periodontal tissues.

8. Acknowledgements

This work was financially sustained by CNCSIS-UEFISCDI, 563 PNII-IDEI/2008, and contract 1137/2009.

9. References

Anusaksathien, O. & Giannobile, W.V. (2002). Growth Factor Delivery to Re-Engineer Periodontal Tissues. *Current Pharmaceutical Biotechnology*, Vol.3, No.2, (May 2002), pp. 129-139

Arikan, F., Buduneli, N., Kütükçüler, N. (2008). Osteoprotegerin levels in peri-implant crevicular fluid. *Clinical Oral Implants Research*, Vol.19, No.3, (March 2008), pp. 283-288

Arikan, F., Buduneli, N., Lappin D.F. (2011). C-telopeptide pyridinoline crosslinks of type I collagen, soluble RANKL, and osteoprotegerin levels in crevicular fluid of dental implants with peri-implantitis: a case-control study. *International Journal of Oral and Maxillofacial Implants*, Vol.26, No.2, pp. 282-298

Armitage, G.C. (1999). Development of a Classification System for Periodontal Diseases and Conditions. *Annals of Periodontology*, Vol.4, no.1, (December 1999), pp. 1-6

Banita, M., Pisoschi, C., Stanciulescu, C., Tuculina, M., Mercut, V. & Caruntu, I.D. (2008). Idiopathic gingival hypertrophy – a morphological study and a review of literature. *Revista Medico- Chirurgicala a Societatii de Medici si Naturalisti Iasi*, Vol.112, No.4, (Octombrie-Decembrie 2008), pp. 1076-1083

Banita, M., Pisoschi, C., Stanciulescu, C., Mercut, V., Scrieciu, M., Hancu, M. & Craitoiu, M. (2011). Phenytoin-induced gingival overgrowth – an immunohistochemical study of TGF-β1 mediated pathogenic pathways, *Farmacia*; Vol.59, No.1, (January-February 2011), pp.24-33

Bartold, P.M. (1993). Platelet-derived Growth Factor Stimulates Hyaluronate but not Proteoglycan Synthesis by Human Gingival Fibroblasts in vitro. Journal of Dental Research, Vol.72, No.11, (November 1993), pp. 1473-1480

Bartold, M., Narayanan, A.S. & Page, R.C. (1992). Platelet-derived growth factor reduces the inhibitory effects of lipopolysaccharide on gingival fibroblast proliferation. *Journal of Periodontal Research*, Vol.27, No.5, (September 1992), pp. 499-505

Bartold, M. & Narayanan, A.S. (2006). Molecular and cell biology of healthy and diseased periodontal tissues, *Periodontology 2000*, Vol.40, pp. 29-49

Beklen, A., Ainola, M., Hukkanen, M., Gurcan, C., Sorsa, T. & Konttinen, Y.T. (2007). MMPs, Il-1 and TNF are Regulated by Il-17 in Periodontitis, *Journal of Dental Research*, Vol. 86, No.4, (April 2007), pp. 347-351

Bildt, M.M., Bloemen, M., Kuijpers-Jagtman, A.M. & Von den Hoff, J.W. (2008). Collagenolytic fragments and active gelatinase complexes in periodontitis. *Journal of Periodontology*, Vol.79, No.9, (September 2008), pp. 1704-1711

Birkedal-Hansen, H., Moore, W.G.I., Bodden, M.K., Windsor, L.J., Birkedal-Hansen, B., DeCarlo, A., Engler, J.A. (1993). Matrix Metalloproteinases: A Review. *Critical Reviews in Oral Biology and Medicine*, Vol.4, No.2, pp. 197-250

Booth, V., Young, S., Cruchley, A., Taichman, N.S. & Paleolog, E. (1998). Vascular endothelial growth factor in human periodontal disease. *Journal of Periodontal Research*, Vol.33, No.8, (November 1998), pp. 491-499

Brigstock, D.R. (2003). The CCN family: a new stimulus package, *Journal of Endocrinology*, Vol. 178, No.2, (August 2003), pp. 169-175

Brew, K., Dinakarpandian, D. & Nagase, H. (2000). Tissue inhibitors of metalloproteinases: evolution, structure and function. *Biochimica Biophysica Acta*, Vol.1477, no.1-2, (March 2000), pp. 267-283

Buduneli, N., Attila, G., Güner, G. & Oktay, G. (2001a). Biochemical analysis of total collagen content and collagen types I, III, IV, V and VI in gingiva of various periodontitis categories. *Journal of International Academy of Periodontology*, Vol.3, No.1, (January 2001), pp. 1-6

Buduneli, N., Kütükçüler, N., Aksu, G. & Attila, G. (2001b). Evaluation of transforming growth factor-beta 1 in crevicular fluid of cyclosporine A-treated patients. *Journal of Periodontology*, Vol. 72, No.4, (April 2001), pp. 526-531

Buduneli, N., Sağol, O., Attila, G., Duman, S. & Holmstrup, P. (2001c). Immunohistochemical analysis of epidermal growth factor receptor in cyclosporin A-induced gingival overgrowth. *Acta Odontologica Scandinavica*, Vol. 59, No.6, (December 2001), pp. 367-371

Buduneli, N., Biyikoglu, B., Sherrabeh, S. & Lappin, D.F. (2008). Saliva concentrations of RANKL and osteoprotegerin in smoker versus non-smoker chronic periodontitis patients. *Journal of Clinical Periodontology*, Vol.35, No.10, (October 2008), pp. 846-852

Buduneli, N. & Kinane, D.F. (2011). Host-derived diagnostic markers related to soft tissue destruction and bone degradation in periodontitis. *Journal of Clinical Periodontology*, Vol.38, Suppl.11, (March 2011), pp. 85-105

Champagne, CM., Buchanan, W., Reddy, M.S., Preisser, J.S., Beck, J.D. & Offenbacher, S. (2003). Potential for gingival crevice fluid markers as predictors of risk for periodontal diseases. *Periodontology 2000*, Vol.31, no1, (February 2003), pp. 167–180

Chang, K.M., Lehrhaupt, N., Lin, L.M., Feng, J., Wu-Wang, C.Y. &Wang, S.L. (1996). Epidermal growth factor in gingival crevicular fluid and its binding capacity in inflamed and non-inflamed human gingiva. *Archives of Oral Biology*, Vol.41, No.7, (July 1996), pp. 719-724

Clokie, C.M. & Bell, R.C. (2003). Recombinant human transforming growth factor β-1 and its effects on osseointegration. *Journal of Craniofacial Surgery*, Vol.14, No.3, (May 2003), pp. 268–277

De Souza, A.P. & Line, S.R.P. (2002). The biology of matrix metalloproteinases. *Revista FOB*, Vol.10, No.1, (March 2002), pp.1-6

Dongari Batzoglou, A. (2004). Academy Report. Drug-Induced Gingival Enlargement. *Journal of Periodontology*, Vol.75, No.10, (October 2004), pp. 1424-1431

Ellis, J.S., Morgan, C.L., Taylor, J.J. & Thomason J.M. (2004). Plasma TGF-β1 as a risk factor for gingival owergrowth, *Journal of Clinical Periodontology*, Vol.31, No.10, (October 2004), pp. 863-868

Emingil, G., Kuula, H., Sorsa, T. & Atilla, G. (2006a). Gingival crevicular fluid matrix metalloproteinase-25 and -26 levels in periodontal disease. *Journal of Periodontology*, Vol.77, No.4, (April 2006), pp. 664-671

Emingil, G., Tervahartiala, T., Mantyla, P., Maatta, M., Sorsa, T. & Atilla, G. (2006b). Gingival crevicular fluid matrix metalloproteinase (MMP)-7, extracellular MMP inducer, and tissue inhibitor of MMP-1 levels in periodontal disease. *Journal of Periodontology*, Vol.77, No.12, (December 2006), pp. 2040-2050

Ferrara, N. (2009). Vascular Endothelial Growth Factor. *Arteriosclerosis, Thrombosis and Vascular Biology*, Vol. 29, pp. 789-791

Frank, S., Madlener, M. & Werner, S. (1996). Transforming growth factors β1, β2 and β3 and their receptors are differentially regulated during normal and impaired wound healing. *Journal of Biological Chemistry*, Vol.271, No.17, (April 1996), pp. 10188-10193

Gao, J., Jordan, T.W. & Cutress, T.W. (1996). Immunolocalisation of basic fibroblast growth factor (bFGF) in human periodontal ligament (PDL) tissue. *Journal of Periodontal Research*, Vol.31, No.4, (May 1996), pp. 260-264

Giannobile, WV. (1996). Committee on Research, Science and Therapy of The American Academy of Periodontology. The Potential Role of Growth and Differentiation Factors in Periodontal Regeneration. *Journal of Periodontology*, Vol.67, 67, No.5, (May 1996), pp. 545-553

Giannobile, W.V., Hernandez, R.A., Finkelman, R.D., Ryan, S., Kiritsy, C.P., D'Andrea, M. & Lynch, S.E. (1996). Comparative effects of platelet-derived growth factor-BB and insulin-like growth factor-I, individually and in combination, on periodontal regeneration in *Macaca fascicularis*. *Journal of Periodontal Research*, Vol.31, No.5, (July 1996), pp. 301–312

Giannobile, W.V., Lee, C.S., Tomala, M.P., Tejeda, K.M. & Zhu, Z. (2001). Platelet-derived growth factor (PDGF) gene delivery for application in periodontal tissue engineering. *Journal of Periodontology*, Vol.72, No.6, (June 2001), pp. 815–23

Giannobile, W.V., Al-Shammari, K.F. & Sarment, D.P. (2003). Matrix molecules and growth factors as indicators of periodontal disease activity. *Periodontology 2000*, Vol.31, No.1, (February 2003), pp. 125-134

Gonçalves, R.P., Damante, C.A., Moura Lima, F.L., Imbronito, A.V., Daumas Nunes, F. & Pustiglioni , F.E. (2009). Detection of MMP-2 and MMP-9 salivary levels in patients with chronic periodontitis before and after periodontal treatment. *Revista Odonto Ciência*, Vol.24, No.3, pp. 264-269

Guneri, P., Unlu, F., Yesilbek, B., Bayraktar, F., Kokuladag, A., Hekimgil, M. & Boyacioglu, H. (2004). Vascular endothelial growth factor in gingival tissues and crevicular fluids of diabetic and healthy periodontal patients. *Journal of Periodontology*, Vol.75, No.1, (January 2004), pp. 91-97

Gurkan, A., Emingil, G., Cinarcik, S. & Berdeli A. (2006). Gingival crevicular fluid transfroming growth factor- $\beta1$ in several forms of periodontal disease. *Archives of Oral Biology*, Vol.51, No.10, (October 2006), pp. 906-912

Havemose-Poulsen, A. & Holmstrup, P. (1997). Factors affecting IL-1-mediated collagen metabolism by fibroblasts and the pathogenesis of periodontal disease: a review of the literature. *Critical Reviews in Oral Biology and Medicine*, Vol.8, No.2, pp. 217-236

Heng, E.C.K., Huang, Y., Black, S.A. Jr., Trackman, P.C. (2006). CCN2, connective Tissue Growth Factor, Stimulates Collagen Deposition by Gingival Fibroblasts via Module 3 and $\alpha6$- and $\beta1$ integrins. *Journal of Cell Biochemistry*, Vol. 98, No.2, (May 2006), pp. 409–420

Hormia, M., Thesleff, I., Perheentupa, J., Pesonen, K. & Saxen, L. (1993). Increased rate of salivary epidermal growth factor secretion in patients with juvenile periodontitis. *European Journal of Oral Sciences*, Vol. 10, no. 3, (June 1993), pp. 138-144

Kaigler, D., Cirelli, J.A. & Giannobile, W.V. (2006). Growth factor delivery for oral and periodontal tissue engineering. *Expert Opinion in Drug Delivery*, Vol.3, No.5, (September 2006), pp. 647–662

Kakimoto, K, Y. & Daiku., Machigashira, M., Ohnishi, t., Kajihara, T., Semba, I., Setoguchi, T., Tamura, M., Izumi hara, Y. (2002). Hepatocyte growth factor in gingival crevicular fluid and the distribution of hepatocyte growth factor-activator in gingival tissue from adult periodontitis. *Archives of Oral Biology*, Vol.47, No.9, (September 2002), pp. 655-663

Kantarci, A., Black, S.A., Xydas, C.E., Murawel, P., Uchida, Y., Yucekal-Tuncer, B., Atilla, G., Emingil, G., Uzel, I.M., Lee, A., Firatli, E., Sheff, M., Hasturk, H., Van Dyke, T.E. & Trackman, P.C. (2006), Epithelial and Connective Tissue Cell CTGF/CCN2 expression in Gingival Fibrosis. *Journal of Pathology*, Vol.210, No.1, (September 2006), pp. 59–66

Kaufman, E. & Lamster, I.B. (2000). Analysis of saliva for periodontal diagnosis: a review. *Journal of Clinical Periodontology*, Vol.27, No.7, (July 2000), pp. 453-465

Keles, G.C., Cetinkaya, B.O., Eroglu, C., Simsek, S.B. &Kahraman, H. (2010). Vascular endothelial growth factor expression levels of gingiva in gingivitis and periodontitis patients with/without diabetes mellitus. *Inflammation Research*, Vol.59, No.7, (July 2010), pp. 543-549

Kinane, D.F., Hart, T.C. (2003). Genes and gene polymorphisms associated with periodontal disease. *Critical Review Oral Biology Medicine* Vol.14, No.6, (November 2003), pp. 430-449

Kinney, J.S., Ramseier, C.A. & Giannobile, W.V. (2007). Oral Fluid-Based Biomarkers of Alveolar Bone Loss in Periodontitis. *Annals of the New York Academy of Sciences*, Vol. 1098, (March 2007), pp. 230–251

Kitamura, M., Nakashima, K., Kowashi, Y., Fujii, T., Shimauchi, H., Sasano, T., Furuuchi, T., Fukuda, M., Noguchi, T., Shibutani, T., Iwayama, Y., Takashiba, S., Kurihara, H., Ninomiya, M., Kido, J., Nagata, T., Hamaci, T., Maeda, K. Hara, Y., Izumil, Y. Hirofuji, T., Imai, E., Omae, M., Watanuki, M. & Murakami, S. (2008). Periodontal Tissue Regeneration Using Fibroblast Growth Factor -2: Randomized Controlled Phase II Clinical Trial. *PLoS ONE*, Vol.3, No.7, (July 2008), e2611, www.plosone.org

Kubota, T., Itagaki, M., Hoshino, C., Nagata, m., Morozumi, T., Kobayashi, T., Takagi, R. & Yoshie, H. (2008). Altered gene expression levels of matrix metalloproteinases and their inhibitors in periodontitis-affected gingival tissue. *Journal of Periodontology*, Vol.79, No.11, (January 2008), pp. 2040-2050

Kumar, M.S., Vamsi, G., Sripriya, R. & Sehgal, P.K. (2006). Expression of matrix metalloproteinases (MMP-8 and -9) in chronic periodontitis patients with and without diabetes mellitus. *Journal of Periodontology*, Vol.77, No.11, (October 2006), pp. 1803-1808

Lambert, E., Dasse, E., Haye, B. & Petitfrere, E. (2004). TIMPs as multifacial proteins. *Critical Review in Oncology/Hematology*, Vol.49, No.3, (March 2004), pp. 187-198

Laurina, Z., Pilmane, M. & Care, R. (2009). Growth factors/cytokines/defensins and apoptosis in periodontal pathologies. *Stomatologija*, Vol.11, No.2, pp. 48-54

Lawrence, D.A (1995). Transforming growth factor-β: an overview. *Kidney Int*, Vol.47, s19-23

Leask, A. & Abraham, D.J. (2003). The role of connective tissue growth factor, a multifunctional matricellular protein, in fibroblast biology. *Biochemistry of Cell Biology*,Vol.81, No.6, (December 2003), pp. 355-363

Lorencini, M., Silva, J.A.F., Almeida, C.A., Bruni-Cardoso, A., Carvalho, H.F. & Stach-Machado, D.R. (2009). A new paradigm in the periodontal disease progression: Gingival connective tissue remodeling with simultaneous collagen degradation and fibers thickening. *Tissue and Cell*, Vol.41, No.1, (February 2009), pp.43-50

Lucarini, G., Zizzi, A., Aspriello, S.D., Ferrante, L., Tosso, E., Lo Muzio, L., Foglini, P., Mattioli-Belmonte, M., DiPrimio, R. & Piemontese, M. (2009). Involvement of vascular endothelial growth factor, CD44 and CD 133 in periodontal disease and diabetes: an immunohistochemical study. *Journal of Clinical Periodontology*, Vol.36, No.1, (January 2009), pp.3-10

Marshall, R.I. & Bartold, P.M. (1998). Medication induced gingival overgrowth. *Oral diseases*, Vol.4, No.2, (June 1998), pp. 130-151

Marshall, R.I.&Bartold, P.M. (1999). A clinical review of drug-induced gingival overgrowths. *Australian Dental Journal*, Vol.44, No.4, (December 1999), pp. 219-232

Massague, J. (1998). TGF-β signal transduction. *Annual Review of Biochemistry*, Vol.67, pp. 753-791

Matsumoto K, Nakamura T (1997) Hepatocyte growth factor (HGF) as a tissue organizer for organogenesis and regeneration. *Biochemistry Biophysics Research Communications*, Vol.239, No.3, (October 1997), pp. 639-644

Miller, C.S., King, C.P., Jr., Chris Langub, M., Kryscio, R.J. & Thomas, M.V. (2006). Salivary biomarkers of existing periodontal disease. A cross-sectional study. *JADA*, Vol.137, (March 2006), pp. 322-329

Mumford, J.H., Carnes, D.L, Cochran, D.L. & Oates, T.W. (2001). The effects of platelet-derived growth factor-BB on periodontal cells in an in vitro wound model. *Journal of periodontology*, Vol.72, No.3, (March 2001), pp. 331-340

Murakami S, Takayama S, Ikezawa K, Shimabukuro Y, Kitamura M, Nozaki T, Terashima, A., Asano, T. & Okada, H. (1999). Regeneration of periodontal tissues by basic fibroblast growth factor. *Journal of Periodontal Research*, Vol.34, No.7, (October 1999), pp. 425–430

Murakami, S., Takayama, S., Kitamura, M., Shimabukuro, Y., Yanagi, K., Ikezawa, K., Saho, T., Nozaki, T. & Okada, H. (2003). Recombinant human basic fibroblast growth factor (bFGF) stimulates periodontal regeneration in class II furcation defects created in beagle dogs. *Journal of Periodontal Research*, Vol.38, No.1, (February 2003), pp. 97–103

Nanci, A.& Bosshardt, D.D. (2006). Structure of periodontal tissues in health and disease. *Periodontology 2000*, Vol.40, No.1, (February 2006), pp. 11-28

Ohnishi, T. & Daikuhara, Y. (2003) Hepatocyte growth factor/scatter factor in development, inflammation and carcinogenesis: its expression and role in oral tissues. *Archives of Oral Biology*, Vol.48, No.12, (December 2003), pp. 797-804

Ohshima, M., Noguchi, Y., Ito, M., Maeno, M. & Otsuka, K. (2001). Hepatocyte growth factor secreted by periodontal ligament and gingival fibroblast is a mjor chemoattractant for gingival epithelial cells. *Journal of Periodontal Research*, Vol.36, No.6, (December 2001), pp. 377-383

Ohshima, M., Yamaguchi, Y., Matsumoto, N., Micke, P., Takenouchi, Y., Nishida, T., Kato, M., Komiyama, K., Abiko, Y., Ito, K., Otsuka, K. & Kappert, K. (2010). TGF-β Signaling in Gingival Fibroblast-Epithelial Interaction. *Journal of Dental Research*, Vol.89, No.11, (December 2010), pp. 1315-1321

Ojima, Y., Mizuno, M., Kuboki, Y. & Komori, T. (2003). In vitro effect of platelet-derived growth factor-BB on collagen synthesis and proliferation of human periodontal ligament cells. *Oral Diseases*, Vol.99, No.3, (May 2003), pp. 144–151

Okuda, K., Murata, M., Sugimoto, M., Saito, Y., Kabasawa, L., Yoshie, H., Saku, T. & Hara, K. (1998). TGF-beta1 influences early gingival wound healing in rats: an immunohistochemical evaluation of stromal remodelling by extracellular matrix molecules and PCNA. *Journal of Oral Pathology &Medicine*, Vol.27, No.10, (November 1998), pp. 463–469

Ozçaka O., Nalbantsoy, A., Buduneli, N. (2011). Salivary osteocalcin levels are decreased in smoker chronic periodontitis. Oral Diseases, Vol.17, No.2, (March 2011), pp. 200-205

Petersen, P.E. (2003). The World Oral Health Report 2003: Continuous improvement of oral health in the 21st century – The approach of the WHO Global Oral Health Programme. *Community Dentistry and Oral Epidemiology*,Vol.31 (Suppl.s1), (December 2003), pp. 3-24,

Pinheiro, M.L., Feres-Filho, E.J., Graves, D.T., Takiya, C.M., Elsas, M.I., Elsas, P.P. & Ruz, R.A. (2003). Quantification and localization of platelet-derived growth factor in gingiva of periodontitis patients. *Journal of Periodontology*, Vol.74, No.3, (March 2003), pp. 323-328

Pisoschi, C., Banita, M., Stanciulescu, C., Fusaru, A.M. & Gheorghita, M. (2009). Influence of some mediators of extracellular matrix remodeling on angiogenesis in diabetic gingival overgrowth. Proceedings of the 34th FEBS Congress, *FEBS Journal*, Vol.276, p. 217, Prague, July 2009

Pisoschi, C., Banita, M., Gheorghita, L., Stanciulescu, C., Craitoiu, M. & Fusaru, A.M. (2010). Salivary Transforming Growth Factor β1 – a possible risk factor for gingival overgrowth. Archives of the Balkan Medical Union, Vol.45, No.1, pp. 18-22

Pisoschi, C., Banita, M., Stanciulescu, C., Fusaru, A.M. & Ene, M. (2011). Correlation between salivary level and tissue expression of connective tissue growth factor in gingival overgrowth. Proceedings of 41st Congress of Turkish Society of Periodontology, p.168, Istanbul, May 2011

Pradeep, A.R., Prapulla, D.V., Sharma, A. & Sujatha, P.B. (2011). Gingival crevicular fluid and serum vascular endothelial growth factor: Their relationship in periodontal health, disease and treatment. Cytokine, Vol.54, No.2, (May 2011), pp. 200-204

Prime, S.S., Pring, M., Davies, M., Paterson, I.C. (2004). TGF beta signal transduction in orofacial health and non-malignant disease (part I).Critical Review Oral Biology Medicine, Vol.1, No.15, (November 2004), pp. 324-336.

Ratcliff, P.A. & Johnson, P.W. (1999). The relationship between oral malodour gingivitis, and periodontitis. A review. Journal of Periodontology, Vol.70, No.5, (May 1999), pp. 485-489.

Reynolds, J.J., Hembry, R.M., Meikle, M.C. (1994). Connective Tissue Degradation in Health and Periodontal Disease and the Roles of Matrix Metalloproteinases and their Natural Inhibitors. Advances in Dental Research, Vol.8, No.2, pp.312-319

Reynolds. JJ., Meikle, M.C. (1997). Mechanisms of connective tissue matrix destruction in periodontitis. Periodontology 2000, Vol.14, No.1, (June 1997), pp. 216-248

Romanos, G.E., Strub, J.R. & Bernimoulin, J.P. (1993). Immunohistochemical distribution of extracellular matrix proteins as a diagnostic parameter in healthy and diseased gingiva, Journal of Periodontology, Vol.64, No.2, (February, 1993), pp. 110-119

Sakallioglu, E.S., Aliyev, E., Lutfioglu, M., Yavuz, U. & Acikgoz, G. (2007). Vascular endothelial growth factor (VEGF) levels of gingiva and gingival crevicular fluid in diabetic and systemically healthy periodontitis patients. Clinical Oral Investigations, Vol.11, No.2, (June 2007), pp. 115-120

Schilephake, H. (2002). Bone growth factors in maxillofacial skeletal reconstruction. International Journal of Oral Maxillofacial Surgery, Vol.31, No.5, (October 2002), pp. 469–484

Seymour, R.A., Ellis, J.S. & Thomason, J.M (2000). Risk factors for drug induced gingival overgrowth. Journal of Clinical Periodontology, Vol.27, No.4, (April 2000), pp. 217-223

Seymour, R.A. (2006). Effects of medications on the periodontal tissues in health and disease. Periodontology 2000, Vol.40, No.1, (February 2006), pp. 120–129

Taba, M. Jr., Jin, Q., Sugai, V. & Giannobile, W.V. (2005). Current concepts in periodontal bioengineering. Orthodontics Craniofacial Research, Vol.8, No.4, (November 2005), pp. 292–302

Takayama, S., Murakami, S., Miki, Y., Ikezawa, K., Tasaka, S., Terashima, A., Asano, T. & Okada, H. (1997). Effects of basic fibroblast growth factor on human periodontal ligament cells. Journal of Periodontal Research, Vol.32, No.8, (November 1997), pp. 667–675

Taylor, BA. (2003). Management of drug-induced gingival enlargement. Australian Prescriber, Vol.26, No.1, pp. 11-13

Taylor, G.W., Borgnakke, W.S. (2008). Periodontal disease: associations with diabetes, glycemic control and complications. Oral Diseases, Vol.14, No.3, (April 2008), pp. 191–203

Terranova, V.P., Odziemiec, C., Tweden, K.S. & Spadone, D.P. (1989). Repopulation of dentin surfaces by periodontal ligament cells and endothelial cells. Effect of basic fibroblast growth factor. Journal of Periodontology, Vol.60, No. 6, (June 1989), pp. 293–301

Trackman, P.C. & Kantarci, A. (2004). Connective tissue metabolism and gingival overgrowth. Critical Review Oral Biology Medicine, Vol.15, No.3, (May 2004), pp. 165-175

Uzel, M.I., Kantarci, A., Hong, H.H., Uygur, C., Sheff, M.C., Firatli, E. & Trackman, P.C. (2001). Connective tissue growth factor in phenytoin-induced gingival overgrowth. Journal of Periodontology, Vol.72, No.7, (July 2001), pp. 921–931

Vestappen, J. & Von den Hoff, J.W. (2006). Tissue Inhibitors of Metalloproteinases (TIMPs): Their Biological Functions and Involvement in Oral Disease. Journal of Dental Research, Vol.85, No.12, (December 2006), pp. 1074-1083

Visse, R. & Nagase, H. (2003). Matrix Metalloproteinases and Tissue Inhibitors of Metalloproteinases. Structure, Function, and Biochemistry. Circulation Research, Vol.92, No.8, (May 2003), pp. 827-839

Werner, H. & Katz, J. (2004). The emerging role of the insulin-like growth factors in oral biology. Journal of Dental Research, Vol.83, No.11, (November 2004), pp. 832-836

Whittaker, M. & Ayscough, A. (2001). Matrix metalloproteinases and their inhibitors – Current Status and Future Challenges. Cell Transmissions, Vol.17, No.1, pp. 3-12

Wilczynska-Borawska, M., Borawski, J., Kovalchuk, O., Chyczewski, L. & Stokowska, W. (2006). Hepatocyte growth factor in saliva is a potential marker of symptomatic periodontal disease. Journal of Oral Science, Vol.48, No.2, (June 2006), pp. 47-50

Wright, H.J., Chapple, I.L. & Matthews, J.B. (2001). TGF-beta isoforms and TGF-beta receptors in drug-induced and hereditary gingival overgrowth. Journal of Oral Pathology&Medicine, Vol.30, No.5, (May 2001), pp.281-289

Wright, H.J., Chapple, I.L., Blair, F. & Matthews, J.B. (2004) Crevicular fluid levels of TGF beta1 in drug-induced gingival overgrowth. Archives of Oral Biology, Vol.49, No.5, (May 2004), pp. 421-425

Yun, Y.R., Won, J.E., Jeon, E., Lee, S., Kang, W., Jo, W., Jang, J.H., Shin, U.E. & Kim, H.W. Fibroblast Growth Factors: Biology, Function, and Application for Tissue Regeneration Journal of Tissue Engineering, Volume 2010, Article ID 218142, 18 pages, doi:10.4061/2010/218142

Zia, A., Khan, S., Bey, A., Gupta, N.D. & Mukhtar-Un-Nisar, S. (2011). Oral biomarkers in the diagnosis and progression of periodontal diseases. Biology and Medicine, Vol.3, No.2, (March 2011), Special Issue, pp. 45-52

5

Effects of Tobacco Smoking on Chronic Periodontitis and Periodontal Treatment

Nurcan Buduneli

Department of Periodontology, School of Dentistry, Ege University, İzmir, Turkey

1. Introduction

Periodontitis is one of the most common oral diseases and is characterised by gingival inflammation and alveolar bone resorption (Savage et al. 2009). Periodontitis is a multifactorial irreversible and cumulative condition, initiated and propagated by bacteria and host factors (Kinane 2001). More than 500 different bacterial species are able to colonise the oral biofilm and up to 150 different species of bacteria are possible in any individual's subgingival plaque. There are two forms of periodontitis; chronic and aggressive periodontitis which differ from each other not only in clinical findings but also age of onset and rate of progression. Chronic periodontitis progresses more slowly compared to the aggressive forms of periodontitis and responds much better to periodontal treatment. According to a report by the World Health Organisation, severe chronic periodontitis leading to tooth loss was found in 5% to 15% of most populations worldwide (Armitage 2004). Hence, it can be considered among the prevalent and important global health problems in terms of quality of life.

The multifactorial nature of periodontitis is based on the complex interactions between microorganisms in the microbial dental plaque, namely dental biofilm, host response mechanisms and environmental factors. Smoking is well known to be the leading environmental factor that is closely related not only with the risk but also the prognosis of periodontitis. Indeed, the harmful effects of smoking on numerous organs have been well-documented for years now. Cigarette smoking is recognised as the major preventable cause of death in the United States (Centres for Disease Control 2002 (CDC 2002)). Smoking is the second strongest modifiable risk factor for periodontal disease after the first one which is the microbial dental plaque. Smokers are more likely to harbour a higher prevalence of potential periodontal pathogens, and smoking impairs various aspects of innate and acquired immune responses. Numerous molecules in the oral fluids namely; gingival crevicular fluid (GCF) and saliva, as well as molecules in blood circulation; serum or plasma have been investigated so far in an attempt to provide a sensitive and specific marker for periodontal tissue destruction (Buduneli & Kinane 2011). The aim of the present literature review is to provide an overview of the evidence for smoking as a risk factor for chronic periodontitis and to discuss the possible mechanisms of action and finally the negative effects of smoking on the outcomes of periodontal treatment in patients with chronic periodontitis.

Smokers are accepted to be more susceptible to advanced and aggressive forms of periodontitis than non-smokers (Haber et al. 1993, Calsina et al. 2002) and former smokers are at decreased disease risk than current smokers (Bostrom et al. 2001). Tobacco smoking modifies the periodontal response to microbial challenge (Barbour et al. 1997, Palmer et al. 2005). Although, smoker and non-smoker patients exhibit more or less the same periodontal pathogens (Preber et al. 1992, Buduneli et al. 2005a) smokers also tend to respond less favourably to periodontal treatment (Ah et al. 1994, Renvert et al. 1998). Smoking was suggested to influence host cytokine levels (Boström et al. 1999, Buduneli et al. 2005b, Buduneli et al. 2006). Furthermore, smoking was reported to reduce salivary osteoprotegerin concentrations in untreated and also treated chronic periodontitis patients (Buduneli et al. 2008). Chronic periodontitis has been associated with various systemic diseases and/or conditions such as cardiovascular diseases and preterm low birth weight. Over the last decade there have been a number of reviews that have considered the biological mechanisms underlying susceptibility to periodontitis in smokers (Barbour et al. 1997, Johnson & Hill 2004, Kinane & Chestnutt 2000, Mullally 2004, Palmer et al. 2005, Scott et al. 2001). Despite that a clear dose-response relationship between chronic periodontitis and smoking was reported (Martinez-Canut et al. 1995) the mechanisms by which smoking contributes to the pathogenesis of periodontitis are not yet clearly understood.

The fundamental mechanisms that lead to the development of chronic periodontitis are closely related to the dynamics of the host immune and inflammatory responses to periodontal pathogens present in the dental biofilm (Gemmell & Seymour 2004). The immune and inflammatory responses are critical to understanding the pathogenesis of periodontal diseases and they are orchestrated by a number of host-related factors, either intrinsic or induced (Taubman et al. 2005). Under normal circumstances, there is a balance between microbial virulence factors and host response. Tissue homeostasis is maintained as long as this balance is preserved. In periodontitis, this balance between the microbial virulence factors and host response is impaired in favour of microbial challenge. Smoking as an environmental factor has been suggested to interact with host cells and affect inflammatory responses to this microbial challenge (Palmer et al. 2005). It is also likely that the toxic components of tobacco smoke, mainly nicotine, may directly or indirectly deteriorate periodontal tissues. Cigarette smoking represents a risk factor for progression of periodontitis, the effect of which may be dose related. Heavy smokers should be considered as high-risk individuals for progression of periodontitis. The clinical implications for this are that smokers should be identified during patient examination and efforts should be made to modify this behavioural risk factor. Furthermore, smoking or molecules related to smoking such as blood cotinine induced by smoking should be considered as important risk markers of periodontal disease that are relevant to the assessment of prognosis (Calsina et al. 2002, Tang et al. 2009).

Smokers are almost four times more likely to have severe periodontitis than non-smokers (Haber et al. 1993). Nicotine and lipopolysaccharide (LPS) effects on the expression of macrophage colony-stimulating factor (M-CSF), osteoprotegerin (OPG), and prostaglandin E_2 (PGE_2) have been evaluated by Tanaka et al. (2006) in osteoblasts and osteoclast-like cells. OPG expression was increased in the initial stages of culture with nicotine and LPS but decreased in the later stages of culture. Apatzidou et al. (2005) stated that smokers with periodontal disease have a suppressed inflammatory response, a significantly less favourable clinical outcome and seem to have an altered host antibody response to antigenic challenge than non-smokers although; the subgingival microflora of smokers appears similar to that of non-smokers. Lappin et al. (2007) reported decreased serum OPG levels and greater soluble receptor activator of nuclear- factor kappa B ligand (sRANKL) sRANKL/OPG ratios in smoker patients in the maintenance program than the non-smoker counterparts. Negative correlation between pack-years and total OPG amount in peri-implant crevicular fluid was detected in clinically healthy implants (Arıkan et al. 2008). Our recent finding of higher sRANKL, lower OPG concentrations in saliva of untreated/treated smokers than non-smokers (Buduneli et al. 2008) confirmed these findings. Furthermore, our saliva data (Buduneli et al. 2008) indicated that treated non-smokers had lower sRANKL levels than untreated non-smokers possibly indicating a more active inflammatory process in untreated patients. Although the exact GCF concentrations of RANKL and OPG varied from study to study, overall RANKL/OPG ratio showed a trend to increase in periodontitis compared to healthy controls (Mogi et al. 2004, Lu et al. 2006, Bostancı et al. 2007, Crotti et al. 2003). This may either be explained by an increase in RANKL or a decrease in OPG levels or both.

Significantly lower plasma OPG concentrations were detected in smoker chronic periodontitis patients than the smoker healthy controls without any significant differences between the smoker and non-smoker study groups (Özçaka et al. 2010). That finding suggests that smoking alone may not be effective on plasma levels of RANKL/OPG system in periodontal disease but when it is coupled with periodontal inflammation the disturbing effect on bone homeostasis may become detectable. Moreover, the significant positive correlations found in the smoker groups between plasma OPG concentrations and probing depth may indicate a tendency towards increased bone metabolism which aims to compensate the increased susceptibility to alveolar bone resorption (Özçaka et al. 2010). Neither the clinical periodontal measurements nor the laboratory data obtained in plasma samples showed significant differences between the smoker and non-smoker chronic periodontitis patients (Özçaka et al. 2010). Indeed, the similarity in clinical periodontal findings between the smoker and non-smoker chronic periodontitis patient groups may explain the lack of significant differences in plasma levels of RANKL and OPG. Darby et al. (2005) suggested that the inferior improvement in probing depth following scaling and root planing in smoker chronic periodontitis patients may reflect the systemic effects of smoking on the host response, the healing process, and the poorer clearance of the microorganisms. The plasma data reported by Özçaka et al. (2010) are in line with the recent study by Tang et al. (2009) reporting similar sRANKL and OPG levels in GCF samples of never smokers, former smokers and current smokers. In that study the only significant difference could be found in GCF OPG levels of the high pack-years group and never smokers.

It has been shown that not only the number of leukocytes is increased but also leukocytes particularly polymorphonuclear neutrophils (PMNs) are significantly activated in smokers, suggesting a systemic inflammatory state. Nicotine has been shown to activate PMNs. Pathogens in microbial dental plaque are capable of stimulating host cells to increase their matrix metalloproteinase (MMP) release which is considered among the indirect mechanisms of tissue destruction seen during periodontitis (Sorsa et al. 2006). Periodontal tissues are infiltrated mainly by neutrophilic granulocytes and PMN which play an important role in the development of inflammatory injury. Tobacco-induced degranulation events in neutrophils, tobacco-induced alterations to the microbial flora, and tobacco-induced increases in pro-inflammatory cytokine burden could each, theoretically, influence MMP-8 levels in the periodontal tissues of smokers. In a recent study (Özçaka et al. 2011), it was hypothesised that smoking may affect MMPs and neutrophil degranulation products in the systemic level eventually leading more severe periodontal tissue destruction and systemic inflammation predisposing to cardiovascular diseases (Pussinen et al. 2007). In that exploratory study, the serum concentrations of MMP-8, MMP-9, TIMP-1, NE, and MPO were evaluated comparatively in smoker versus non-smoker patients with chronic periodontitis as well as periodontally healthy subjects. The clinical periodontal measurements were recorded and serum samples were analyzed in 55 patients with the clinical diagnosis of chronic periodontitis (16 smoker and 39 non-smoker) and 56 periodontally healthy subjects (17 smoker and 39 non-smoker). The findings of significantly elevated serum MMP-9, MPO, NE together with decreased TIMP-1 in smoker patients with chronic periodontitis than non-smoker counterparts support the idea that smoking together with periodontal destruction may expose/predispose to cardiovascular diseases.

MMP-8 activity has been found to be modified in various organs and body fluids in tobacco smokers. Knuutinen et al. (2002) noted an increased MMP-8 concentration in the resulting fluid infiltrate in smokers compared to that in the non-smokers following the induction of suction blisters on the upper arm. Furthermore, Betsuyaku et al. (1999) have shown increased MMP-8 and MMP-9 activity in the bronchial alveolar lavage fluids of smokers with emphysema compared to those without emphysema. A significant correlation between increased MMP-8 levels and periodontal disease severity has been suggested. Liu et al. (2006) have reported increased local MMP-8 expression in the periodontal tissues of smokers compared to the non-smokers and a slight increase in the serum MMP-8 concentration, although the difference between the smoker and non-smoker groups did not reach the level of significance.

On the other hand, Söder et al. (2002) found a positive correlation between elastase complexed to α1-antitrypsin and MMP-8 concentrations in the gingival crevicular fluid (GCF) of smokers in individuals with various persistent periodontal diseases. However, they did not observe any difference in GCF MMP-8 levels between smokers and non-smokers. Persson et al. (2003) reported that GCF MMP-8 levels remained unchanged in the smokers following surgical treatment for periodontitis, whereas decreased levels were observed in the non-smokers, suggesting a tobacco-induced MMP-8 burden. Liede et al. (1999) examined salivary MMP-8 concentrations in 327 smokers and 82 quitters and found lower MMP-8 levels in the current smokers than the ex-smokers. According to our recent data (Özçaka et al. 2011), serum MMP-8 concentrations did not differ significantly between the smokers and non-smokers. It should be kept in mind that self-reports of non-smoking people can sometimes be unreliable (Buduneli et al. 2006). Therefore, confirmation of the smoking status by serum and/or salivary cotinine analysis may result in changing the accurate group of individual subjects which may eventually affect the results. Therefore, apart from the relatively small numbers of smokers in some of the studies, lack of cotinine analysis may explain the discrepancies between the findings of different clinical studies.

MPO was suggested as an early marker of systemic inflammation in smokers without severe airway symptoms in a study aiming to relate smoking and chronic obstructive pulmonary disease (Andelid et al. 2007). The authors reported significant increases in serum MPO concentrations in smokers than never smokers at 6th year of follow-up. Enhanced serum levels of MPO indicate increased degranulation of specific granules of neutrophils (Rautelin et al. 2009). Accordingly, our recent data indicated significant increases in serum concentrations of MPO in smoker chronic periodontitis patients, although the clinical periodontal measurements did not differ from those of the non-smoker counterparts (Özçaka et al. 2011a). This increase in serum MPO concentration may be regarded as an indicator of increased risk for local and systemic inflammation such as periodontal tissue destruction or an early sign of atherosclerosis.

NE, which is a serine protease, can also accelerate MMP-cascades by activating latent proMMPs and inactivating TIMP-1 (Sorsa et al. 2006). NE was suggested to be involved in the degradation of non-collagenous protein-covered collagen fibrils in the early destructive stages of periodontal diseases (Ujiie et al. 2007). To our best of knowledge, serum NE levels as a systemic inflammatory parameter reflecting effects of smoking on chronic periodontitis has been evaluated only in our recent study (Özçaka et al. 2011) which revealed significantly higher serum NE concentrations in smoker chronic periodontitis patients than those of non-smokers.

Significantly increased serum concentrations of MMP-9 together with significant decreases in TIMP-1 concentrations in smoker chronic periodontitis patients deserve further investigation and suggest that chronic periodontitis together with smoking can predispose the development of cardiovascular diseases (Pussinen et al. 2007). Persistent smoking and periodontal inflammation predispose the patients for enhanced systemic inflammation in addition to enhanced periodontal destruction.

Carboxyterminal-telopeptide pyridinoline cross-links of type I collagen (ICTP) is released into the periodontal tissues as a consequence of collagen degradation and alveolar bone resorption (Seibel 2003). Type I collagen composes 90 % of the organic matrix of bone and is the most abundant collagen in osseous tissue (Narayanan & Page 1983). Studies assessing the role of ICTP levels in GCF or peri-implant crevicular fluid as a diagnostic marker of periodontal disease activity have reported promising results so far (Oringer et al. 1998, 2002). ICTP was suggested to predict future bone loss, to correlate with clinical parameters and putative periodontal pathogens and also to reduce following periodontal therapy (Giannobile 1999). Apart from the direct cigarette smoke-mediated effects, tissue damage mediated by impaired balance of bone turnover markers originating from tobacco smoke and tobacco-induced inflammation may be a potential mechanism.

Osteocalcin (OC) is a calcium-binding protein of bone and the most abundant non-collagenous protein of the mineralized tissue (Lian & Gundberg 1988). Serum level of OC is considered as a marker of bone formation (Christenson 1997). Serum levels of OC were reported to be lower in periodontitis patients compared with healthy subjects suggesting lower osteoblastic activity and bone formation ability (Shi et al. 1996).

In a recent study, we investigated possible effects of smoking on saliva ICTP and OC concentrations comparatively in patients with chronic periodontitis and periodontally healthy subjects (Özçaka et al. 2011b). Smoker periodontitis patients revealed similar clinical periodontal index values with non-smoker counterparts, whereas salivary OC levels were lower in smokers than non-smokers. ICTP levels in non-smoker chronic periodontitis patients were higher than non-smoker controls and smoker healthy control group revealed higher ICTP levels than non-smoker counterparts. The data suggested that suppression of salivary OC level by smoking may at least partly explain the deleterious effects of smoking on periodontal status. In another recent study by our group (Gürlek et al. 2009) similar salivary ICTP levels were detected in smoker, non-smoker and ex-smoker patient groups with similar clinical periodontal findings. Smoking status was confirmed by salivary cotinine analysis but there was no clinically healthy control group in that study and the number of teeth present, average probing depths and attachment levels were all similar in the three study groups. There were no significant differences in saliva ICTP concentrations between the smoker and non-smoker patient groups. It may be suggested that the similarity in clinical periodontal disease parameters may explain the similar salivary ICTP levels obtained in these studies.

Significantly lower salivary OC concentrations in both healthy and diseased smokers than their non-smoker counterparts were reported by Özçaka et al. (2011b). The detrimental effects of smoking may explain these decreases in salivary levels of OC in smokers also indicating a deficiency in tissue response to the injuries in smoker subjects. The differences in patient numbers and/or the possible differences in the disease activity states may explain the differences in findings of the present study and the previous ones. On the other hand, significantly lower salivary OC concentrations in the smoker patients than the non-smokers as well as the ex-smokers may at least partly explain the mechanisms of negative effects of smoking on periodontal health.

Lymphocyte functions including antibody production may also be affected by smoking. However, such affects seem to be complex and some components of cigarette such as nicotine are immunosuppressive (Geng et al. 1996) whereas some others are immunostimulatory such as tobacco glycoprotein and metals (Francus et al. 1988, Brooks et al. 1990). Serum immunoglobulin G (IgG) levels were reduced in smoker patients with periodontitis (Quinn et al. 1998). On the other hand, the number of B lymphocytes seemed to be similar in smokers and non-smokers but their function in peripheral blood was impaired in smokers, as reflected in proliferative response to polyclonal B cell activators and antigens (Sopori et al. 1989).

Interleukin-1 (IL-1), tumour necrosis factor (TNF), and prostaglandin E_2 (PGE2) are among the major inflammatory mediators that play significant role in alveolar bone resorption. Increased GCF levels of TNF-alpha were detected in current and former smokers (Bostrom et al. 1998). Moreover, it was reported that the expressions of inflammatory mediators such as IL-1, IL-6, IL-8, TNF-α, and cyclooxygenase-2 (COX-2) in response to lipopolysaccharide (LPS) of gram negative bacteria were increased in smokers (Bostrom et al. 1999, Tappia et al. 1995, Kuschner et al. 1996).

Tobacco smoking mostly in the form of cigarette smoking has been accused of impairing microcirculatory system and the relevant changes in vascular formations and functions may have a negative influence on the immune and inflammatory reactions in periodontal tissues. Smokers were reported to have significantly less number of vessels in inflamed gingival tissue compared to non-smokers (Rezavandi et al. 2002). Long-term smoking has an established negative effect on the vasculature of periodontal tissues. Acute exposure to cigarette smoke induces gingival hyperaemia, which is caused by the concomitant increase in blood pressure against a small but significant sympathetically induced vasoconstriction in healthy gingiva (Mavropoulos et al. 2003). Smoking even one cigarette has been suggested to have the potential to cause a decrease in gingival blood flow (Mavropoulos et al. 2007). Such small but repeated vasoconstrictive attacks and impairment of revascularization due to cigarette smoking may contribute to disruption of immune response and delay in the healing response, leading to an increased risk of periodontal disease (Ojima & Hanioka 2010). Vascular dysfunction may also reduce oxygen delivery to gingival tissue. Pocket oxygen tension was reported to be significantly lower in smokers than non-smokers providing support for the negative effects of smoking on vascular system (Hanioka et al. 2000). Evidence from both human and experimental studies suggests that smoking has a long-term chronic effect, and its effect is not simply a vasoconstriction. Its suppressive effects on the vascular system of gingiva can be observed through less gingival redness, lower bleeding on probing and fewer vessels visible clinically and histologically.

A better understanding of the influence of tobacco smoke on the host response to periodontal infection has been the major concern in numerous studies whereas, limited research has been published aiming to identify the influence of tobacco smoke on the dental biofilm. Tobacco smoke has been shown to cause shifts in the microbial species that comprise dental plaque (Haffajee & Socransky 2001, Kamma et al. 1999, Shiloah et al. 2000, Umeda et al. 1998, van Winkelhoff et al. 2001, Zambon et al. 1996). In a recent study by our group (Buduneli et al. 2011), it was hypothesized that tobacco may induce alterations to the molecular structure of lipid A in a manner consistent with reduced inflammatory potential. Therefore, the ratios of 3-OH fatty acids in smoking and non-smoking chronic periodontitis patients were investigated. The findings suggested that smoking induces specific structural alterations to the lipid A-derived 3-OH fatty acid profile in saliva that are consistent with an oral microflora of reduced inflammatory potential. Such data may explain increased infection with periodontal pathogens but reduced clinical inflammation in smokers. However, further studies are warranted to better clarify this issue.

In a systematic review, Bergstrom (2006) concluded that 100% of 70 cross-sectional studies and 100% of 14 case-control studies indicate an association between smoking and an impaired periodontal health condition, and 95% of 21 cohort studies indicate a greater periodontal health impairment rate in smokers than in non-smokers. Therefore, he suggested that there is good evidence to recommend smoking to be specifically considered in a periodontal health examination. Indeed, in a review by Hilgers & Kinane (2004) it was concluded that smoking cessation is indicated in the promotion of better general health and in the improvement of periodontal health. Considering the existing evidences, the authors suggested that dentists should offer to refer patients for smoking cessation counselling.

In conclusion, smoking is accepted as a strong risk factor for destructive periodontal disease. Gelskey (1999) stated that smoking meets most of the criteria for causation proposed by Hill (1965). This statement is based on the consistency and strength of association between smoking and periodontal disease severity demonstrated by multiple cross-sectional as well as longitudinal studies. Further evidence comes from the dose effect of smoking on periodontal disease severity and a slowing of disease progression in patients who quit smoking. Furthermore, smoking has a negative impact on periodontal treatment outcomes. Smoking is harmful virtually to every tissue in the body. The basis for these deleterious effects is related to the adverse impact of smoking on microbial and host factors.

The proposed mechanisms for the negative effects of smoking on periodontal health were summarised by Johnson & Guthmiller (2007) as follows; decreased immunoglobulin G2 production, chronic reduction in blood flow and vascularity, increased prevalence of potential periodontal pathogens, shift in neutrophil function towards destructive activities, negative effects on cytokine and growth factor production and inhibition of fibroblast growth, attachment and collagen production.

In addition to be accepted as an important risk factor for destructive periodontal disease, smoking has been suggested to interfere with the outcomes of various periodontal therapies. Bostrom (2006) systematically reviewed the intervention studies both in terms of non-surgical and surgical periodontal therapy. It was concluded that the results of the intervention studies suggest an inferior therapeutic outcome in smoker patients compared to non-smoker counterparts. The author reports that in 80% of studies the results were statistically significant. When measured in terms of mean probing depth reduction or mean clinical attachment level gain after a maximum of 9 months, the outcome on the average is less efficient in smokers than in non-smokers (Bostrom 2006). However, none of the non-surgical intervention studies has evaluated the effect of smoking in terms of a successful versus a non-successful outcome following predetermined criteria. Furthermore, it was stated that it is still not known whether or not a negative short-term effect of smoking observed in terms of probing depth or clinical attachment level holds true in the long run as tooth loss. Most of the intervention studies have a rather short follow-up period and therefore unable to provide an answer in terms of the rate of tooth loss. It is quite clear that further intervention studies with larger scales and longer follow-ups are required to better clarify this issue. Smoking more than 10 cigarettes per day is considered as heavy smoking and heavy smokers have a poorer treatment response than non-smokers or ex-smokers (Kaldahl et al. 1996, Norderyd 1998).

A meta-analysis by Labriola et al. (2005) evaluated the impact of smoking on non-surgical periodontal therapy and reported that probing depth reduction in sites where probing depth was initially equal to or more than 5 mm was significantly greater in non-smokers than in smokers in eight studies (Grossi et al. 1997, Mongardini et al. 1999, Palmer et al. 1999, Preber et al. 1995, Pucher et al. 1997, Renvert et al. 1998, Ryder et al. 1999, Williams et al. 2001).

In a recent intervention study (Buduneli et al. 2009), effects of initial periodontal treatment on GCF levels of interleukin-17 (IL-17), sRANKL, and OPG in smoker versus non-smoker patients with chronic periodontitis. All clinical periodontal measurements decreased significantly after the initial periodontal treatment in both the smoker and non-smoker patient groups. There were no significant differences between the smoker and non-smoker patients in regards with the changes in clinical periodontal data following initial periodontal treatment. Data indicated that GCF volume, OPG total amount and concentration decreased in both smokers and non-smokers after scaling and root planning (SRP), whereas IL-17 concentration increased. sRANKL levels did not differ between groups or with SRP. Significant correlations were found between baseline IL-17 and RANKL levels, baseline papilla bleeding on probing and OPG levels. According to the findings, it was suggested that neither smoking nor periodontal inflammation appears to influence GCF RANKL levels in systemically healthy patients with chronic periodontitis. Smoker and non-smoker patients with chronic periodontitis seem to be affected indifferently by the initial periodontal treatment in regards with GCF IL-17 and OPG concentrations. Smoking seems to suppress OPG synthesis and might be contributory to increased bone destruction often seen in smokers.

Surgical periodontal therapy aims to eliminate periodontal pockets and obtain physiological contours in both soft and hard periodontal tissues. As with the non-surgical intervention studies, the primary outcome measures in surgical intervention studies are probing depth and clinical attachment level. On the basis of a systematic review, Bostrom (2006) reported that 91% of 10 non-surgical and 93% of 14 surgical therapy intervention studies indicate an untoward effect of smoking on the therapeutic outcome. The author concluded that there is limited but consistent evidence to suggest that smoking negatively interferes with the therapy outcomes of nonsurgical as well as surgical periodontal interventions.

Haesman et al. (2006) also reviewed the clinical evidence for the relative clinical responses to periodontal treatment in smokers, non-smokers and ex-smokers. The authors concluded that data from epidemiological, cross-sectional and case-control studies strongly suggest that quitting smoking is beneficial to patients following periodontal treatments. The response of ex-smokers to periodontal treatment suggests that quitting smoking helps to improve the clinical periodontal status but there are only limited data from long-term longitudinal clinical trials to demonstrate unequivocally the periodontal benefit of quitting smoking. It is clear that long-term, longitudinal clinical trial that monitors over several years the response to treatment in a cohort of smokers with chronic periodontitis will provide valuable data on the detrimental effects of smoking. However, such a study is definitely not easy to conduct both from the practical and financial points of view. At present, the dental profession can rely on the strong evidence base of the epidemiological, cross-sectional, and case-control studies concluding that quitting smoking is likely to be beneficial to oral and in particular periodontal health.

Johnson & Guthmiller (2007) suggested that smoking cessation cannot reverse the negative past effects of smoking; however, the rate of bone and attachment loss slows after patients quit smoking. Periodontal disease severity in former smokers falls between that of current smokers and never smokers (Bergstrom et al. 2000, Jansson & Lavstedt 2002, Tomar & Asma 2000, Torrunggruang et al. 2005). Preshaw et al. (2005) evaluated the effect of smoking cessation on non-surgical periodontal treatment in 49 smokers who wanted to quit smoking. Therapy included individualised cessation interventions, scaling and root planning and oral hygiene instructions followed by maintenance phase of periodontal treatment. Only 26 patients completed the study; 10 successfully stopped smoking, 10 continued smoking, and six stopped but relapsed during the study period. The authors reported that the patients who successfully quit smoking had the best response to therapy; the "oscillators" had an intermediate response to the non-smokers and quitters. These results underscore the challenges of cessation of tobacco smoking. Counselling on the benefits of smoking cessation by dentists may encourage the patients to seek periodontal therapy and eventually lead to improved periodontal health. Likewise, Borrell & Papapanou (2005) suggested that smoking cessation is a key in the prevention and control of periodontal disease because it affects both the bacterial and host etiological components in the disease process.

In conclusion, the data from both cross-sectional and epidemiological studies over the past 15 years evaluating the relationship between smoking and periodontal diseases suggest that there is strong evidence of a positive association between smoking and clinical and biochemical signs of periodontitis, as well as an increased risk of periodontitis in smokers. Furthermore, the evidence for smoking having a deleterious effect on periodontal treatment outcomes is quite convincing but still needs more data from longitudinal intervention studies.

2. Source of funding

The author declares no conflict of interest.

3. References

Ah MK, Johnson GK, Kaldahl WB, Patil KD, Kalkwarf KL. (1994) The effect of smoking on the response to periodontal therapy. *Journal of Clinical Periodontology* 21:91-97.

Al-Ghamdi HS, Anıl S. (2007) Serum antibody levels in smoker and non-smoker Saudi subjects with chronic periodontitis. *Journal of Periodontology* 78: 1043-1050.

Andelid K, Bake B, Rak S, Lindén A, Rosengren A, Ekberg-Jansson A. (2007) Myeloperoxidase as a marker of increasing systemic inflammation in smokers without severe airway symptoms. *Respiratory Medicine* 101:888-895.

Apatzidou DA, Riggio MP, Kinane DF. (2005) Impact of smoking on the clinical, microbiological and immunological parameters of adult patients with periodontitis. *Journal of Clinical Periodontology* 32:973-983.

Arıkan F, Buduneli N, Kütükçüler N. (2008) Osteoprotegerin levels in peri-implant crevicular fluid. *Clinical Oral Implants Research* 19:283-288.

Armitage GC. (2004) Analysis of gingival crevice fluid and risk of progression of periodontitis. *Periodontology 2000* 34: 109-119.

Barbour SE, Nakashima K, Zhang JB, Tangada S, Hahn CL, Schenkein HA, Tew JG. (1997) Tobacco and smoking: environmental factors that modify the host response (immune system) and have an impact on periodontal health. *Critical Reviews in Oral Biology and Medicine* 8:437-460.

Betsuyaku T, Nishimura M, Takeyabu K, et al. (1999) Neutrophil granule proteins in bronchoalveolar lavage fluid from subjects with subclinical emphysema. *American Journal of Respiratory and Critical Care Medicine* 159:1985-1991.

Bergstrom J, Eliasson S, Dock J. (2000) A 10-year prospective study of tobacco smoking and periodontal health. *Journal of Periodontology* 71:1338-1347.

Bergstrom J. (2006) Periodontitis and smoking: An evidence-based appraisal. *Journal of Evidence Based Dental Practice* 6:33-41.

Borrell LN, Papapanou PN. (2005) Analytical epidemiology of periodontitis. *Journal of Clinical Periodontology* 32 (Suppl.6): 132-158.

Bostanci N, İlgenli T, Emingil G, Afacan B, Han B, Töz H, Atilla G, Hughes FJ, Belibasakis GN. (2007) Gingival crevicular fluid levels of RANKL and OPG in periodontal diseases: Implications of their relative ratio. *Journal of Clinical Periodontology* 34: 370-376.

Boström L, Linder LE, Bergstrom J. (1999) Smoking and crevicular fluid levels of IL-6 and TNF-alpha in periodontal disease. *Journal of Clinical Periodontology* 26:352-357.

Boström L, Bergström J, Dahlen G, Linder LE. (2001) Smoking and subgingival microflora in periodontal disease. *Journal of Clinical Periodontology* 28: 212-219.

Brooks SM, Baker DB, Gann PH, et al. (1990) Cold air challenge and platinum skin reactivity in platinum refinery workers. Bronchial reactivity precedes skin prick response. *Chest* 97:1401-1407.

Buduneli N, Baylas H, Buduneli E, Türkoğlu O, Dahlen G. (2005a) Evaluation of the relationship between smoking during pregnancy and subgingival microbiota. *Journal of Clinical Periodontology* 32: 68-74.

Buduneli N, Buduneli E, Kardeşler L, Lappin D, Kinane DF. (2005b) Plasminogen activator system in smokers and non-smokers with and without periodontal disease. *Journal of Clinical Periodontology* 32: 417-424.

Buduneli N, Kardeşler L, Işik H, Willis CS 3rd, Hawkins SI, Kinane DF, Scott DA. (2006) Effects of smoking and gingival inflammation on salivary antioxidant capacity. *Journal of Clinical Periodontology* 33:159-164.

Buduneli N, Bıyıkoğlu B, Sherrabeh S, Lappin D. (2008) Saliva concentrations of RANKL and osteprotegerin in smoker versus non-smoker chronic periodontitis patients. *Journal of Clinical Periodontology* 35: 846-852.

Buduneli N, Buduneli E, Kütükçüler N. (2009) Interleukin-17, RANKL, osteoprotegerin levels in gingival crevicular fluid from smoker versus non-smoker chronic periodontitis patients during initial periodontal treatment. *Journal of Periodontology* 80: 1274-1280.

Buduneli N, Kinane DF. (2011) Host-derived diagnostic markers related to soft tissue destruction and bone degradation in periodontitis. *Journal of Clinical Periodontology* Mar;38 Suppl 11:85-105.

Buduneli N, Larsson L, Biyikoglu B, Renaud DE, Bagaitkar J, Scott DA. (2011) Fatty acid profiles in smokers with chronic periodontitis. *Journal of Dental Research* 90:47-52.

Calsina G, Ramon JM, Echeverria JJ. (2002) Effects of smoking on periodontal tissues. *Journal of Clinical Periodontology* 29: 771-776.

Centres for Disease Control and Prevention. (2002) Annual smoking- attributable mortality, years of potential life lost, and economic costs-United States, 1995-1999. *Morbidity and Mortality Weekly Reports* 51:300-303.

Christenson RH. (1997) Biochemical markers of bone metabolism: an overview. *Clinical Biochemistry* 30: 573-593.

Crotti T, Smith MD, Hirsch R, Soukoulis S, Weedon H, Capone M, Ahern MJ, Haynes D. (2003) Receptor activator NF kappaB ligand (RANKL) and osteoprotegerin (OPG) protein expression in periodontitis. *Journal of Periodontal Research* 38: 380-387.

Darby IB, Hodge PJ, Riggio MP, Kinane DF. (2005) Clinical and microbiological effect of scaling and root planing in smoker and non-smoker chronic and aggressive periodontitis patients. *Journal of Clinical Periodontology* 32:200-206.

Francus T, Klein RF, Staiano-Coico L, Becker CG, Siskind GW. (1988) Effects of tobacco glycoprotein (TGP) on the immune system. II.TGP stimulates the proliferation of human T cells and the differentiation of human B cells into Ig secreting cells. *Journal of Immunology* 140:1823-1829.

Fredriksson MI, Figueredo CM, Gustafsson A, Bergström KG, Asman BE. (1999) Effect of periodontitis and smoking on blood leukocytes and acute-phase proteins. *Journal of Periodontology* 70: 1355-1360.

Gelskey SC. (1999) Cigarette smoking and periodontitis: methodology to assess the strength of evidence in support of a causal association. *Community Dentistry and Oral Epidemiology* 27:16-24.

Gemmell E, Seymour GJ. (2004) Immunoregulatory control of Th1/Th2 cytokine profiles in periodontal disease. *Periodontology 2000* 35:21-41.

Geng Y, Savage SM, Razani-Boroujerdi S, Sopori ML. (1996) Effects of nicotine on the immune response.II.Chronic nicotine treatment induces T cell anergy. *Journal of Immunology* 156:2384-2390.

Giannobile WV. (1999) C-telopeptide pyridinoline cross-links. Sensitive indicators of periodontal tissue destruction. *Annals of New York Academy of Sciences* 878, 404-412.

Grossi SG, Zambon J, Machtei EE, Schifferle R, Andreana S, Genco RJ, Cummins D, Harrap G. (1997) Effects of smoking and smoking cessation on healing after mechanical periodontal therapy. *Journal of American Dental Association* 128:599-607.

Gürlek Ö, Lappin DF, Buduneli N. (2009) Effects of smoking on salivary C-telopeptide pyridinoline cross-links of type I collagen and osteocalcin levels. *Archives of Oral Biology* 54, 1099-1104.

Haber J, Wattles J, Crowley M, Mandell R, Joshipura K, Kent RL. (1993) Evidence for cigarette smoking as a major risk factor periodontitis. *Journal of Periodontology* 64:16-23.

Haffajee AD, Socransky SS. (2001) Relationship of cigarette smoking to the subgingival microbiota. *Journal of Clinical Periodontology* 28: 377-388.

Haesman L, Stacey F, Preshaw PM, McCracken GI, Hepburn S, Haesman PA. (2006) The effect of smoking on periodontal treatment response: a review of clinical evidence. *Journal of Clinical Periodontology* 33:241-253.

Hanioka T, Tanaka M, Ojima M, Takaya K, Matsumori Y, Shizukuishi S. (2000) Oxygen sufficiency in the gingival of smokers and non-smokers with periodontal disease. *Journal of Periodontology* 71:1846-1851.

Hilgers KK, Kinane DF. (2004) Smoking, periodontal disease and the role of the dental profession. *International Journal of Dental Hygiene* 2:56-63.

Hill AB. (1965) The environment and disease: association or causation? *Proceedings of the Royal Society of Medicine* 58:295-300.

Jansson L, Lavstedt S. (2002) Influence of smoking on marginal bone loss and tooth loss-a prospective study over 20 years. *Journal of Clinical Periodontology* 29:75-756.

Johnson GK, Hill M. (2004) Cigarette smoking and the periodontal patient. *Journal of Periodontology* 75:196-209.

Johnson GK, Guthmiller JM. (2007) The impact of cigarette smoking on periodontal disease and treatment. *Periodontology 2000* 44:178-194.

Kaldahl WB, Johnson GK, Patil KD, Kalkwarf KL. (1996) Levels of cigarette consumption and response to periodontal therapy. *Journal of Periodontology* 67:675-681.

Kamma JJ, Nakou M, Baehni PC. (1999) Clinical and microbiological characteristics of smokers with early onset periodontitis. *Journal of Periodontal Research* 34: 25-33.

Kinane DF. (2001) Causation and pathogenesis of periodontal disease. *Periodontology 2000* 25, 8-20.

Kinane DF, Chestnutt IG. (2000) Smoking and periodontal disease. *Critical Reviews in Oral Biology and Medicine* 11, 356-365.

Knuutinen A, Kokkonen N, Risteli J, et al. (2002) Smoking affects collagen synthesis and extracellular matrix turnover in human skin. *British Journal of Dermatology* 146:588-594.

Labriola A, Needleman I, Moles DR. (2005) Systematic review of the effect of smoking on non-surgical periodontal therapy. *Periodontology 2000* 37:124-137.

Lappin DF, Sherrabeh S, Jenkins WM, Macpherson LM. (2007) Effect of smoking on serum RANKL and OPG in sex, age and clinically matched supportive-therapy periodontitis patients. *Journal of Clinical Periodontology* 34:271-277.

Lian JB, Gundberg CM. (1988) Osteocalcin: biochemical considerations and clinical applications. *Clinical Orthopedia Related Research* 226: 267-291.

Liede KE, Haukka JK, Hietanen JH, Mattila MH, Ronka H, Sorsa T. (1999) The association between smoking cessation and periodontal status and salivary proteinase levels. *Journal of Periodontology* 70:1361-1368.

Liu KZ, Hynes A, Man A, Alsagheer A, Singer DL, Scott DA. (2006) Increased local matrix metalloproteinase-8 expression in the periodontal connective tissues of smokers with periodontal disease. *Biochim Biophys Acta* 1762:775-780.

Lu HK, Chen YL, Chang HC, Li CL, Kuo MY. (2006) Identification of the osteoprotegerin/receptor activator of nuclear factor-kappa B ligand system in gingival crevicular fluid and tissue of patients with chronic periodontitis. *Journal of Periodontal Research* 41: 354-360.

Martinez-Canut P, Lorca A, Magan R. (1995) Smoking and periodontal disease severity. *Journal of Clinical Periodontology* 22: 743-749.

Mavropoulos A, Aars H, Brodin P. (2003) Hyperaemic response to cigarette smoking in healthy gingiva. *Journal of Clinical Periodontology* 30:214-221.

Mavropoulos A, Brodin P, Rosing CK, Aass AM, Aars H. (2007) Gingival blood flow in periodontitis patients before and after periodontal surgery assessed in smokers and non-smokers. *Journal of Periodontology* 78:1774-1782.

Mogi M, Otogoto J, Ota N, Togari A. (2004) Difefrential expression of RANKL and osteoprotegerin in gingival crevicular fluid of patients with periodontitis. *Journal of Dental Research* 83: 166-169.

Mongardini C, van Steenberghe D, Dekeyser C, Quirynen M. (1999) One stage full- versus partial-mouth disinfection in the treatment of chronic adult or generalised early-onset periodontitis I. Long-term clinical observations. *Journal of Periodontology* 70:632-645.

Mullally BH. (2004) The influence of tobacco smoking on the onset of periodontitis in young persons. *Tobacco Induced Diseases* 2:53-65.

Narayanan AS, Page RC. (1983) Connective tissues of the periodontium: A summary of current work. *Collagen Related Research* 3: 33-64.

Norderyd O. (1998) Risk for periodontal disease in a Swedish adult population. Cross-sectional and longitudinal studies over two decades. *Swedish Dental Journal* Suppl. 132:1-67.

Offenbacher S, Odle BM, Van Dyke TE. (1984) The use of crevicular fluid prostaglandin E2 levels as a predictor of periodontal attachment loss. *Journal of Periodontal Research* 21: 101-112.

Ojima M, Hanioka T. (2010) Destructive effects of smoking on molecular and genetic factors of periodontal disease. *Tobacco Induced Diseases* 8:4.

Oringer RJ, Palys MD, Iranmanesh A, Fiorellini JP, Haffajee AD, Socransky SS, Giannobile WV. (1998) C-telopeptide pyridinoline cross-links (ICTP) and periodontal pathogens associated with endosseous oral implants. *Clinical Oral Implants Research* 9: 365-373.

Oringer RJ, Al-Shammari KF, Aldredge WA, Iacono VJ, Eber RM, Wang HL, Berwald B, Nejat R, Giannobile WV. (2002) Effect of locally delivered minocycline microspheres on markers of bone resorption. *Journal of Periodontology* 73: 835-842.

Özçaka Ö, Nalbantsoy A, Köse T, Buduneli N. (2010) Plasma osteoprotegerin levels are decreased in smoker chronic periodontitis patients. *Australian Dental Journal* 55:405-410.

Özçaka Ö, Bıçakçı N, Pussinen P, Sorsa T, Köse T, Buduneli N. (2011a) Smoking and matrix metalloproteinases, neutrophil elastase, and myeloperoxidase in chronic periodontitis. *Oral Diseases* 17:68-76.

Özçaka Ö, Nalbantsoy A, Buduneli N. (2011b) Salivary osteocalcin levels are decreased in smoker chronic periodontitis patients. *Oral Diseases* 17:200-205.

Palmer RM, Matthews JP, Wilson RF. (1999) Non-surgical periodontal treatment with and without adjunctive metronidazole in smokers and non-smokers. *Journal of Clinical Periodontology* 26:158-163.

Palmer RM, Wilson RF, Hasan AS, Scott DA. (2005) Mechanisms of action of environmental factor-tobacco smoking. *Journal of Clinical Periodontology* 32:180-195

Persson L, Bergstrom J, Gustafsson A. (2003) Effect of tobacco smoking on neutrophil activity following periodontal surgery. *Journal of Periodontology* 74:1475-1482.

Preber H, Bergstrom J, Linder LE. (1992) Occurrence of periopathogens in smoker and non-smoker patients. *Journal of Clinical Periodontology* 19:667-671.

Preber H, Linder L, Bergström J. (1995) Periodontal healing and periopathogenic microflora in smokers and non-smokers. *Journal of Clinical Periodontology* 22: 946-952.

Preshaw PM, Haesman L, Stacey F, Steen N, McCracken GI, Haesman PA. (2005) The effect of quitting smoking on chronic periodontitis. *Journal of Clinical Periodontology* 32:869-879.

Pucher JJ, Shibley O, Dentino AR, Ciancio SG. (1997) Results of limited initial periodontal therapy in smokers and non-smokers. *Journal of Periodontology* 68:851-856.

Pussinen PJ, Paju S, Mantyla P, Sorsa T. (2007) Serum microbial- and host-derived markers of periodontal diseases: A review. *Current Medical Chemistry* 14, 2407-2412.

Rautelin HI, Oksanen AM, Veijola LI, et al. (2009) Enhanced systemic matrix metalloproteinase response in Helicobacter pylori gastritis. *Annals of Medicine* 41:208-215.

Renvert S, Dahlen G, Wikstrom M. (1998) The clinical and microbiological effects of non-surgical periodontal therapy in smokers and non-smokers. *Journal of Clinical Periodontology* 25:153-157.

Rezavandi K, Palmer RM, Odell EW, Scott DA, Wilson RF. (2002) Expression of ICAM-1 and E-selectin in gingival tissues of smokers and non-smokers with periodontitis. *Journal of Oral Pathology and Medicine* 31:59-64.

Ryder MI, Pons B, Adams D, Beiswanger B, Blanco V, Bogle G, Donly K, Hallmon W, Hancock EB, Hanes P, Hawley C, Johnson L, Wang HL, Wolinsky L, Yukna R,

Polson A, Carron G, Garrett S. (1999) Effects of smoking on local delivery of controlled-release doxycycline as compared to scaling and root planning. *Journal of Clinical Periodontology* 26:683-691.

Savage A, Eaton KA, Moles DR, Needleman I. (2009) A systematic review of definitions of periodontitis and methods that have been used to identify this disease. *Journal of Clinical Periodontology* 36:458-467.

Scott DA, Palmer RM, Stapleton JA. Validation of smoking status in clinical research into inflammatory periodontal disease. *Journal of Clinical Periodontology* 2001; 28:715-722.

Seibel MJ. (2003) Biochemical markers of bone metabolism in the assessment of osteoporosis: useful or not? *Journal of Endocrinology Investment* 26: 464-471.

Shi F, Yu S, Xu L. (1996) Analysis of serum osteocalcin of patients with periodontitis. *Zhonghua Kou Qiang Yi Xue Za Zhi* 31: 300-302. (Article in Chinese)

Shiloah J, Patters MR, Waring MB. (2000) The prevalence of pathogenic periodontal microflora in healthy young adult smokers. *Journal of Periodontology* 71:562-567.

Sopori ML, Cherian S, Chilukuri R, Shopp GM. (1989) Cigarette smoke causes inhibition of the immune response to intratracheally administered antigens. *Toxicology Applications in Pharmacology* 97:489-499.

Sorsa T, Tjaderhane L, Konttinen YT, Lauhio A, Salo T, Lee H-M, Golub LM, Brown DL, Mantyla P. (2006) Matrix metalloproteinases: Contribution to pathogenesis, diagnosis and treatment of periodontal inflammation. *Annals of Medicine* 38: 306-321.

Söder B, Jin LJ, Wickholm S. (2002) Granulocyte elastase, matrix metalloproteinase-8 and prostaglandin E2 in gingival crevicular fluid in matched clinical sites in smokers and non-smokers with persistent periodontitis. *Journal of Clinical Periodontology* 29:384-391.

Tanaka H, Tanabe N, Shoji M, et al. (2006) Nicotine and lipopolysaccharide stimulate the formation of osteoclast-like cells by increasing macrophage colony-stimulating factor and prostaglandin E2 production by osteoblasts. *Life Sciences* 78:1733-1740.

Tang TH, Fitzsimmons TR, Bartold M. (2009) Effect of smoking on concentrations of receptor activator of nuclear factor κB ligand and osteoprotegerin in human gingival crevicular fluid. *Journal of Clinical Periodontology* 36: 713-718.

Tappia PS, Troughton KL, Langley-Evans SC, Grimble RF. (1995) Cigarette smoking influences cytokine production and antioxidant defences. *Clinical Sciences* 88:485-489.

Taubman MA, Valverde P, Han X, Kawai T. (2005) Immune response: The key to bone resorption in periodontal disease. *Journal of Periodontology* 76 Suppl.: 2033-2041.

Tomar SL, Asma S. (2000) Smoking-attributable periodontitis in the United States: findings from NHANES III. National Health and Nutrition Examination Survey. *Journal of Periodontology* 71:743-751.

Torrungruang K, Nisapakultorn K, Sutdhibhisal S, Tamsailom S, Rojanasomsith K, Vanichjakvong O, Prapakamol S, Premsirinirund T, Pusiri T, Jaratkulangkoon O, Kusump S, Rajatanavin R. (2005) The effect of cigarette smoking on the severity of periodontal disease among older Thai adults. *Journal of Periodontology* 76:566-572.

Quinn SM, Zhang JB, Gunsolley JC, Schenkein HA, Tew JG. (1998) The influence of smoking and race on adult periodontitis and serum IgG2 levels. *Journal of Periodontology* 69:171-177.

Ujiie Y, Oida S, Gomi K, Arai T, Fukae M. (2007) Neutrophil elastase is involved in the initial destruction of human periodontal ligament. *Journal of Periodontal Research* 42:325-330.

Umeda M, Chen C, Bakker I, Contreras A, Morrison J, Slots J. (1998) Risk indicators for harbouring periodontal pathogens. Journal of Periodontology 69:1111-1118.

van Winkelhoff AJ, Bosch-Tijhof CJ, Winkel EG, van der Reijden WA. (2001) Smoking affects the subgingival microflora in periodontitis. *Journal of Periodontology* 72: 666-671.

Williams RC, Paquette DW, Offenbacher S, Adams DF, Armitage GC, Bray K, Caton J, Cochran DL, Drisko CH, Fiorellini JP, Giannobile WV, Grossi S, Guerrero DM, Johnson GK, Lamster IB, Magnusson I, Oringer RJ, Persson GR, Van Dyke TE, Wolff LF, Santucci EA, Rodda BE, Lessem J. (2001) Treatment of periodontitis by local administration of minocycline microspheres: a controlled trial. *Journal of Periodontology* 72:1535-1544.

Zambon JJ, Grossi SG, Machtei EE, Ho AW, Dunford R, Genco RJ. (1996) Cigarette smoking increases the risk for subgingival infection with periodontal pathogens. *Journal of Periodontology* 67: 1050-1054.

6

Advanced Glycation End Products: Possible Link Between Metabolic Syndrome and Periodontal Diseases

Maria Grazia Cifone, Annalisa Monaco,
Davide Pietropaoli, Rita Del Pinto and Mario Giannoni
University of L'Aquila – Department of Health Sciences
San Salvatore Hospital Building Delta 6 – 67100 - L'Aquila,
Italy

1. Introduction

At a planetary scale, the Metabolic Syndrome (MetS) is the third cause of inability after malnutrition and nicotinism, even higher than water shortage and sedentariness. In the USA, the prevalence is estimated at over 25% of the population; in Italy, it involves approximately 25% of men and even 27% of women (Ford et al. 2002). These are very high figures, corresponding to approximately 14 million affected individuals. The prevalence is alarming and must not be underestimated, particularly in the dental field, where more than one patient out of four sitting in a dentist's chair is affected. The aetiology of periodontal disease has not been clarified yet, and recently the idea to consider it as a multifactor pathology has been developed. Cofactors such as the formation of reactive oxygen species (ROS), oxidative stress, lipid peroxidation, and formation of glycation end-products (AGEs) probably play an important role in the onset of periodontal disease (Pietropaoli et al. 2010). The AGEs are compounds physiologically produced by all metabolically active cells. However, they accumulate and cause pro-inflammatory statuses, when the cellular clearance fails, or in hyperglycaemic and oxidative statuses (Peppa et al. 2008). All these conditions can be clinically summarized as Metabolic Syndrome.

The purpose of this literature review is to establish a relationship between two pathologies with very high prevalence: Metabolic Syndrome and Periodontal Diseases.

The literature seems to have clarified that the Metabolic Syndrome involves a pro-oxidation status, which induces AGE formation. AGEs play a very important role in the course and severity of periodontal diseases.

2. The Metabolic Syndrome

The Metabolic Syndrome (MetS) (also known as X-syndrome, insulin-resistance syndrome, or Reaven's syndrome) refers to a clinical condition involving a high cardio- cerebrovascular (CVD) risk, which includes a number of risk factors and symptoms of simultaneous appearance in individuals. These are often related to the individual's life style (overweight, sedentary habits), or existing pathological conditions (e.g. obesity and hypercholesterolemia) (Lakka et al. 2002).

The studies confirm that individuals affected by Metabolic Syndrome, who do not dramatically change their life style, have a high mortality related to CVD (Lakka et al. 2002).

The accepted definition of MetS, which is broadly applied at the international level, is given by the Third Report of the National Cholesterol Education Program (NCEP-III). According to the NCEP-III, a diagnosis of Metabolic Syndrome is applicable when at least 3 out of 5 of the following elements are identified:

- Abdominal Obesity (abdomen circumference >102 cm in Men, >88 cm in Women)
- Triglyceridemia ≥ 150 mg/dl
- Plasma HDL cholesterol <40 mg/dl in Men, <50 mg/dl in Women
- Arterial blood pressure ≥130 and/or ≥85 mm Hg
- Fasting plasmatic glycaemia ≥110 mg/dl Expert Panel on Detection and of High Blood Cholesterol in Adults (2001).

More recently (2005), the International Diabetes Federation has reviewed the diagnostic criteria, proposing the presence of two of the following disorders in the same patient as a method to identify the disease:

- Triglyceridemia ≥150 mg/dl
- Plasma HDL cholesterol <40 mg/dl in Men, <50 mg/dl in Women, or hypolipemizing treatment
- Arterial blood pressure ≥130 and/or ≥85 mm Hg, or anti-hypertension treatment
- Fasting plasmatic glycaemia ≥110 mg/dl (IFG stage),

associated with waist circumference of more than 94 cm in men and 80 cm in women for Caucasian patients (the parameters vary, based on the patient's ethnic group) (Alberti et al. 2005).

Substantially, these two definitions are the same. However, in the most recent review, the International Diabetes Federation associated the diagnostic factors with above-normal waist circumference and classified it as a required condition for diagnosis.

Despres et al. (2000) assessed the lipid profile (total cholesterol, HDL cholesterol, triglycerides, plasmatic values of apolipoprotein B) and glucide profile (fasting insulin haematic values) of 2103 male patients, aged 45-76 years, representative as a sample population of Québec. The analysis was carried out to determine the association between cardiovascular risk factors and ischemic cardiopathy during a five-year period (Després et al. 2000). During the study, significantly higher fasting insulinemia (p < 0.001) was observed in patients affected by ischemic events. The hyperinsulinemia-artherosclerotic cardiopathy association kept this high rate also after a correction of triglycerides, apolipoprotein B, LDL cholesterol, and HDL cholesterol levels. Therefore, high insulin plasmatic concentrations in non-diabetic individuals – who can be classified as 'insulin-resistant' – were associated with an ischemic cardiopathy increase, independently from the lipid profile (although a lipid profile alteration in pro-atherogen sense has a synergic effect with hyperinsulinemia) (Després et al. 2000).

In addition to the role played in glucidic metabolism, insulin contributes to regulating lipid and protein metabolism and arterial blood pressure, interfering with platelet function and the balance between pro-thrombotic factors and endogenous fibrinolysis modulators. It also regulates the proliferative stimuli on smooth muscle cells of vascular walls and influences the endothelial function: all this explains the possible role played by insulin- resistance in determining the Metabolic Syndrome (Harano et al. 2002).

The mechanisms of insulin resistance, or the insulin-cell surface-intracellular compartment interaction sites, in which the chain of signals produced by the hormones stops, preventing an appropriate use of circulating glucose, are not known yet. Insulin-resistance almost certainly develops much before the Metabolic Syndrome and other more advanced clinical diseases, such as type-2 diabetes mellitus and atherosclerosis, appearing in all contexts as a multifactor reality in terms of both its onset and potential harm (Harano et al. 2002).

It is clear that, in a person affected by MetS, a hyperglycaemia status triggers cellular damage with repercussions at the systemic level and also on periodontal tissue. Periodontal diseases of diabetic origin are a clear example of this (Bensley et al. 2011).

New studies focus on the aetiology of periodontal diseases and the role of oxidative stress, starting a cascade of molecular signals from inflammation mediators, which cause loss of attachment, reabsorption of alveolar bone, and, ultimately, tooth loss, through activation of osteoclasts (Pietropaoli et al. 2010). As a source of oxidative stress, the MetS could provide an alternative etiological explanation to the development of periodontal disease, as suggested by Bullon et al. (2009).

The purpose of this study is to extend this vision, which includes the residual products of non-enzymatic glycosylation, originated from oxidative metabolism conditions, as factors promoting periodontal disease.

3. Metabolic Syndrome and oxidative stress

It is known that all MetS triggering factors play a clear role in the onset of oxidative stress, in the subsequent formation of Reactive Oxygen Species (ROS), and probably also in the activation of the pro-oxidising, pro-inflammatory AGE-RAGE system (Koyama et al. 2005). Many inflammatory pathways are activated by these conditions. The excess of visceral fat (high waist circumference) is certainly one of the most important factors in activating these signalling molecular cascades through the TNF-alfa pathway (Boden 2006).

Visceral fat, unlike subcutaneous fat, induces lipolysis increase, when stimulated, with release of Free Fatty Acids (FFA) in the blood circulation. Excess FFAs significantly contribute to inducing hyperinsulinemia, as they reduce insulin clearance, increase hepatic gluconeogenesis, reduce glucose uptake in the muscle tissues, and facilitate a pro-inflammatory status (Liu et al. 2011).

TNF-alfa increase, in turn, contributes to triggering the molecular processes that lead to the development of insulin-resistance, which would apparently play a key pathogenetic role in all MetS conditions (Odrowaz-Sypniewska 2007). When calorie intake is higher than body consumption, ROS excess is created, due to hyper-activity of the citric acid cycle, hence oxidative stress (Maddux et al. 2001). This oxidative stress alters intracellular signalling and contributes to the development of insulin-resistance (Evans et al. 2003). On the other hand, Ceriello et al. (2000) showed that insulin-sensitivity improves after administration of anti-oxidizing substances (Ceriello and Motz 2004).

Soory et al. (2009) claim that ROS increase causes a hyper-inflammation status in its most aggressive forms of periodontal disease and causes an unbalance of redox status, outcome of which is damage. In accordance with this vision, the hyper-inflammation status associated with periodontal disorder could overload the body with Reactive Oxygen Species, which are in turn able to contribute to the development of other pathologies, such as metabolic, articular, neoplastic, or geriatric diseases (Soory, 2009). In addition to lipid peroxidation, the AGEs are another emerging marker of oxidative stress. The AGEs are a set of heterogeneous products constantly formed in physiological conditions, but significantly increasing in the presence of hyperglycaemia and excessive oxidative stress (Peppa et al., 2008). The recent literature suggests that the AGEs are the cause of a large number of adverse conditions established in systemic diseases, where the oxidative component is strong, as in diabetes (Xue et al., 2011).

The activation of these pathways is not restricted to limited areas of the body, but their signalling triggers systemic responses, which are also visible at the level of teeth supporting tissues. Since the 1970s, it is known that obesity and hypertension increase the severity of the periodontal disease (Perlstein and Bissada, 1977). It is also suggested that overweight individuals have a worse periodontal status than individuals with a normal body weight, with evident histological changes on dental tissues (Suvan et al., 2011). To support this suggestion, Pischon et al. (2007) clearly emphasised that inflammation caused by obesity markedly affects the status of periodontal tissues. In these cases, the activation of pro-inflammatory cytokines has been broadly supported by scientific literature. In fact, TNF-alfa, Interleukin-6 and -10 (IL-6, IL-10), and C-Reactive Protein (CRP) are certainly involved in individuals with high Body Mass Index (BMI) (Pischon et al., 2007).

The activation of these complexes leads to the interaction between AGEs and RAGE cellular receptors (found in many cell populations), which amplify the release of cytokines, metalloproteinases (MMPs), and ROS.

It is worth stressing that the nature of an individual's diet certainly contributes to the action of inflammatory cytokines. Obese individuals eat several times during the day, without caring too much for oral hygiene, thus facilitating accumulation of dental plaque and dental calculus. This condition is the basis of periodontal problems in these subjects.

4. Advanced Glycation End-Products (AGEs)

The AGEs are a heterogeneous group of physiologically formed compounds, which accumulate when cellular clearance fails, and in hyperglycaemia and oxidative stress conditions (Peppa et al., 2008).

The accumulation of AGEs may also be dependent on environmental sources, such as tobacco smoking (Yamagishi et al., 2008), vegetarian diet (Sebeková et al., 2006), alcohol (Kalousová et al., 2004), consumption of browned foods, and high lipid/glucide quantities (Krajcovicová-Kudláčková et al., 2002). Approximately one third of AGEs intake through diet is excreted with urine, whereas the remaining part is supposedly incorporated in tissues (Bohlender et al., 2005).

These compounds are produced through enzymatic pathway from monosaccharide substances, such as glucose and fructose, but also dicarbonyls originating from Maillard's reaction, sugar self-oxidation, and other molecular pathways, such as glycolysis, which involves the formation of glyoxal and methylglyoxal (Fu et al., 1996).The non-enzymatic post-translational glycosilations of proteins occur through reductive amination reaction between the non-reducing end of a carbohydrate and primary amino groups located on macromolecules containing lysine or arginine residues (amino acids, proteins, phospholipids, lipids, and nucleic acids). These reactions lead to the formation of a number of reversible intermediate products called Schiff's bases and Amadori products (e.g. Glycated haemoglobin; HbA1C). Any subsequent rearrangement of these complexes lead to the formation of much more stable products, the AGEs, which affect the functionality and properties of proteins, lipids, and DNA (Thornalley, 2005; Fu et al., 1996).A key role in the formation of these adducts can be referred to oxidative stress and aging (Baynes, 2001). Oxidising conditions and Reactive Oxygen Species (ROS) facilitate the formation of AGEs, which in turn increase the production of free radicals (Wen et al., 2002; Yin et al., 2001). Schiff's bases and Amadori products increase ROS production, and hyperglycaemia promotes glucose self-oxidation, which involves OH radicals (Noiri and Tsukahara, 2005). Several studies clearly show that the AGEs are involved in the development of diabetes problems, andin CVD and renal and neurodegenerative disease pathogenesis (Goldin et al., 2006; Zhang et al., 2009).

Throughout life, AGEs produced accumulate in the tissues and can be found in plasma (Ulrich and Cerami, 2001). The pathogenetic action of these compounds performs directly, damaging the tissues, or indirectly, binding a specific receptor, called RAGE, which belongs to the family of immunoglobulins (Ramasamy et al., 2005).

This receptor is physiologically found in small quantities in many cells, but it is over-expressed in conditions such as diabetes, vasculopathy, and cancer (Ramasamy et al., 2005). The AGE-RAGE bond involves a cascade of pro-inflammatory signalling with subsequent activation of redox-sensitive transcription factors, such as nuclear factor kappa B (NF-κB) (Schmidt and Stern, 2000). This interaction involves hyper-permeability, at the level of endothelial cells, and activates the vascular cell adhesion molecule-1 (VCAM-1) molecule, whereas on monocytes it involves chemotaxis and cytokine increase, such as the tumour necrosis factor (TNF), and interleukins IL-1 and IL-6 (Vlassara et al., 1988). Collagen synthesis by fibroblasts is also reduced (Hollá et al., 2001).

In addition to persistent hyperglycaemia statuses, transient hyperglycaemia is also a risk condition, as it induces pro-inflammatory signalling and activates the long-lasting expression of p65, which is a fraction of the above-mentioned NF-κB (Siebel et al., 2010). Recently, the interest in this condition has grown, as a few studies report that the 'cell memory' – thus, pro-inflammatory signalling – continues up to 16 hours after the end of the hyperglycaemic condition (El-Osta et al., 2008).

Long-survival proteins, such as collagen, are the most vulnerable molecules exposed to cross-links and forming AGEs, with subsequent subtraction to proteolysis and tissue remodelling (Verzijl et al., 2000). Collagen irreversibly modified by the AGEs is also the vascular collagen, which contributes to the formation of atherosclerosis and development of kidney failure (Bohlender et al., 2005). The AGEs have a higher predictive value of microvascular complication development than the value of other risk predictors, such as the duration of diabetes and HbA1c.

On the other hand, reduced clearance of serum AGEs can further increase the accumulation of AGEs in tissues and their new formation, which worsens kidney failure (Miyata et al., 1997).

5. Aetiology and pathogenesis of periodontitis

The aetiology of periodontitis has not been fully clarified yet. However, it is commonly accepted that it may result from an opportunistic infection. The bacteria cross the epithelial barrier and invade the sub-epithelial connective tissue. A crucial role is played by the increase in the number of dental plaque microorganisms, their capacity to penetrate the tissues, and the host's immunological status. The damage is only partially reversible, even after professional treatment (Needleman et al., 2006).

The hyper-inflammation following these events determines the failure of the immunological response: it does not only remove the pathogens, but it also involves the prolonged release of proteolytic enzymes by the neutrophils, pro-inflammatory mediators, and ROS (Sheikhi et al., 2000). These elements determine periodontal attachment destruction (Chapple and Matthews, 2007). *Fusobacterium nucleatum* and the other oral pathogens induce an increase in intracellular production and ROS release in neutrophils (Sheikhi et al., 2000). Higher ROS levels are, in fact, found in saliva and gingival crevicular fluid of patients with chronic periodontitis as compared with healthy controls (Tsai et al., 2005).

Lee et al. (2008) suggest that hydrogen peroxide (oxygenated water) deposited in periodontal tissues to reduce the inflammation caused by bacteria accelerates their destruction by activating the IL-8 pathway in periodontal cells (Lee et al., 2008). This event should not be underestimated and should be taken into consideration during periodontal surgery.

Soory et al. (2009) proposed that during periodontal disease, increased ROS production may worsen an inflammatory condition, causing an alteration of the redox status and inducing damage from oxidative stress, which involves a more rapid evolution of the disease (Soory, 2008). A broad body of literature documenting a link between periodontal diseases and other pro-oxidative inflammatory diseases support this hypothesis. In fact, it has been confirmed that diseases inducing oxidative metabolic changes, such as diabetes, arthritis, neoplasias, and aging, are associated with periodontal disease, increasing its severity (Soory, 2009).

Based on these observations, it is clear that many conditions may worsen periodon- tal disorders or promote new onset. Contemporary literature supports the assumption that, in addition to inflammation and oxidative stress, other conditions such as cigarette smoking (Bagaitkar et al., 2009), vitamin deficits, alcohol abuse, diet (Dye, 2010; Hujoel, 2009), and other pro-oxidation conditions, such as MetS, play a key role in the activation of signalling pathways, which act in promoting ROS development and probably also in worsening or producing new onset of a periodontal disease (Liu et al., 2011; Soory, 2009; Boden, 2006).

SO, WHY IS METS INVOLVED IN PERIODONTAL DISEASES?

Certainly this is because a pathological range including all pro-oxidation conditions (hyperglycaemia, hyperlipaemia, obesity, and hypertension), which coexist in a vicious circle, and establish and support the onset of free radicals and products from non-enzymatic glycosilation. As yet, there is not much in literature to support this assumption, except for a note- worthy epidemiological analysis, which helps to provide the background on the relationship between MetS and periodontal diseases, i.e. the analysis of the American study NHANES III (D'Aiuto et al., 2008). NHANES III (Third National Health and Nutrition

Examination Survey) analysed 13,994 individuals (men and women) aged over 17. The study assessed their periodontal condition through plaque and bleeding indexes, and testing depth, as well as the Metabolic Syndrome parameters. The patients aged over 45 affected by MetS had a risk 2.31 times higher than healthy individuals of being affected by periodontal diseases. The study authors concluded that serious periodontal disease is associated with middle-aged individuals affected by MetS (D'Aiuto et al., 2008). Further investigations are required to support and extend this hypothesis. However, it is clear enough that the MetS negatively influences the health of tissues supporting the teeth.

6. Metabolic Syndrome, AGEs, and periodontal diseases

Hypertension, obesity, dyslipidemia, and hyperglycaemia, which coexist in MetS, play an incremental role in ROS and AGEs production (Turco et al., 2011). This is probably on the basis of a potential MetS role in the destruction of periodontal tissues. In fact, the AGEs create damage by directly modifying proteins (Verzijl et al., 2000), or indirectly, activating signalling through its RAGE receptors (Schmidt et al., 2000). The interaction AGE-RAGE results in pro-inflammatory signalling and in generation of intracellular oxidative stress and subsequent activation of the redox-sensitive transcription factors such as NF-κB (Schmidt and Stern, 2000). Formation of AGEs is a way to maintain the signal of a short oxidative burst in a much longer-lived post translational modified proteins (Andrassy et al., 2006). Interaction of RAGE with AGEs in endothelial cells results in hyperpermeability and enhanced expression of adhesion molecules such as vascular cell adhesion molecule-1 (VCAM-1). This interaction on monocytes induces chemotaxis, as well as an increased generation of cytokines such as tumour necrosis factor (TNF), interleukin-1 (IL-1), or IL-6 (Vlassara et al., 1988).

Furthermore, the engagement of RAGE results in diminished collagen synthesis in fibroblasts (Hollá et al., 2001). Recent observations suggest that RAGE is a central cell-surface receptor also for EN-RAGE (extracellular newly identified RAGE binding proteins) and other members of the S100/calgranulin family of pro-inflammatory cytokines (Hofmann et al., 1999). These intracellular proteins may gain access to extracellular space in the inflammatory milieu. Upon release, their ability to interact with cellular RAGE appears to be an important means by which to propagate inflammatory cellular perturbation and chronic tissue injury (Schaefer and Heizmann, 1996). It is important to note that a study with diabetic rats shows that RAGE inhibition prevents the progression of periodontal disease, improving the prognosis, and reduces the formation of pro-inflammatory cytokines, such as IL-6, TNF-alfa, and metalloproteinases, significantly reducing the loss of alveolar bone (Schmidt et al., 1996). The authors have also observed that the beneficial effect of the RAGE block is independent from glycaemic control, thus supporting the importance of signalling RAGE in periodontal disease. Observations based on the involvement of RAGEs in periodontal disease are not valid to support the hypothesis that the AGEs are involved in the onset of periodontal disease. However, this aspect has been recently studied by Murillo et al. (2008) and Ren et al. (2009), who assessed the in vitro effect of AGEs on human gingival and periodontal fibroblasts. Both of these studies started from the premise that an important role in periodontal physiology is played by cell interaction with molecules of the extracellular matrix (Steffensen et al., 2001). In an *in vitro* model of periodontal cells, the behaviour of human gingival fibroblasts (hGFs) and human periodontal fibroblasts (hPDLs) is deeply influenced by changes in the surrounding environment (Lackler et al., 2000). The glycated proteins of the extracellular matrix can also have their pathogenic effects interacting with RAGE. The observation that the AGEs can regulate the cellular function and hGFs' collagen metabolism supports this assumption. It was also found that the AGEs reduce the mobility of these cells and significantly inhibit the expression of type I and III collagen (Ren et al., 2009). The importance of these mechanisms in the pathogenesis of periodontal disease is emphasised by the observation according to which the reduction of periodontal integrity, which occurs physiologically with age, could be referred to a reduced expression of type I collagen caused by age-dependent hypermethylation in the gene-promoting area (Ohi et al., 2006).

In concurrence with the above-mentioned data, it seems that the AGEs participate in the pathogenesis of periodontal disease, independently from the mechanisms provoking their accumulation. This hypothesis is supported by a recent study, which has investigated the existing relationship between the development of periodontal disease and glycosylated haemoglobin (HbA1c) levels in non-diabetic individuals. The periodontal health status, analysed in these patients using modified CPI (Community Periodontal Index), was significantly correlated with HbA1c levels. After the normalisation of data, the authors observed that mean HbA1c was significantly increased in the case of periodontal deterioration (Hayashida et al., 2009).

7. Final considerations and future developments

The literature analysed clearly shows that all the conditions and pathologies causing oxidative stress, production of AGEs, and activation of RAGE, are potentially involved in the aetiology and severity of periodontal diseases, and particularly in the development of chronic periodontitis.

As the MetS is defined by the presence of hyperglycaemia, dyslipidemia, obesity, hypertension – all these conditions determine ROS increase and AGEs production – it is clear that the MetS may worsen an existing state, or cause a new periodontal pathology, with mechanisms like those described for diabetes, where the AGEs play a key role in the onset of microangiopathy, retinopathy, nephropathy, neuropathy, and general tissue degeneration conditions (Ramasamy et al., 2005). Considered individually, the conditions defining the MetS play an important role. However, their role is certainly at a lower level as compared with synergic action. It is now described by clinical evidence and scientific literature that neglecting a high BMI involves a cascade of other compensatory and dysfunctional conditions promoted by humoral signalling; whose sum defines the MetS (Martin-Cordero et al., 2011; Martínez-Clemente et al., 2011).

The AGEs that may irreversibly accumulate in periodontal tissue with age, prolonged hyperglycaemia and/or chronic inflammation statuses, such as those that may be observed in the MetS, can damage the tissues and affect the functional status of collagen fibres and increase ROS and inflammation mediator levels through the interaction with RAGE. The formation of AGEs in the extracellular matrix may contribute to increasing ROS production and release from phagocytes and periodontal ligament cells, with subsequent induction of pro-inflammatory cytokines and metalloproteinases, leading to osteoclast activation and bone loss.

Since AGEs are products of accumulation, all these conditions have more significance in a condition which needs long time to develop, just as chronic periodontitis.

Therefore, we believe periodontal diseases , and particularly chronic periodontitis, should be considered by a multidisciplinary approach, bearing in mind that the periodontal tissues exposed not only to local bacterial onslaught, but also to systemic conditions damaging them through the same mechanisms provoking damage in other tissues.

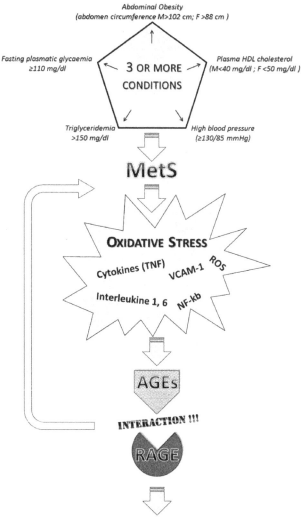

Fig. 1. In this figure has been represented the hypothesis supported in this article. MetS promote a self supporting ROS and AGEs accumulation that result in chronic inflammation signalling. This condition also promotes the osteoclast activation that result in alveolar bone loss.

8. References

Alberti, K. G. M. M., Zimmet, P., Shaw, J., and Group, I. D. F. E. T. F. C. (2005). The metabolic syndrome–a new worldwide definition. *Lancet*, 366(9491):1059–1062.

Andrassy, M., Igwe, J., Autschbach, F., Volz, C., Remppis, A., Neurath, M. F., Schleicher, E., Humpert, P. M., Wendt, T., Liliensiek, B., Morcos, M., Schiekofer, S., Thiele, K., Chen, J., Kientsch-Engel, R., Schmidt, A.-M., Stremmel, W., Stern, D. M., Katus, H. A., Nawroth, P. P., and Bierhaus, A. (2006). Posttranslationally modified proteins as mediators of sustained intestinal inflammation. *Am J Pathol*, 169(4):1223–1237.

Bagaitkar, J., Williams, L. R., Renaud, D. E., Bemakanakere, M. R., Martin, M., Scott, D. A., and Demuth, D. R. (2009). Tobacco-induced alterations to porphyromonas gingivalis-host interactions. *Environ Microbiol*, 11(5):1242–1253.

Baynes, J. W. (2001). The role of ages in aging: causation or correlation. *Exp Gerontol*, 36(9):1527–1537.

Bensley, L., VanEenwyk, J., and Ossiander, E. M. (2011). Associations of self-reported periodontal disease with metabolic syndrome and number of self-reported chronic con- ditions. *Prev Chronic Dis*, 8(3):A50.

Boden, G. (2006). Fatty acid-induced inflammation and insulin resistance in skeletal muscle and liver. *Curr Diab Rep*, 6(3):177–181.

Bohlender, J. M., Franke, S., Stein, G., and Wolf, G. (2005). Advanced glycation end products and the kidney. *Am J Physiol Renal Physiol*, 289(4):F645–F659.

Bullon, P., Morillo, J. M., Ramirez-Tortosa, M. C., Quiles, J. L., Newman, H. N., and Battino, M. (2009). Metabolic syndrome and periodontitis: is oxidative stress a common link? *J Dent Res*, 88(6):503–518.

Ceriello, A. and Motz, E. (2004). Is oxidative stress the pathogenic mechanism underlying insulin resistance, diabetes, and cardiovascular disease? the common soil hypothesis revisited. *Arterioscler Thromb Vasc Biol*, 24(5):816–823.

Chapple, I. L. C. and Matthews, J. B. (2007). The role of reactive oxygen and antioxidant species in periodontal tissue destruction. *Periodontol 2000*, 43:160–232.

D'Aiuto, F., Sabbah, W., Netuveli, G., Donos, N., Hingorani, A. D., Deanfield, J., and Tsakos, G. (2008). Association of the metabolic syndrome with severe periodontitis in a large u.s. population-based survey. *J Clin Endocrinol Metab*, 93(10):3989–3994.

Després, J. P., Lemieux, I., Dagenais, G. R., Cantin, B., and Lamarche, B. (2000). Hdl-cholesterol as a marker of coronary heart disease risk: the québec cardiovascular study. *Atherosclerosis*, 153(2):263–272.

Dye, B. A. (2010). The relationship between periodontitis and alcohol use is not clear. *J Evid Based Dent Pract*, 10(4):225–227.

El-Osta, A., Brasacchio, D., Yao, D., Pocai, A., Jones, P. L., Roeder, R. G., Cooper, M. E., and Brownlee, M. (2008). Transient high glucose causes persistent epigenetic changes and altered gene expression during subsequent normoglycemia. *J Exp Med*, 205(10):2409–2417.

Evans, J. L., Goldfine, I. D., Maddux, B. A., and Grodsky, G. M. (2003). Are oxida- tive stress-activated signaling pathways mediators of insulin resistance and beta-cell dysfunction? *Diabetes*, 52(1):1–8.

Expert Panel on Detection, E. and of High Blood Cholesterol in Adults, T. (2001). Exec- utive summary of the third report of the national cholesterol education program (ncep) expert panel on detection, evaluation, and treatment of high blood cholesterol in adults (adult treatment panel iii). *JAMA*, 285(19):2486–2497.

Ford, E. S., Giles, W. H., and Dietz, W. H. (2002). Prevalence of the metabolic syndrome among us adults: findings from the third national health and nutrition examination survey. *JAMA*, 287(3):356–359.

Fu, M. X., Requena, J. R., Jenkins, A. J., Lyons, T. J., Baynes, J. W., and Thorpe, S. R. (1996). The advanced glycation end product, nepsilon-(carboxymethyl)lysine, is a product of both lipid peroxidation and glycoxidation reactions. *J Biol Chem*, 271(17):9982–9986.

Goldin, A., Beckman, J. A., Schmidt, A. M., and Creager, M. A. (2006). Advanced glycation end products: sparking the development of diabetic vascular injury. *Circulation*, 114(6):597–605.

Han, S.-H., Kim, Y. H., and Mook-Jung, I. (2011). Rage: the beneficial and deleterious effects by diverse mechanisms of actions. *Mol Cells*, 31(2):91–97.

Harano, Y., Suzuki, M., Koyama, Y., Kanda, M., Yasuda, S., Suzuki, K., and Takamizawa, I. (2002). Multifactorial insulin resistance and clinical impact in hypertension and cardiovascular diseases. *J Diabetes Complications*, 16(1):19–23.

Hayashida, H., Kawasaki, K., Yoshimura, A., Kitamura, M., Furugen, R., Nakazato, M., Takamura, N., Hara, Y., Maeda, T., and Saito, T. (2009). Relationship between periodontal status and BbA1c in nondiabetics. *J Public Health Dent*, 69(3):204–206.

Hofmann, M. A., Drury, S., Fu, C., Qu, W., Taguchi, A., Lu, Y., Avila, C., Kambham, N., Bierhaus, A., Nawroth, P., Neurath, M. F., Slattery, T., Beach, D., McClary, J., Nagashima, M., Morser, J., Stern, D., and Schmidt, A. M. (1999). Rage mediates a novel proinflammatory axis: a central cell surface receptor for s100/calgranulin polypeptides. *Cell*, 97(7):889–901.

Hollá, L. I., Kanková, K., Fassmann, A., Bucková, D., Halabala, T., Znojil, V., and Vanek, J. (2001). Distribution of the receptor for advanced glycation end products gene polymorphisms in patients with chronic periodontitis: a preliminary study. *J Periodontol*, 72(12):1742–1746.

Hujoel, P. (2009). Dietary carbohydrates and dental-systemic diseases. *J Dent Res*, 88(6):490–502.

Kalousová, M., Zima, T., Popov, P., Spacek, P., Braun, M., Soukupová, J., Pelinkova, K., and Kientsch-Engel, R. (2004). Advanced glycation end-products in patients with chronic alcohol misuse. *Alcohol Alcohol*, 39(4):316–320.

Koyama, H., Shoji, T., Yokoyama, H., Motoyama, K., Mori, K., Fukumoto, S., Emoto, M., Shoji, T., Tamei, H., Matsuki, H., Sakurai, S., Yamamoto, Y., Yonekura, H., Watanabe, T., Yamamoto, H., and Nishizawa, Y. (2005). Plasma level of endogenous secretory rage is associated with components of the metabolic syndrome and atherosclerosis. *Arterioscler Thromb Vasc Biol*, 25(12):2587–2593.

Krajcovicová-Kudláčková, M., Sebeková, K., Schinzel, R., and Klvanová, J. (2002). Advanced glycation end products and nutrition. *Physiol Res*, 51(3):313–316.

Lackler, K. P., Cochran, D. L., Hoang, A. M., Takacs, V., and Oates, T. W. (2000). Development of an in vitro wound healing model for periodontal cells. *J Periodontol*, 71(2):226–237.

Lakka, H.-M., Laaksonen, D. E., Lakka, T. A., Niskanen, L. K., Kumpusalo, E., Tuomile- hto, J., and Salonen, J. T. (2002). The metabolic syndrome and total and cardiovascular disease mortality in middle-aged men. *JAMA*, 288(21):2709–2716.

Lee, Y.-S., Bak, E. J., Kim, M., Park, W., Seo, J. T., and Yoo, Y.-J. (2008). Induction of il-8 in periodontal ligament cells by h(2)o (2). *J Microbiol*, 46(5):579–584.

Liu, J., Jahn, L. A., Fowler, D. E., Barrett, E. J., Cao, W., and Liu, Z. (2011). Free fatty acids induce insulin resistance in both cardiac and skeletal muscle microvasculature in humans. *J Clin Endocrinol Metab*, 96(2):438–446.

Maddux, B. A., See, W., Lawrence, J. C., Goldfine, A. L., Goldfine, I. D., and Evans, J. L. (2001). Protection against oxidative stress-induced insulin resistance in rat l6 muscle cells by mircomolar concentrations of alpha-lipoic acid. *Diabetes*, 50(2):404–410.

Martin-Cordero, L., Garcia, J. J., Hinchado, M. D., and Ortega, E. (2011). The interleukin-6 and noradrenaline mediated inflammation-stress feedback mechanism is dysregulated in metabolic syndrome: Effect of exercise. *Cardiovasc Diabetol*, 10(1):42.

Martínez-Clemente, M., Clària, J., and Titos, E. (2011). The 5-lipoxygenase/leukotriene pathway in obesity, insulin resistance, and fatty liver disease. *Curr Opin Clin Nutr Metab Care*, in press:in press.

Miyata, T., Ueda, Y., Yoshida, A., Sugiyama, S., Iida, Y., Jadoul, M., Maeda, K., Kurokawa, K., and van Ypersele de Strihou, C. (1997). Clearance of pentosidine, an advanced glycation end product, by different modalities of renal replacement therapy. *Kidney Int*, 51(3):880–887.

Murillo, J., Wang, Y., Xu, X., Klebe, R. J., Chen, Z., Zardeneta, G., Pal, S., Mikhailova, M., and Steffensen, B. (2008). Advanced glycation of type i collagen and fibronectin modifies periodontal cell behavior. *J Periodontol*, 79(11):2190–2199.

Needleman, I. G., Worthington, H. V., Giedrys-Leeper, E., and Tucker, R. J. (2006). Guided tissue regeneration for periodontal infra-bony defects. *Cochrane Database Syst Rev*, 19(2):CD001724.

Noiri, E. and Tsukahara, H. (2005). Parameters for measurement of oxidative stress in di- abetes mellitus: applicability of enzyme-linked immunosorbent assay for clinical eval- uation. *J Investig Med*, 53(4):167–175.

Odrowaz-Sypniewska, G. (2007). Markers of pro-inflammatory and pro-thrombotic state in the diagnosis of metabolic syndrome. *Adv Med Sci*, 52:246–250.

Ohi, T., Uehara, Y., Takatsu, M., Watanabe, M., and Ono, T. (2006). Hypermethylation of cpgs in the promoter of the col1a1 gene in the aged periodontal ligament. *J Dent Res*, 85(3):245–250.

Peppa, M., Uribarri, J., and Vlassara, H. (2008). Aging and glycoxidant stress. *Hormones (Athens)*, 7(2):123–132.

Perlstein, M. I. and Bissada, N. F. (1977). Influence of obesity and hypertension on the severity of periodontitis in rats. *Oral Surg Oral Med Oral Pathol*, 43(5):707–719.

Pietropaoli, D., Tatone, C., D'Alessandro, A. M., and Monaco, A. (2010). Possible involvement of advanced glycation end products in periodontal diseases. *Int J Im- munopathol Pharmacol*, 23(3):683–691.

Pischon, N., Heng, N., Bernimoulin, J.-P., Kleber, B.-M., Willich, S. N., and Pischon, T. (2007). Obesity, inflammation, and periodontal disease. *J Dent Res*, 86(5):400–409.

Ramasamy, R., Vannucci, S. J., Yan, S. S. D., Herold, K., Yan, S. F., and Schmidt, A. M. (2005). Advanced glycation end products and rage: a common thread in aging, dia- betes, neurodegeneration, and inflammation. *Glycobiology*, 15(7):16R–28R.

Ren, L., Fu, Y., Deng, Y., Qi, L., and Jin, L. (2009). Advanced glycation end prod- ucts inhibit the expression of collagens type i and iii by human gingival fibroblasts. *J Periodontol*, 80(7):1166–1173.

Schaefer, B. W. and Heizmann, C. W. (1996). The s100 family of ef-hand calcium-binding proteins: functions and pathology. *Trends Biochem Sci*, 21(4):134–140.

Schmidt, A. M. and Stern, D. M. (2000). Hyperinsulinemia and vascular dysfunction: the role of nuclear factor-kappab, yet again. *Circ Res*, 87(9):722–724.

Schmidt, A. M., Weidman, E., Lalla, E., Yan, S. D., Hori, O., Cao, R., Brett, J. G., and Lamster, I. B. (1996). Advanced glycation endproducts (ages) induce oxidant stress in the gingiva: a potential mechanism underlying accelerated periodontal disease associ- ated with diabetes. *J Periodontal Res*, 31(7):508–515.

Schmidt, A. M., Yan, S. D., Yan, S. F., and Stern, D. M. (2000). The biology of the receptor for advanced glycation end products and its ligands. *Biochim Biophys Acta*, 1498(2-3):99–111.

Sebeková, K., Boor, P., Valachovicová, M., Blazícek, P., Parrák, V., Babinská, K., Hei- dland, A., and Krajcovicová-Kudlácková, M. (2006). Association of metabolic syn- drome risk factors with selected markers of oxidative status and microinflammation in healthy omnivores and vegetarians. *Mol Nutr Food Res*, 50(9):858–868.

Sheikhi, M., Gustafsson, A., and Jarstrand, C. (2000). Cytokine, elastase and oxygen radical release by fusobacterium nucleatum-activated leukocytes: a possible pathogenic factor in periodontitis. *J Clin Periodontol*, 27(10):758–762.

Siebel, A. L., Fernandez, A. Z., and El-Osta, A. (2010). Glycemic memory associated epigenetic changes. *Biochem Pharmacol*, 80(12):1853–1859.

Soory, M. (2008). A role for non-antimicrobial actions of tetracyclines in combating oxidative stress in periodontal and metabolic diseases: a literature review. *Open Dent J*, 2:5–12.

Soory, M. (2009). Redox status in periodontal and systemic inflammatory conditions including associated neoplasias: antioxidants as adjunctive therapy? *Infect Disord Drug Targets*, 9(4):415–427.

Steffensen, B., Häkkinen, L., and Larjava, H. (2001). Proteolytic events of wound- healing- coordinated interactions among matrix metalloproteinases (mmps), integrins, and extracellular matrix molecules. *Crit Rev Oral Biol Med*, 12(5):373–398.

Suvan, J., D'Aiuto, F., Moles, D. R., Petrie, A., and Donos, N. (2011). Association between overweight/obesity and periodontitis in adults. a systematic review. *Obes Rev*, 12(5):e381–e404.

Thornalley, P. J. (2005). Dicarbonyl intermediates in the maillard reaction. *Ann N Y Acad Sci*, 1043:111–117.

Tsai, C. C., Chen, H. S., Chen, S. L., Ho, Y. P., Ho, K. Y., Wu, Y. M., and Hung, C. C. (2005). Lipid peroxidation: a possible role in the induction and progression of chronic periodontitis. *J Periodontal Res*, 40(5):378–384.

Turco, S. D., Navarra, T., Gastaldelli, A., and Basta, G. (2011). Protective role of adiponectin on endothelial dysfunction induced by ages: A clinical and experimental approach. *Microvasc Res*, 22:[in press].

Ulrich, P. and Cerami, A. (2001). Protein glycation, diabetes, and aging. *Recent Prog Horm Res*, 56:1–21.

Verzijl, N., DeGroot, J., Thorpe, S. R., Bank, R. A., Shaw, J. N., Lyons, T. J., Bijlsma, J. W., Lafeber, F. P., Baynes, J. W., and TeKoppele, J. M. (2000). Effect of colla- gen turnover on the accumulation of advanced glycation end products. *J Biol Chem*, 275(50):39027–39031.

Vlassara, H., Brownlee, M., Manogue, K. R., Dinarello, C. A., and Pasagian, A. (1988). Cachectin/tnf and il-1 induced by glucose-modified proteins: role in normal tissue re- modeling. *Science*, 240(4858):1546–1548.

Wen, Y., Skidmore, J. C., Porter-Turner, M. M., Rea, C. A., Khokher, M. A., and Singh, B. M. (2002). Relationship of glycation, antioxidant status and oxidative stress to vascular endothelial damage in diabetes. *Diabetes Obes Metab*, 4(5):305–308.

Xue, J., Rai, V., Singer, D., Chabierski, S., Xie, J., Reverdatto, S., Burz, D. S., Schmidt, A. M., Hoffmann, R., and Shekhtman, A. (2011). Advanced glycation end product recognition by the receptor for ages. *Structure*, 19(5):722–732.

Yamagishi, S., Matsui, T., and Nakamura, K. (2008). Possible involvement of tobacco-derived advanced glycation end products (ages) in an increased risk for developing cancers and cardiovascular disease in former smokers. *Med Hypotheses*, 71(2):259–261.

Yin, M., Gäbele, E., Wheeler, M. D., Connor, H., Bradford, B. U., Dikalova, A., Rusyn, I., Mason, R., and Thurman, R. G. (2001). Alcohol-induced free radicals in mice: direct toxicants or signaling molecules? *Hepatology*, 34(5):935–942.

Zhang, Q., Ames, J. M., Smith, R. D., Baynes, J. W., and Metz, T. O. (2009). A perspec- tive on the maillard reaction and the analysis of protein glycation by mass spectrometry: probing the pathogenesis of chronic disease. *J Proteome Res*, 8(2):754–769.

Part 2

Treatment Approaches in Periodontitis

7

Clinical Considerations
of Open Gingival Embrasures

Jae Hyun Park, Kiyoshi Tai, John Morris and Dorotea Modrin

Arizona School of Dentistry & Oral Health, A. T. Still University
U.S.A.

1. Introduction

Gingival embrasures are defined as the embrasure cervical to the interproximal contact.[1] If the embrasure space is not completely filled by the gingiva, it is considered open. Open gingival embrasures contribute to retention of food debris and can adversely affect the health of the periodontium. They are more common in adult patients with bone loss.[2] Black triangles occur in more than 1/3 of all adults and should be discussed with patients prior to initiating dental treatment.[1,3] Key considerations in restorative and orthodontic treatment are preserving papilla and avoiding black triangles in the gingival embrasures of the esthetic zone (Figure 1). Open embrasures are best managed with a team work involving restorative, orthodontic and periodontal parts (Figure 2).

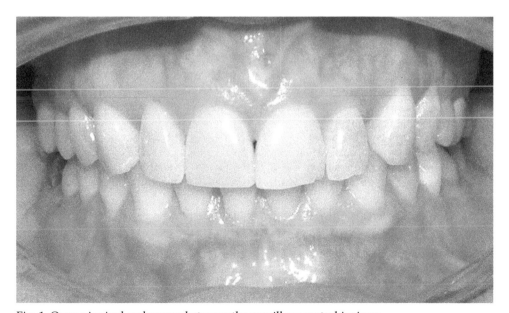

Fig. 1. Open gingival embrasure between the maxillary central incisors.

Open gingival embrasures are visibly unesthetic and negatively affect a person's smile. In a study by Kokich et al.,[4] orthodontists considered a 2 mm open gingival embrasure as noticeably less attractive than an ideal smile with normal gingival embrasure. Open gingival embrasures slightly greater than 3 mm were considered less attractive by both general dentists and the general population.

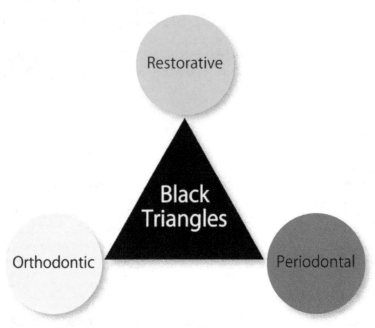

Fig. 2. Interdisciplinary approach to overcome black triangles.

To better manage open gingival embrasures, the dental clinician must be aware of the underlying etiology and make an individualized treatment plan for each patient. Many embrasures may be corrected with restorative procedures, but if the underlying etiology is not addressed correctly, the result may not be as esthetic as expected.[5] Open gingival embrasures are more frequently encountered in adults undergoing orthodontic treatment (38%) than adolescents in treatment (15%).[3] However, 41.9% of adolescent patients who are treated for maxillary incisor crowding have gingival embrasures.[6] The higher prevalence in adults is related to periodontal disease and periodontal or orthognathic surgery.[1,7] Gingival embrasures change over time, and once filled, embrasures may become open again.[8,9]

2. Etiology and prevalence of open gingival embrasures

Etiologic factors for open gingival embrasures include; dimensional changes of papilla during orthodontic treatment, long lasting orthodontic treatment, loss of periodontal attachment resulting in recession, loss of height of the alveolar bone relative to interproximal contact, length of embrasure area, root angulations, age, contact position, and triangular-shaped crowns.[10-12] Patients may present with one or more etiologic factor; thus, managing each patient requires an individual assessment and treatment plan.

The occurrence of open gingival embrasures is found to be age related. Studies[1,13] have demonstrated that patients over 20 are more susceptible than those under 20. Open gingival embrasures were reported in 67% of the population over 20 compared with 18% in the population under 20.[1] This is due to the thinning of oral epithelium, a decrease in keratinization, and a reduction in papilla height as a result of the aging process. Therefore, age is a significant factor leading to wide and long embrasure spaces in adults. Embrasure and tooth morphology also is another etiologic factor. Open embrasures occur more frequently in short narrow, long narrow, long wide, and short wide embrasure morphologies.[11,13]

3. Periodontal disease and open gingival embrasures

Periodontal disease leads to loss of alveolar bone which also affects the interdental papilla. If the distance from the alveolar crest to interdental contact point exceeds 5 mm, it is more likely that the papilla is insufficient to fill the embrasure.[2] The distance between the contact point and the alveolar crest is less than 5 mm in healthy periodontium whereas, pocket depths greater than 3 mm will lead to increased plaque retention, inflammation, and possibly gingival recession.[14] For those with periodontal diseases, it is the bone loss that increases the distance between the contact points and alveolar crest and eventually creates open gingival embrasures.

The distance from the base of the contact point to the alveolar crest in central incisors is a strong indicator of the presence of open gingival embrasures (Figure 3a). Tarnow et al.[2] reported an association between black triangles and the distance from the contact point to the alveolar crest of the bone. Another study found that a distance of 5, 6, and 7 mm resulted in an open embrasure in 2, 44, and 73% of the cases, respectively.[15] These observations indicated that papilla was present in almost 100% of the cases if the distance from the alveolar crest to the contact point was 5 mm or less. When the distance was more than 7 mm, most cases had an open gingival embrasure. At 6 mm, the papilla was present in half of the cases.[15] Other studies[14,16] have reported similar results (Figure 3b).

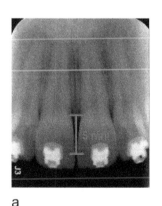

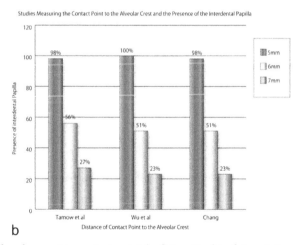

a   b

Fig. 3. (a) The distance between the alveolar crest to contact point (red) is critical in determining the extent of an open embrasure. A distance greater than 5 mm is considered to be a black triangle. (b) Summary of several studies measuring the distance from the alveolar crest to the contact point. Increasing the distance will increase the likelihood of an open embrasure.

The prevalence of plaque accumulation and gingivitis is probably higher in people with crowding, but host susceptibility and other factors may also play a role in the occurrence of open gingival embrasures, especially in patients who have been previously treated for periodontal disease.[17] For these patients, there needs to be an increased effort to enhance periodontal maintenance and oral hygiene to prevent bone loss and recession.

Adult patients with open gingival embrasures have an increased alveolar bone crest-interproximal contact distance of 5.5 mm or more.[3] An increase of 1 mm in the distance between the alveolar bone crest and interproximal contact increases the possibility of an open gingival embrasure from 78 to 97%. As a rule, 5-6 mm distance from the contact point to the alveolar crest is the most critical in determining the presence or absence of an open gingival embrasure.[15]

Chronic periodontitis and tooth brush trauma are other factors that may cause open embrasures. If tooth brushing is causing gingival recession, interproximal tooth brushing should be discontinued until the tissue can recover if it causes loss of interdental papilla.[18] At present, there are no surgical procedures to augment papilla with a predictable outcome.[19-25] Surgical papillary reconstruction often results in contraction and necrosis of the grafted tissue due to tissue fragility and the low blood supply to interdental papilla.[15] However, case studies[26,27] have reported some degree of success with subepithelial connective tissue grafts and orthodontic therapy. Pedicle flaps have provided better results than free gingival grafts.[15]

Presence of a thick biotype gingiva and no loss of insertion at the periodontal attachment are important for the successful outcome of the surgery.[18] Patients with a thin biotype of gingiva are more susceptible to recession and consequently, to open gingival embrasures. Patients with thin periodontium are shown to have long narrow maxillary central incisors, whereas patients with a thick biotype have short and wide central incisors.[28] In addition, the thick periodontal biotype has a thick osseous structure with flat morphology and a thick gingival tissue with short wide papilla. Thick biotype is associated with less open embrasures especially around implants.[29] In contrast, thin biotype is characterized by a scalloped appearance with long interdental papilla.[30] Typically thick biotype has a better vascular supply and biological tissue memory that helps the tissue to rebound, whereas the thin biotype usually results in permanent recession.[24] Once interdental gingival recession has occurred, there is a reduced height and thickness of free gingiva that results in a long clinical crown. This recession is aggravated by plaque and toothbrush trauma. Atraumatic plaque control is highly recommended for patients susceptible to black triangles.[31]

4. Orthodontic correction of open gingival embrasures

Root divergency of adjacent teeth is strongly associated with open gingival embrasures. This either occurs naturally or is caused by improper bracket placement during orthodontic treatment. Kurth et al.[3] showed that the mean root angulation in normal gingival embrasures converge at 3.65° and an increase in root divergence by just 1° increases the probability of an open gingival embrasure from 14 to 21%. Orthodontic treatment can be performed to converge maxillary incisor roots to reduce or eliminate open gingival embrasures (Figure 4).

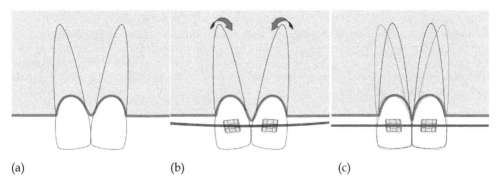

(a)   (b)   (c)

Fig. 4. Paralleling divergent roots will decrease the severity of a black triangle. (a) Divergent roots with an open black triangle. (b) Bracket positioning to follow the long axis of the tooth and correct for black triangle. (c) Converged roots with a closed black triangle after orthodontic treatment.

The bracket slots must be perpendicular to the long axis of the tooth and not parallel to the incisal edges during bracket placement, especially in adults with worn incisal edges. It is important to evaluate the periapical radiograph prior to bracket placement, especially in patients with attrition.[15] If brackets are placed based on incisal edges, greater root divergence may cause an open gingival embrasure. Bonding brackets with slots perpendicular to the long axis of the teeth will allow roots to converge, and may require the worn distoincisal edges to be restored or contoured. As roots become more parallel, the contact point will lengthen and move apically toward the papilla, thus reducing open gingival embrasures.[15] The crowns of each incisor will move closer, causing the stretched transseptal fibers to relax and fill in the gingival embrasure.[2]

Patients with triangular crown morphology are more susceptible to open gingival embrasures (Figure 5a). In this case, the crowns of the central incisors are much wider incisally than cervically, resulting in a high contact point. Interproximal reduction (IPR) of enamel between triangular crowns will broaden the point contact area which will reduce open gingival embrasures. Reduction of interproximal enamel with a reducing diamond strip is one way to correct the black triangle. Typically, 0.5 - 0.75 mm of enamel is removed with IPR.[15] Orthodontic space closure after IPR will lengthen the contact point and move the contact gingivally, thus reducing open gingival embrasures (Figures 5b-5d).

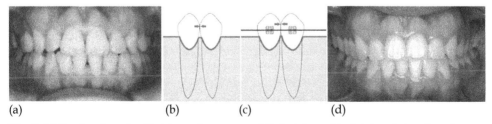

(a)   (b)   (c)   (d)

Fig. 5. (a) Pre-treatment with triangular crowns. Minimizing a black triangle by changing point contact (b) to a broader surface (c) through interproximal reduction (IPR). (d) Post-treatment.

After orthodontic treatment, the direction of orthodontic tooth movement and labiolingual thickness of the supporting bone and soft tissue determines whether gingival embrasures will be present. Interestingly, maxillary incisor imbrication and rotation have a controversial association with open gingival embrasure spaces.[3,6,31] It would be wise to inform patients with imbricated maxillary incisors that they may be predisposed to an open gingival embrasure following orthodontic treatment.

The amount of crowding plays only a limited role in the prevalence of open gingival embrasures. Ko-Kimura et al.[1] reported that open embrasures occur in a similar percentage of patients with incisor crowding of less than 4 mm and those with 4 - 8 mm of incisor crowding. When crowding was more than 8 mm, the occurrence of open gingival embrasures increased by 7%. However, these results revealed no statistically significant differences. The authors also found that the length of orthodontic treatment had insignificant effect on occurrence of open gingival embrasures.

The volume of soft tissue in the gingival embrasure depends on the existing tissue, bone levels, and the severity of diastema. Closing a diastema by orthodontic treatment compresses the soft tissue, making it fill the embrasure area. Minor diastema closure can be simplified with a removable orthodontic appliance (Figure 6). However, large diastema closure may require more complex treatment with additional orthodontic and/or restorative measures.

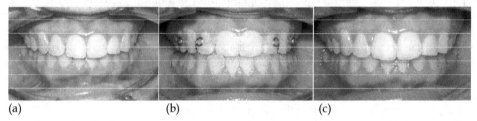

(a)   (b)   (c)

Fig. 6. Limited orthodontic treatment to close a diastema. (a) Pre-treatment of diastema. (b) A modified maxillary Hawley retainer with extended arms. 3/8″, 3.5 oz elastics (3M Unitek, Monrovia, CA, USA) are worn across the teeth from the right arm to the left arm of the retainer. (c) Post-treatment after 4 weeks of treatment.

5. Restorative correction of open gingival embrasures

Prosthetic alterations of crown forms by mesiocervical restorations or full veneers will reduce the unaesthetic appearance of open gingival embrasures. To guide the shape of the interdental papilla, composite resin can be extended into the gingival sulcus, much like a provisional crown for an implant.[5] When restorative measures are used, care must be taken not to impinge on the interdental tissue or harbor plaque. Typically, maxillary central incisors have 80% width to height ratio, which is considered to be ideal. Simply using a restorative treatment to reduce a large space may cause a divergence of this ratio, resulting in an unaesthetic crown appearance. In this case, an interdisciplinary approach may be necessary.

A connector is the point where teeth appear to contact, and the contact point is the place where they actually do. For restorative treatment to be successful, an appropriate ratio of crown height between the connector and central incisor is required. The connector of maxillary anterior teeth has a proportional relationship to the height of the central incisors. The ratio of connector to tooth height for the central, lateral, and canine is 50, 40, and 30%, respectively.[32] Teeth with longer crown height will have longer connectors (Figure 7). Furthermore, embrasures are smaller between the central incisors and increase progressively toward the posterior region. The application of pink-colored porcelain or a removable appliance is recommended to hide severe tissue defects.[2] A comprehensive understanding of anterior esthetics is critical in determining the appropriate treatment for any individual patient.[33-37]

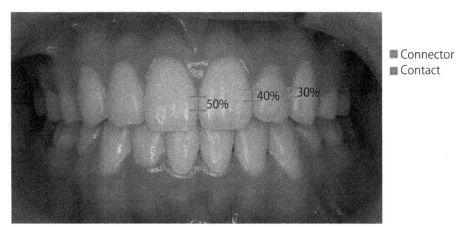

Fig. 7. Connectors and interproximal contact. Connectors (red) are where teeth appear to meet. Contact (blue) between teeth is where they actually meet. The appropriate ratio for a connector between maxillary central incisors is 50% of the central incisor height. The ratio between central–lateral connectors is 40% of the central incisor height, and ratio between lateral-canine connectors is 30% of central incisor height.

6. Considerations for open gingival embrasures with single tooth implants

Currently, the single tooth implant is one of the most common treatment alternatives for the replacement of missing teeth. During the treatment planning of single tooth implants to replace congenitally missing lateral incisors, an interdisciplinary approach is preferred to provide the most predictable treatment outcome. Studies have documented successful osseointegration and long term function of restorations supported by single tooth implants.[38-41] One of the main advantages of this type of restoration is the ability to keep the adjacent teeth intact. However, orthodontic treatment is often necessary to provide adequate room both in the coronal and apical areas.

The biological width of periimplant mucosa is about 2-3 mm; and a similar amount of supracrestal soft tissue is required to allow for the formation of a stable soft tissue attachment and to prevent bone resorption.[39] Orthodontic treatment should be designed to minimize extrusion of the adjacent teeth because any such movement will have the effect of an apical migration of the implant.[38] To preserve the interdental papilla and allow for adequate oral hygiene, 1.5 - 2.0 mm of space is needed between the implant and the tooth on each side. Therefore, 7 mm of mesiodistal space must be created between the adjacent teeth.[41] After the appropriate amount of coronal space has been determined, it is necessary to evaluate the interradicular spacing. The minimum interradicular distance required is generally 5-7 mm for a single implant placement. Problems with inadequate space between the root apices are generally due to improper mesiodistal root angulation. When patients with a missing tooth undergo orthodontic treatment, it is important to take a periapical radiograph of the edentulous area prior to removing orthodontic appliances to confirm the ideal root position of the adjacent teeth and adequate spacing for a future implant placement.[38]

A provisional restoration should be placed on the implant to prosthetically guide the soft tissue into its final position.[41] When a provisional restoration is placed, the subgingival contours and shape of this provisional will influence the position of the soft tissue.[42] Adding more contour to the facial aspect of the provisional causes the facial free gingival margin to move apically, whereas adding interproximal contour to the provisional helps create a more ideal papillary form. The provisional restoration is generally allowed to remain in place for 4-6 weeks.

The correct buccolingual position of an anterior implant is another important esthetic factor. The head of the implant should be placed inside an imaginary line connecting the incisal margins of the adjacent teeth, so the longitudinal axis of the implant should be 4 mm from a line tangent to the adjacent occlusal surfaces (Figure 8). In the horizontal plane, the center of the crown placed on the implant should be no farther than half of the abutment radius from the center of the implant — that is approximately 1 mm in the case of a standard abutment. This location may help to prevent resorption of the thinner cortical buccal bone and consequent recession.[43] Vertically, the implant platform should be 3-5 mm apical to the gingival margins of the adjacent teeth to provide a harmonious smile line (Figure 9). An adequate band of attached gingiva also helps reduce the risk of gingival recession.

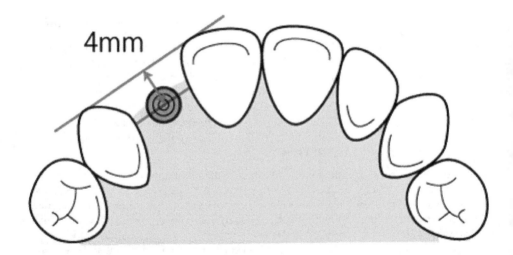

Fig. 8. The longitudinal axis of the implant should be approximately 4 mm away from an imaginary line connecting the incisal surfaces of the adjacent teeth.

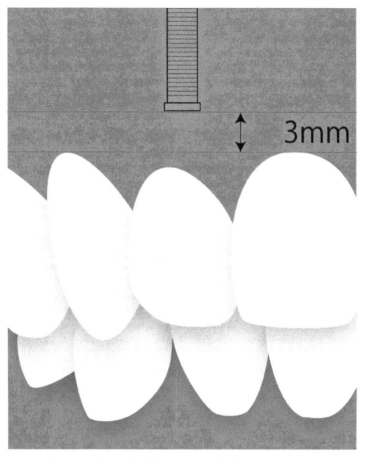

Fig. 9. The implant platform should be 3-5 mm apical to the gingival margins of the adjacent teeth to provide a harmonious smile line.

Single tooth implants have a significant possibility of papilla loss because of an increase in the distance between the contact point and the alveolar crest.[44-46] It is important to keep the distance between the contact point and bone level as 5 mm or less to preserve papilla around implants. The distance of the adjacent natural teeth to the alveolar crests is the most critical factor, whereas the height of the implant contact to the bone is less important.[44] Choquet et al.[45] showed the presence of papilla at 100% and 50% level in healthy teeth when the distance from the alveolar crest to the contact point of single implant in the maxillary anterior region was 5 and 6 mm, respectively. A significant increase in black triangles was observed at distances above 7 mm.[28] Some clinicians believe that tissue healing around an immediate provisional abutment helps in proper tissue contouring. However, Ryser et al.[44] stated that there was no difference in papilla loss even if an implant had a provisional placed immediately. Extrusion of a tooth prior to implant placement allows the bone to extrude with the tooth, resulting in an increase in soft tissue dimensions. Tooth extrusion can be performed with intermaxillary elastics and a clear removable appliance such as an

Essix.[47] However, existing tissue loss prior to implant placement usually results in an open embrasure following final restoration. Grunder et al.[48] reported a 0.375 mm increase in soft tissue volume after 1 year, although 0.6 mm of soft tissue shrinkage occurred on the buccal side of the implant crown. Jemt[49] also suggested that the volume of soft tissue around anterior single tooth implants can be expected to undergo soft tissue shrinkage on the buccal; whereas, an increase in soft tissue volume occurs in 80% of cases after 1.5 years.

7. Considerations for open gingival embrasure with adjacent implants

In cases where two implants are placed adjacent to each other, open gingival embrasures are more pronounced. Up to 4 mm of vertical alveolar bone may be lost in such cases.[50] Fibers are stretched vertically instead of perpendicularly from the implant surface and there is reduced blood supply, further complicating papilla restoration.[51] A soft tissue deficiency of 1-2 mm occurs because the biological width around an implant is apical to the platform for the abutment.[52] As a result, the biological width of implants is located subcrestally rather than the supracrestal location with natural teeth.[43] The distance between the implant shoulder and alveolar crest should be at least 4 mm in the maxillary anterior region. To prevent bone loss and subsequent papilla loss, it is important that the distance between two adjacent implants exceeds 3 mm.[44] This helps to maintain interproximal bone above the implant shoulder. In the anterior region, it is usually difficult to achieve this ideal mesiodistal distance between implants. One way to compensate for the loss of interproximal bone is to augment the buccal bone in the papillary area,[53,54] but it is not possible to ensure a complete papilla with distances greater than 3 mm. There are several procedures that may help to prevent additional interproximal bone loss but they won't allow papilla regeneration. When placing and restoring adjacent immediate implants, papilla is better preserved if the distance is 2-4 mm.[55] To prevent unaesthetic open embrasures in the esthetic zone, adjacent implants should better be avoided. Options for two missing teeth in the esthetic zone include orthodontic movement of teeth, placing an implant with a cantilever pontic and performing a soft tissue graft, interproximal bone augmentation, or a three unit bridge involving one implant.[46]

8. Summary

The distance between the alveolar crest and interproximal contact point together with periodontal bone loss appear to be the most significant factors contributing to occurrence of open gingival embrasures. The etiology of open gingival embrasures is multifactorial, so to determine the ideal treatment for the patient, the clinician should first evaluate whether the problem is caused by soft or hard tissue problem. An interdisciplinary team approach including a general dentist, an orthodontist, a periodontist, and a prosthodontist should be considered for the optimum restoration of open gingival embrasures.

9. References

[1] Ko-Kimura N, Kimura-Hayashi M, Yamaguchi M, et al. Some factors associated with open gingival embrasures following orthodontic treatment. *Aust Orthod J.* 2003;19(1):19-24.

[2] Tarnow DP, Magner AW, Fletcher P. The effect of the distance from the contact point to the crest of bone on the presence or absence of the interproximal dental papilla. *J Periodontol*. 1992;63(12):995-996.

[3] Kurth JR, Kokich VG. Open gingival embrasures after orthodontic treatment in adults: prevalence and etiology. *Am J Orthod Dentofacial Orthop*. 2001;120(2):116-123.

[4] Kokich VO Jr, Kiyak HA, Shapiro PA. Comparing the perception of dentists and lay people to altered dental esthetics. *J Esthet Dent*. 1999;11(6):311-324.

[5] Clark D. Correction of the "black triangle": restoratively driven papilla regeneration. *Dent Today*. 2009;28(2):150, 152, 154-155.

[6] Burke S, Burch JG, Tetz JA. Incidence and size of pretreatment overlap and posttreatment gingival embrasure space between maxillary central incisors. *Am J Orthod Dentofacial Orthop*. 1994;105(5):506-511.

[7] Chang LC. Effect of bone crest to contact point distance on central papilla height using embrasure morphologies. *Quintessence Int*. 2009;40(6):507-513.

[8] Becker W. Commentary. Esthetic considerations in interdental papilla: remediation and regeneration. *J Esthet Restor Dent*. 2010;22(1):29-30.

[9] Theytaz GA, Kiliaridis S. Gingival and dentofacial changes in adolescents and adults 2 to 10 years after orthodontic treatment. *J Clin Periodontol*. 2008;35(9):825-830.

[10] Sharma AA, Park JH. Esthetic considerations in interdental papilla: remediation and regeneration. *J Esthet Restor Dent*. 2010;22(1):18-28.

[11] Ikeda T, Yamaguchi M, Meguro D, Kasai K. Prediction and causes of open gingival embrasure spaces between the mandibular central incisors following orthodontic treatment. *Aust Orthod J*. 2004;20(2):87-92.

[12] Cardaropoli D, Re S. Interdental papilla augmentation procedure following orthodontic treatment in a periodontal patient. *J Periodontol*. 2005;76(4):655-661.

[13] Chang LC. The association between embrasure morphology and central papilla recession. *J Clin Periodontol*. 2007;34(5):432-436.

[14] Zetu L, Wang HL. Management of inter-dental/inter-implant papilla. *J Clin Periodontol*. 2005;32(7):831-839.

[15] Wu YJ, Tu YK, Huang SM, Chan CP. The influence of the distance from the contact point to the crest of bone on the presence of the interproximal dental papilla. *Chang Gung Med J*. 2003;26(11):822-828.

[16] Chang LC. Assessment of parameters affecting the presence of the central papilla using a non-invasive radiographic method. *J Periodontol*. 2008;79(4):603-609.

[17] Prato GPP, Rotundo R, Cortellini P, Tinti C, Azzi R. Interdental papilla management: a review and classification of the therapeutic approaches. *Int J Periodontics Restorative Dent*. 2004;24(3):246-255.

[18] Tanaka OM, Furquim BD, Pascotto RC, et al. The dilemma of the open gingival embrasure between maxillary central incisors. *J Contemp Dent Pract*. 2008;9(6):92-98.

[19] Ravon NA, Handelsman M, Levine D. Multidisciplinary care: periodontal aspects to treatment planning the anterior esthetic zone. *J Calif Dent Assoc*. 2008;36(8):575-584.

[20] Lee DW, Kim CK, Park KH, Cho KS, Moon IS. Non-invasive method to measure the length of soft tissue from the top of the papilla to the crestal bone. *J Periodontol.* 2005;76(8):1311-1314.

[21] Azzi R, Takei HH, Etienne D, Carranza FA. Root coverage and papilla reconstruction using autogenous osseous and connective tissue grafts. *Int J Periodontics Restorative Dent.* 2001;21(2):141-147.

[22] Oringer RJ, Iacono VJ. Current periodontal plastic procedures around teeth and dental implants. *N Y State Dent J.* 1999;65(6):26-31.

[23] Blatz MB, Hürzeler MB, Strub JR. Reconstruction of the lost interproximal papilla-presentation of surgical and nonsurgical approaches. *Int J Periodontics Restorative Dent.* 1999;19(4):395-406.

[24] van der Velden U. Regeneration of the interdental soft tissues following denudation procedures. *J Clin Periodontol.* 1982;9(6):455-459.

[25] Roy BJ. Improving prosthetic results through periodontal procedures. *J Indiana Dent Assoc.* 1998;77(1):17-20, 33-35.

[26] Checchi L, Montevecchi M, Checchi V, Bonetti GA. A modified papilla preservation technique, 22 years later. *Quintessence Int.* 2009;40(4):303-311.

[27] Nemcovsky CE. Interproximal papilla augmentation procedure: a novel surgical approach and clinical evaluation of 10 consecutive procedures. *Int J Periodontics Restorative Dent.* 2001;21(6):553-559.

[28] Olsson M, Lindhe J, Marinello CP. On the relationship between crown form and clinical features of the gingiva in adolescents. *J Clin Periodontol.* 1993;20(8):570-577.

[29] Chow YC, Wang H-L. Factors and techniques influencing peri-implant papillae. *Implant Dent.* 2010;19(3):208-219.

[30] Chang L-C. The association between embrasure morphology and central papilla recession: a noninvasive assessment method. *Chang Gung Med J.* 2007;30(5):445-452.

[31] Kandasamy S, Goonewardene M, Tennant M. Changes in interdental papillae heights following alignment of anterior teeth. *Aust Orthod J.* 2007;23(1):16-23.

[32] Raj V, Heymann HO, Hershey HG, Ritter AV, Casko JS. The apparent contact dimension and covariates among orthodontically treated and nontreated subjects. *J Esthet Restor Dent.* 2009;21(2):96-111.

[33] Cardaropoli D, Re S, Corrente G. The Papilla Presence Index (PPI): a new system to assess interproximal papillary levels. *Int J Periodontics Restorative Dent.* 2004;24(5):488-492.

[34] Martegani P, Silvestri M, Mascarello F, et al. Morphometric study of the interproximal unit in the esthetic region to correlate anatomic variables affecting the aspect of soft tissue embrasure space. *J Periodontol.* 2007;78(12):2260-2265.

[35] Sarver DM. Principles of cosmetic dentistry in orthodontics: Part 1. Shape and proportionality of anterior teeth. *Am J Orthod Dentofacial Orthop.* 2004;126(6):749-753.

[36] Kokich VG. Esthetics and vertical tooth position: orthodontic possibilities. *Compend Contin Educ Dent.* 1997;18(12):1225-1231.

[37] Kokich V. Esthetics and anterior tooth position: an orthodontic perspective. Part III: Mediolateral relationships. *J Esthet Dent.* 1993;5(5):200-207.

[38] Thilander B, Odman J, Jemt T. Single implants in the upper incisor region and their relationship to the adjacent teeth. An 8-year follow-up study. *Clin Oral Implants Res*. 1999;10(5):346-355.

[39] Goldberg PV, Higginbottom FL, Wilson TG. Periodontal considerations in restorative and implant therapy. *Periodontol 2000*. 2001;25(1):100-109.

[40] Noack N, Willer J, Hoffmann J. Long-term results after placement of dental implants: longitudinal study of 1,964 implants over 16 years. *Int J Oral Maxillofac Implants*. 1999;14(5):748-755.

[41] Zuccati G. Implant therapy in cases of agenesis. *J Clin Orthod*. 1993;27(7):369-373.

[42] Senty EL. The maxillary cuspid and missing lateral incisors: esthetics and occlusion. *Angle Orthod*. 1976;46(4):365-371.

[43] Adell R, Eriksson B, Lekholm U, Brånemark PI, Jemt T. Long-term follow-up study of osseointegrated implants in the treatment of totally edentulous jaws. *Int J Oral Maxillofac Implants*. 1990;5(4):347-359.

[44] Ryser MR, Block MS, Mercante DE. Correlation of papilla to crestal bone levels around single tooth implants in immediate or delayed crown protocols. *J Oral Maxillofac Surg*. 2005;63(8):1184-1195.

[45] Choquet V, Hermans M, Adriaenssens P, et al. Clinical and radiographic evaluation of the papilla level adjacent to single-tooth dental implants. A retrospective study in the maxillary anterior region. *J Periodontol*. 2001;72(10):1364-1371.

[46] Tarnow D, Elian N, Fletcher P, et al. Vertical distance from the crest of bone to the height of the interproximal papilla between adjacent implants. *J Periodontol*. 2003;74(12):1785-1788.

[47] Park JH, Kim TW. Open-bite treatment utilizing clear removable appliances with intermaxillary and intramaxillary elastics. *World J Orthod*. 2009;10(2):130-134.

[48] Grunder U, Gracis S, Capelli M. Influence of the 3-D bone-to-implant relationship on esthetics. *Int J Periodontics Restorative Dent*. 2005;25(2):113-119.

[49] Jemt T. Regeneration of gingival papillae after single-implant treatment. *Int J Periodontics Restorative Dent*. 1997;17(4):326-333.

[50] Lekovic V, Kenney EB, Weinlaender M, et al. A bone regenerative approach to alveolar ridge maintenance following tooth extraction. Report of 10 cases. *J Periodontol*. 1997;68(6):563-570.

[51] Pradeep AR, Karthikeyan BV. Peri-implant papilla reconstruction: realities and limitations. *J Periodontol*. 2006;77(3):534-544.

[52] Tarnow DP, Cho SC, Wallace SS. The effect of inter-implant distance on the height of inter-implant bone crest. *J Periodontol*. 2000;71(4):546-549.

[53] Grunder U. Stability of the mucosal topography around single-tooth implants and adjacent teeth: 1-year results. *Int J Periodontics Restorative Dent*. 2000;20(1):11-17.

[54] Grunder U, Spielman HP, Gaberthüel T. Implant-supported single tooth replacement in the aesthetic region: a complex challenge. *Pract Periodontics Aesthet Dent*. 1996;8(9):835-842.

[55] Degidi M, Novaes AB Jr, Nardi D, Piattelli A. Outcome analysis of immediately placed, immediately restored implants in the esthetic area: the clinical relevance of different interimplant distances. *Periodontol.* 2008;79(6):1056-1061.

Interdisciplinary Treatment of Aggressive Periodontitis: Three-Dimensional Cone-Beam X-Ray Computed Tomography Evaluation

Tetsutaro Yamaguchi[1], Kazushige Suzuki[2],
Yoko Tomoyasu[1], Matsuo Yamamoto[2] and Koutaro Maki[1]
[1]*Department of Orthodontics, Showa University School of Dentistry, Tokyo,*
[2]*Department of Periodontology, Showa University School of Dentistry, Tokyo,*
Japan

1. Introduction

Periodontitis is characterized by an inflammatory reaction that affects tooth attachment tissues and can be classified as chronic periodontitis or aggressive periodontitis (AgP) according to clinical characteristics and rate of progression. The current classification of periodontal disease describes two clinically distinct forms of periodontitis. AgP is characterized by rapid progression and severe periodontal destruction, mainly seen in younger individuals (Meng et al., 2007). Chronic periodontitis is characterized by a lower rate of progression (Schätzle et al., 2009). AgP constitutes a group of rare and rapidly progressing forms of periodontitis that are frequently characterized by an early age of clinical onset (Genco et al., 1986). AgP is defined as a destructive periodontal disease affecting more than 14 teeth in young individuals. Its etiology has been linked to the presence of *Aggregatibacter actinomycetemcomitans* (Fine et al., 2007; Haraszthy et al., 2000; Di Rienzo et al., 1994), host response defects (Page et al., 1984, 1985; Lavine et al., 1979), and possibly to genetic inheritance (Hart & Kornman, 1997; Kinane et al., 2000; Boleghman et al., 1992; Beaty et al., 1987; Hart et al., 1992; Melnick et al., 1976; Page et al., 1985). In contrast, chronic periodontitis is characterized by a lower rate of progression (Schätzle et al., 2009), although like AgP it can reach a severe stage, leading to tooth loss and edentualism. Many clinicians report difficulty in establishing a differential diagnosis for AgP and chronic periodontitis due to an overlapping "gray area" that often negates a clear-cut diagnosis. Such issues raise the question of whether these are actually two distinct clinical entities.

In AgP, comprehensive mechanical/surgical and antimicrobial therapy is usually required for long-term stabilization of periodontal health (Buchmann et al., 2002). Enamel matrix proteins have been proposed to promote regeneration of the lost periodontal tissues when used during periodontal surgery (Gestrelius et al., 2000; Hammarström, 1997). Indeed, clinical studies showed that applying the commercially available enamel matrix derivative (EMD) to deep intrabony defects during periodontal flap surgery promotes a favorable clinical outcome in terms of clinical attachment gain and probing depth reduction (Heijl et al., 1997; Heden & Wennström, 2006). Other treatment alternatives for bone defects include grafting or extraction of the affected teeth, with possible orthodontic movement into the involved sites (McLain et al., 1983). AgP has the potential to cause tooth mobility and pathological tooth movement, and thus orthodontic treatment might become necessary. It is well established that despite bone loss, teeth can be moved orthodontically if the remaining bone and the periodontium can be brought back to a healthy state (Boyd et al., 1989).

Although the use of conventional computed tomography (CT) is well established in oral surgery (Gold et al., 2003), three-dimensional (3D) CT imaging can provide particularly useful information that may assist in diagnosis and planning of treatment strategies (Ferrario et al., 1996). Furthermore, computational simulations that include 3D image processing and biomechanical calculations show promise as useful tools for orthodontic research and assist in clinical decision-making (Maki et al., 2003).

This report describes the multidisciplinary treatment of AgP patient with progressing full-mouth bone resorption. Orthodontic treatment was performed after completion of periodontal treatment including regenerative surgery using EMD.

2. Diagnosis and etiology

An 18-year-old female patient was referred by a general practitioner to the Department of Periodontology at Showa University Dental Hospital for treatment of AgP (Fig. 1A). A review of her medical history did not reveal any systemic disease. Familial aggregation of AgP was denied. An initial examination revealed probing depths of 7 to 10 mm at teeth numbers 16, 15, 14, 13, 11, 21, 23, 24, 25, 26, 36, 35, 42, 43, 44, and 46, with bleeding on probing (Table 1A). Suppuration was registered at teeth numbers 15, 14, and 21. Full-mouth periapical radiographs revealed an overall pattern of severe horizontal bone loss with localized cratering (Fig. 1B).

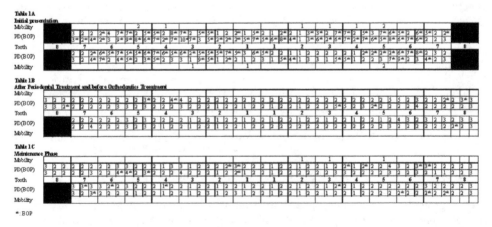

Table 1. (A-C). Probing depths (PD) and bleeding on probing (BOP) in the patient before, during, and after periodontal treatment.

A

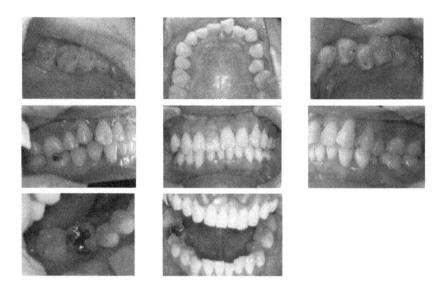

B

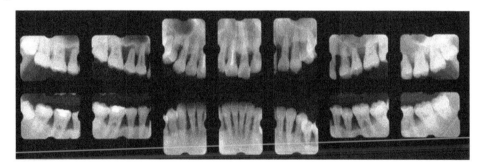

Fig. 1. Oral photographs at initial presentation (A) and dental X-rays at initial presentation (B).

Prior to commencing orthodontic treatment, the patient underwent periodontal treatment. Periodontal treatment involved oral hygiene instructions, scaling, root planing, temporary fixation using 4-META/MMA-TBB resin, occlusal adjustment, and periodontal surgery. After periodontal treatment the patient was introduced to the Department of Orthodontics at Showa University School of Dentistry for tooth alignment. She presented with a Class II malocclusion. Cone-beam CT (CBCT) imaging confirmed aggressive horizontal and vertical alveolar bone resorption throughout the whole area. Facial photographs before orthodontic treatment are presented in Fig. 2A. The maxillary central incisors were crowded (Fig. 2B). The patient's chief concerns for orthodontic treatment were the longevity of her front teeth and the possibility of enhancing aesthetics.

A

B

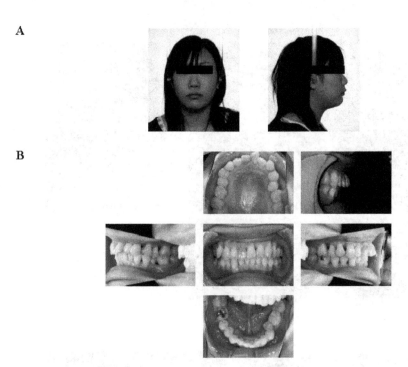

Fig. 2. Facial photographs before orthodontic treatment (A) and oral photographs before orthodontic treatment (B).

3. Treatment objectives

The clinical objectives of treatment were as follows: (1) to achieve adequate daily plaque control and clinically healthy gingiva, (2) to avoid occlusal trauma, and (3) to correct the planarization of the alveolar bone level. Furthermore, orthodontic treatment was also planned with the patient's expectations regarding with the longevity of her teeth and enhanced aesthetics.

4. Treatment results

Prior to commencing orthodontic treatment, the patient underwent periodontal treatment by a periodontist for 20 months. The primary goal in the treatment of this patient was to control her periodontal infection. Periodontal treatment was started by oral hygiene instruction and subsequent scaling and root planing under local anesthesia. Manual and ultrasonic instruments were used for scaling and root planing. Then, temporary fixation using 4-META/MMA-TBB resin (teeth numbers 16, 15, 14, 13, 23, 24, 25, 26, 33, 34, 35, 36, and 37) and occlusal adjustment were performed with the goals of reducing occlusal interferences in lateral excursions and improving canine guidance. Following the reevaluation after this initial treatment phase, periodontal surgery was performed. The bone defects at the maxillary right second premolar were subjected

to regenerative periodontal surgery. Intrabony defects and root surfaces were
degranulated and cleaned with curettes, rinsed with saline, and dried with cotton
swabs. The exposed root surfaces were demineralized using EDTA for 2 minutes. After
thorough rinsing with saline, EMD (Emdogain; Institut Straumann, Basel, Switzerland)
was applied to the root surfaces. The autogenous bone was then blended with EMD, and
the osseous defect was grafted. The autogenous bone was harvested using a trephine bar
from the extraction fossa around the right third molar in the mandible and crushed using
a bone mill (Fig. 3A, B). Radiographs obtained 3 years after surgery showed marked
filling of the defects and sharp contours of the hard tissue that had developed (Fig. 4A, B).

A   B

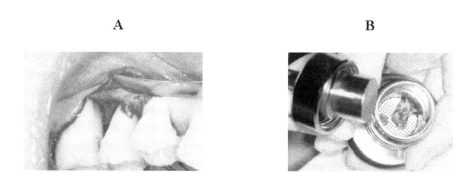

Fig. 3. Buccal view of the surgical wound after a full-thickness flap was reflected,
granulation tissue was removed, and the root surfaces and bone defect were conditioned
with EDTA. After thorough rinsing with saline, EMD was applied (A). The autogenous bone
was harvested using a trephine bar from the extraction fossa around the right third molar in
the mandible and crushed using a bone mill (B).

A   B

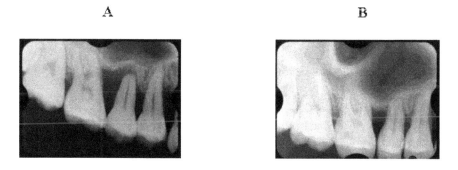

Fig. 4. Radiographs obtained 3 years after surgery showing a marked filling of the defects
and sharp contours of hard tissues gained through therapy.

The right first molar in the mandible had class I furcation involvement at the lingual sites. The furcation involvement was treated by a flap operation with furcation plasty (odontoplasty and osteoplasty) (Fig. 5). Clinical examination showed improved probing depths after periodontal treatment (Table 1B).

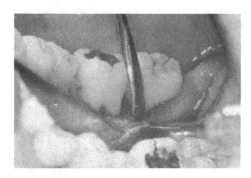

Fig. 5. The mandibular right first molar had class I furcation lesion at the lingual site. The furcation lesion was treated with furcation plasty.

All teeth were sequentially bonded or banded with 0.018- × 0.025-in standard edgewise brackets. For the upper teeth, a 0.012-in round stainless steel archwire was initially placed, followed by a 0.014-in round stainless steel archwire. By 6 months, the incisors were leveled by the use of a 0.016-in round stainless steel archwire. The alignment proceeded until a 0.016- × 0.016-in rectangular archwire was placed. For the lower teeth, the initial archwires consisted of the following: 0.012-in round stainless steel, 0.013- and 0.014-in nickel titanium, followed by 0.016- × 0.016-in nickel titanium archwires by the 9th month of treatment. The alignment proceeded until a 0.016- × 0.016-in rectangular archwire was placed. The patient was instructed to carefully clean around the orthodontic appliances and was monitored for gingival and tooth mobility changes at every orthodontic visit. The patient compliance was good throughout the orthodontic treatment period with regular periodontal maintenance appointments. Scaling, localized root planing, polishing, and follow-up examinations of plaque control were performed at each maintenance visit. After 12 months of orthodontic treatment, a removable Hawley retainer for the maxilla and mandible was recommended for nighttime use over the course of a year.

Post-treatment facial photographs are shown in Fig. 6A. Intraoral views (Fig. 6B) showed an acceptable occlusion in which a normal overbite and overjet were achieved. However, the intraoral view also showed that the midlines of the incisors were not coincident. We avoided aggressive tooth movement concerning to the damage of tooth root and periodontal tissue. This resulted in dis-coincident of midline. Cephalometric superimpositions (Fig. 7, Table 2) showed that the incisors were retracted 2 to 3 mm with a slight reduction in protrusion. After full orthodontic treatment, the left central incisor and canine in the maxilla were treated with a connective tissue graft (Fig. 8).

Interdisciplinary Treatment of Aggressive Periodontitis: Three-Dimensional Cone-Beam X-Ray Computed Tomography Evaluation

133

A

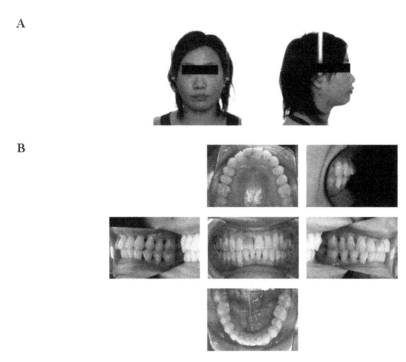

B

Fig. 6. Facial photographs (A) intraoral photographs (B) after orthodontic treatment.

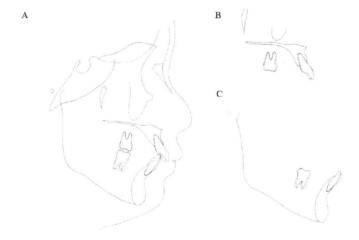

Fig. 7. Superimposed cephalometric tracings, pretreatment (solid line) and post-treatment (dotted line). (A) Superimposed on the SN plane registered at S. (B) Superimposed on the palatal plane registered at ANS. (C) Superimposed on the mandibular plane registered at Me.

Angular (°)	PRE-Tx		POST-Tx	
	Mean	SD	Mean	SD
SNA	83.1	+1	82.9	+1
SNB	78.1	−1	78.2	−1
ANB	5.0	+1	4.7	+1
Mandibular plane angle	33.4	−1	33.5	−1
Gonial angle	121.4	+1	121.7	+1
Ramus inclination	85.2	−1	85.3	−1
U1 to FH plane angle	121.5	+2	117.1	−1
L1 to Mandibular plane angle	102.8	+2	106.1	+2
FMIA	50.7	−1	54.0	−1

The data indicate mean and standard deviation (SD).

Table 2. Cephalometric analysis of patient pre- and post-treatment.

A   B

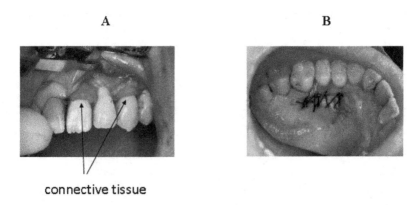

connective tissue

Fig. 8. Connective tissue graft for root coverage.

The satisfactory clinical results including the reduction in mean pocket depth from 3.9 ± 2.3 mm to 2.1 ± 0.6 mm and flattening of the alveolar bone level were achieved. Clinical examination showed appreciable gains in clinical attachment levels and improved probing depths from 1 to 4 mm at all sites after periodontal and orthodontic treatment (Table 1C). Radiographic analysis showed improvement in bone height at all sites. Overall, full mouth radiographs showed significant changes in the crater-like bone defects on teeth numbers 21, 23, 35, and 46 (Fig. 9A), and intraoral views showed aesthetic improvement by prosthetic treatment of the central incisor on the upper right side. Tooth mobility was also significantly reduced compared with pretreatment values. A complete blood count including differential blood counts also improved compared with pretreatment levels.

3D CT allows for precise assessment of bone defects caused by periodontal disease (Naito et al., 1998). In this study, CBCT (CB MercuRay; Hitachi Medical Technology, Tokyo, Japan) was performed prior to orthodontic treatment (Fig. 10, Fig. 12A) and during retention phases (Fig. 11, Fig. 12B). It was confirmed that all teeth were positioned appropriately in alveolar bone.

A

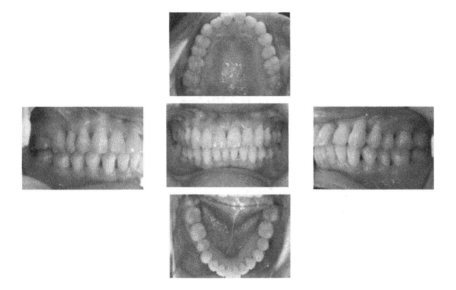

B

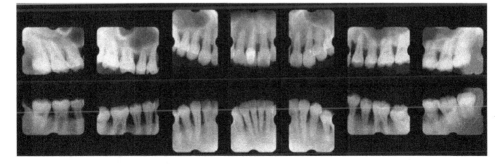

Fig. 9. Oral photographs after prosthetic treatment (A) and dental X-rays at retention (B).

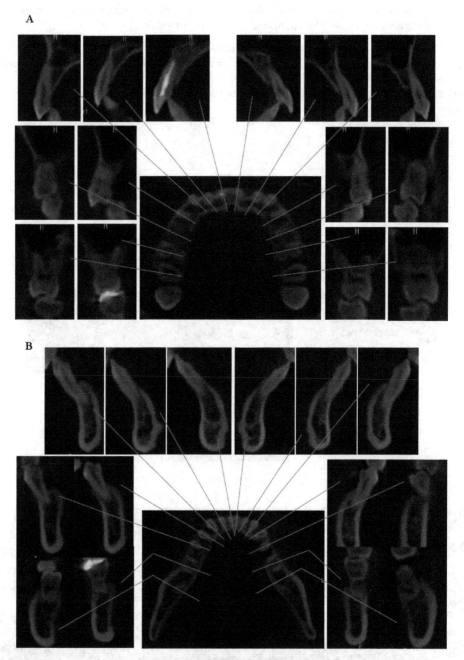

Fig. 10. Cone-beam X-ray computed tomography (CBCT) images of the upper arch in pre-orthodontic treatment (A) and CBCT images of the lower arch in pre-orthodontic treatment (B).

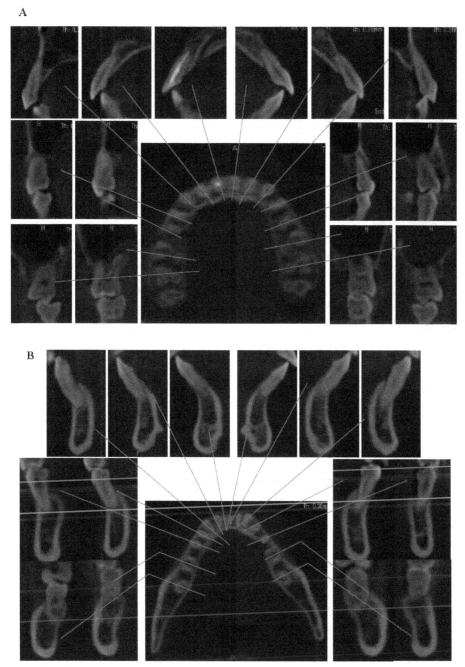

Fig. 11. Cone-beam X-ray computed tomography (CBCT) images of the upper arch during retention phases (A) and CBCT images of the lower arch during retention phases (B).

A

B

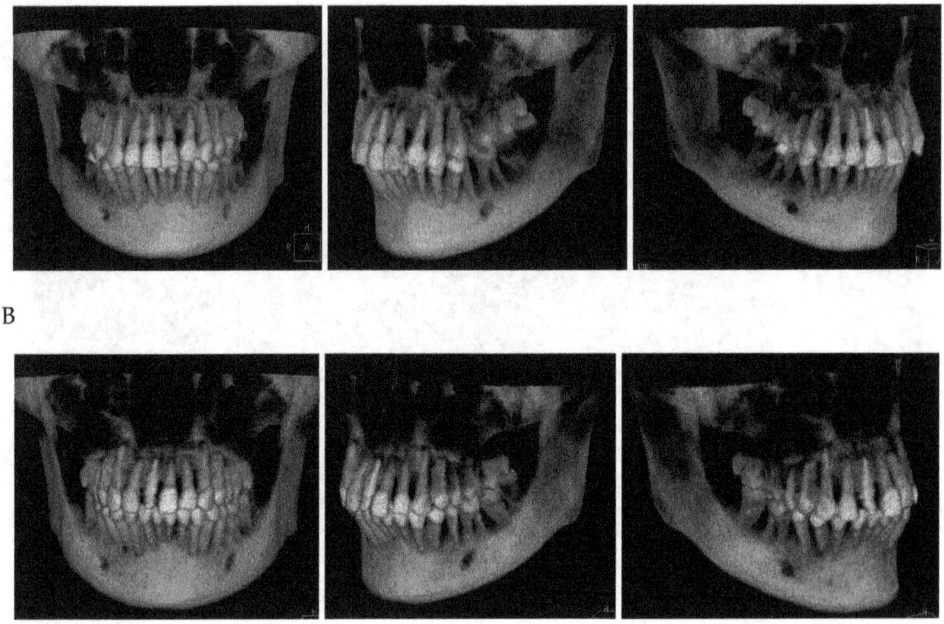

Fig. 12. Volumetric rendering in pre-orthodontic treatment (A) and in pre-orthodontic treatment (B)

5. Discussion

Rescala et al. (2010) reported similar microbiological and immunological parameters for subjects with chronic periodontitis and AgP who showed comparable periodontal disease severity. Herein we report dental management of an otherwise healthy patient diagnosed with generalized AgP and rapidly progressing bone loss throughout the mouth. Generalized AgP features loss of supporting tissues in addition to changes in tooth mobility and pathological tooth movement that are associated with sustained periodontal tissue destruction. In such cases, a comprehensive and effective treatment plan often includes periodontal therapy to relieve inflammation and orthodontic treatment to correct malocclusion. Comprehensive periodontal therapy is also often necessary in severe chronic periodontitis. The present patient showed a successful periodontal response with no progressive bone loss during or after treatment.

The strategy of treatment planning for periodontitis patients with aggressive or chronic periodontitis is well established. For patients with aggressive or chronic periodontitis, phases of treatment - systemic, initial, re-evaluation, surgical, maintenance, and restorative – are generally accepted. The amount of active planning required at each step may be greater for the patient with aggressive periodontal disease. To retain teeth cannot help but complicate the treatment-planning process. Therefore, the patient with aggressive periodontitis to have experienced attachment loss would be expected at a younger age, at a

faster rate and to a greater extent than the patient with chronic periodontitis (Deas et al.,
2010).

Some authors reported that tooth intrusion might deepen the defect and improve blood
circulation (Vandevska-Radunovic et al., 1994; Ericsson et al., 1977), suggesting that this
provides a better environment for guided tissue regeneration procedures (Rabie et al., 1996).
In the presence of osteoinductive factors, mesenchymal cells differentiate into cells capable
of regenerating the periodontal structures. This procedure is an alternative to rebuilding the
bone and the original periodontal architecture. It therefore seems reasonable to manage a
patient with compromised periodontal dentition using an interdisciplinary approach
consisting of both orthodontic and periodontal treatment strategies.

In this study, the initial periodontal treatment was followed by periodontal regeneration
therapy using EMD for the maxillary right second premolar. The bone defect involved one
to two wall defects and the radiographic bone gain was 4-5 mm in the 3 year follow-up
evaluationafter surgery. In prospective controlled clinical trials using EMD therapy, clinical
attachment gains of 2.2-3.4 mm have been observed in addition to bone growth (Pontoriero
et al., 1999; Sculean et al., 2001; Heijl et al., 1997). Thus, the clinical findings presented herein
are equal to or better than those in previous reports, and there are a number of clinical
scenarios associated with this therapy: (1) EMD only, if the defect is well contained, i.e., two-
and three-walled intrabony defects and craters; (2) a combination of EMD and graft
material, as in cases of moderate to deep, non-contained intraosseous defects; and (3) a
combination of EMD, graft material, and barrier membrane, as in supracrestal cases with
shallow intraosseous defects. In each case, a coronally advanced flap procedure must be
performed (Froum et al., 2001). Because the patient in this report presented with a non-
contained intraosseous bone defect of the maxillary right second premolar, we performed
combination therapy of EMD and autogenous grafting, which resulted in a satisfactory and
uneventful treatment outcome.

Meticulous initial therapy and good oral hygiene are considered prerequisites for successful
regenerative periodontal surgery (Cortellini et al., 1994). In studies reporting the best
regenerative outcomes, patients with chronic periodontitis were carefully selected regarding
oral hygiene performance, the proportion of bleeding sites remaining after initial
periodontal therapy, as well as smoking habits (Cortellini & Tonetti, 2005; Wachtel et al.,
2003). In agreement with these reports, the present patient with AgP qualified for
periodontal regeneration therapy using EMD as a nonsmoker with low plaque levels and
minimal bleeding scores.

Early comparisons of imaging techniques have shown that CT yields more detailed
information than conventional radiography for visualizing bone (Sarikaya et al., 2002;
Ericson & Kurol, 1988). Consequently, CT is now frequently used to qualitatively and
quantitatively assess potential implant sites (Fuhrmann et al., 1995), instead of conventional
dental radiographs, which do not allow for the evaluation of dehiscence at the implant site.
Cone Beam CT (CBCT) and other such 3D technologies compare well with traditional
methods, with the additional advantage that periodontal defects can be observed in all
directions (Misch et al., 2006). It is clinically important to determine the direction of
orthodontic movement and the groups of teeth with higher risks of dehiscence and

fenestration. In the present case, all teeth were appropriately maintained in alveolar bone, and the recovery of such bone in molar regions was also investigated using CBCT.

An important factor underlying the successful periodontal outcome and lack of progressive bone loss during and after treatment in the present case was the patient's strict adherence to regular periodontal maintenance at 3-monthly intervals. A recent longitudinal study indicated that patients with reduced, but healthy periodontal tissues (after successful periodontal treatment) undertook a full course of orthodontic treatment with fixed appliances without the occurrence of additional bone loss, provided that plaque removal was effective and a 3-monthly periodontal maintenance schedule was followed (Boyd et al., 1989). Periodontal disease progression was successfully arrested in 95% of the initially compromised lesions, while 2-5% of patients experienced discrete or recurrent episodes of loss of periodontal support (Buchmann et al., 2002). It is therefore clear that periodontal follow-up is crucial for successful treatment. In many patients with a periodontally involved dentition, pathological tooth migration can create serious functional and aesthetic problems. The coordination of proper orthodontic and periodontal therapies has proven to be effective in such situations, with long-term stability of the results obtained. A key point for achieving therapeutic success is therefore the patient's periodontal health status prior to and during the orthodontic treatment. Because periodontal health is essential for any form of dental treatment, good oral hygiene at home and professional maintenance care are important during and after active orthodontic treatment.

6. Conclusion

Prior to the commencement of orthodontic treatment, periodontal inflammation should be appropriately addressed by eliminating calculus and overhanging restorations, scaling, root planing, and instructing patients on proper oral hygiene. Deep pockets must be eliminated before orthodontic treatment to avoid apical displacement of plaque to avoid establishing progressive periodontal lesions.

Unlike other imaging methods, CBCT allows detailed imaging of periodontal defects to be gathered from a number of directions. The application of this technology is highly relevant for oral health professionals because it potentially provides the necessary information on tooth movement to the treating orthodontist and allows the periodontist to make treatment plans for periodontal disease.

7. Acknowledgment

We would like to acknowledge the clinically relevant technical advice given by Professor Hajime Miyashita.

8. References

Beaty, T.H., Boleghman, J.A., Yang, P., et al. (1987). Genetic analysis of juvenile periodontitis in families ascertained through an affected proband. *Am J Hum Genet*, Vol.40, No.5, (May 1987), pp. 443-452, ISSN 0002-9297

Boleghman, J.A., Astemborski, J.A., Suzuki, J.B. (1992). Phenotypic assessment of early onset periodontitis in sibships. *J Clin Periodontol*, Vol.19, No.4, (April 1992), pp. 233-239, ISSN 0303-6979

Boyd, R.L., Leggott, P.J., Quinn, R.S., et al. (1989). Periodontal implications of orthodontic treatment in adults with reduced or normal periodontal tissues versus those of adolescents. *Am J Orthod Dentofacial Orthop*, Vol.96, No.3, (September 1989), pp. 191-198, ISSN 0889-5406

Buchmann, R., Nunn, M.E., Van Dyke, T.E., et al. (2002). Aggressive periodontitis: 5-year follow-up of treatment. *J Periodontol*, Vol.73, No.6, (June 2002), pp. 675-683, ISSN 0022-3492

Cortellini, P., Pini-Prato, G., Tonetti, M. (1994). Periodontal regeneration of human infrabony defects (V). Effect of oral hygiene on long-term stability. *J Clin Periodontol*, Vol.21, No.9, (October 1994), pp. 606-610, ISSN 0303-6979

Cortellini, P., Tonetti, M.S. (2005). Clinical performance of a regenerative strategy for intrabony defects: Scientific evidence and clinical experience. *J Periodontol*, Vol.76, No.3, (March 2005), pp. 341-350, ISSN 0022-3492

Deas, D.E., Mealey, B.L. (2010). Response of chronic and aggressive periodontitis to treatment. *Periodontol 2000*, Vol.53, (June 2010), pp. 154-166, ISSN 1600-0757

Di Rienzo, J.M., Slots, J., Sixou, M., et al. (1994). Specific genetic variants of *Actinobacillus actinomycetemcomitans* correlate with disease and health in a regional population of families with localized juvenile periodontitis. *Infect Immun*, Vol.62, No.8, (August 1994), pp. 3058-3065, ISSN 0019-9567

Ericsson, I., Thilander, B., Lindhe, J., et al. (1977). The effect of orthodontic tilting movements on the periodontal tissues of infected and non-infected dentitions in dogs. *J Clin Periodontol*, Vol.4, No.4, (November 1977), pp. 278-293., ISSN 0303-6979

Ericson, S., Kurol, J. (1988) CT diagnosis of ectopically erupting maxillary canines--a case report. *Eur J Orthod*, Vol.10, No.2, (May 1988), pp. 115-121, ISSN 0141-5387

Ferrario, V.F., Sforza, C., Puleo, A., et al. (1996). Three-dimensional facial morphometry and conventional cephalometrics: a correlation study. *Int J Adult Orthodon Orthognath Surg*, Vol.11, No.4, (1996), pp. 329-338, ISSN 0742-1931

Fine, D., Markowitz, K., Furgang, D., et al. (2007). *Aggregatibacter actinomycetemcomitans* and its relationship to initiation of localized aggressive periodontitis: Longitudinal cohort study of initially healthy adolescents. *J Clin Microbiol*, Vol.45, No.12, (December 2007), pp. 3859-3869, ISSN 0095-1137

Froum, S., Lemler, J., Horowitz, R., et al. (2001). The use of enamel matrix derivative in the treatment of periodontal osseous defects: a clinical decision tree based on biologic principles of regeneration. *Int J Periodontics Restorative Dent*, Vol.21, No.5, (October 2001), pp. 437-449, ISSN 0198-7569

Fuhrmann, R.A., Wehrbein, H., Langen, H.J., et al. (1995). Assessment of the dentate alveolar process with high resolution computed tomography. *Dentomaxillofac Radiol*,Vol.24, No.1, (February 1995), pp. 50-54, ISSN 0250-832X

Genco, R.J., Christersson, L.A., Zambon, J.J. (1986). Juvenile periodontitis. *Int Dent J*, Vol.36, No.3, (September 1986), pp. 168-176, ISSN 0020-6539

Gestrelius, S., Lyngstadaas, S.P., Hammarström, L. (2000). Emdogain--periodontal regeneration based on biomimicry. *Clin Oral Investig*, Vol.4, No.2, (June 2000), pp. 120-125, ISSN 1432-6981

Gold, L., Nazarian, L.N., Johar, A.S., et al. (2003). Characterization of maxillofacial soft tissue vascular anomalies by ultrasound and color Doppler imaging: an adjuvant to computed tomography and magnetic resonance imaging. *J Oral Maxillofac Surg*, Vol.61, No.1, (January 2003), pp. 19-31, ISSN 0278-2391

Hammarström, L. (1997). Enamel matrix, cementum development and regeneration. *J Clin Periodontol*, Vol.24, No.9 Pt 2, (September 1997), pp. 658-668, ISSN 0303-6979

Haraszthy, V.I., Hariharan, G., Tinoco, E.M., et al. (2000). Evidence for the role of highly leukotoxic *Actinobacillus actinomycetemcomitans* in the pathogenesis of localized juvenile and other forms of early-onset periodontitis. *J Periodontol*, Vol.71, No.6, (June 2000), pp. 912-922, ISSN 0022-3492

Hart, T.C., Kornman, K.S. (1997). Genetic factors in the pathogenesis of periodontitis. *Periodontol 2000*, Vol.14, (June 1997), pp. 202-215, ISSN 0906-6713

Hart, T.C., Marazita, M.L., Schenkein, H.A., et al. (1992). Re-interpretation of the evidence for X-linked dominant inheritance of juvenile periodontitis. *J Periodontol*. Vol.63, No.3, (March 1992), pp. 169-173, ISSN 0022-3492

Heden, G., Wennström, J.L. (2006). Five-year follow-up of regenerative periodontal therapy with enamel matrix derivative at sites with angular bone defects. *J Periodontol*, Vol.77, No.2, (February 2006), pp. 295-301, ISSN 0022-3492

Heijl, L., Heden, G., Svärdström, G., et al.. (1997) Enamel matrix derivative (EMDOGAIN) in the treatment of intrabony periodontal defects. *J Clin Periodontol*. Vol.24, No.9 Pt 2, (September 1997), pp. 705-714, ISSN 0303-6979

Kinane, D.F., Shiba, H., Hart, T.C. (2005). The genetic basis of periodontitis. *Periodontol 2000*, Vol.39, (2005), pp. 91-117, ISSN 0906-6713

Lavine, W.S., Maderazo, E.G., Stolman, J., et al. (1979). Impaired neutrophil chemotaxis in patients with juvenile and rapidly progressing periodontitis. *J Peridontal Res*, Vol.14, No.1, (January 1979), pp. 10-19, ISSN 0022-3484

Maki, K., Inou, N., Takanishi, A., et al. (2003). Computer-assisted simulations in orthodontic diagnosis and the application of a new cone beam X-ray computed tomography. *Orthod Craniofac Res*, Vol.6, Suppl 1, (2003), pp. 95-101, ISSN 1601-6335

McLain, J.B., Proffit, W.R., Davenport, R.H. (1983). Adjunctive orthodontic therapy in the treatment of juvenile periodontitis: report of a case and review of the literature. *Am J Orthod*, Vol.83, No.4, (April 1983), pp. 290-298, ISSN 0002-9416

Melnick, M., Shields, E.D., Bixler, D. (1976). Periodontosis: A phenotypic and genetic analysis. *Oral Surg Oral Med Oral Pathol*, Vol.42, No.1, (July 1976), pp. 32-41, ISSN 0030-4220

Meng, H., Xu, L., Li, Q., et al. (2007). Determinants of host susceptibility in aggressive periodontitis. Periodontol 2000, Vol.43, (2007), pp. 133-159, ISSN 0906-6713

Misch, K.A., Yi, E.S., Sarment, D.P. (2006). Accuracy of cone beam computed tomography for periodontal defect measurements. *J Periodontol*, Vol.77, No.7, (July 2006), pp. 1261-1266, ISSN 0022-3492

Naito, T., Hosokawa, R., Yokota, M. (1998). Three-dimensional alveolar bone morphology analysis using computed tomography. *J Periodontol*. Vol.69, No.5, (May 1998), pp. 584-589, ISSN 0022-3492

Page, R.C., Sims, T.J., Geissler, F., et al. (1984). Abnormal leukocyte motility in patients with early-onset periodontitis. *J Peridontal Res*, Vol.19, No.6, (November 1984), pp. 591-594, ISSN 0022-3484

Page, R.C., Sims, T.J., Geissler, F., et al. (1985). Defective neutrophil and monocyte motility in patients with early onset periodontitis, *Infect Immun*, Vol.47, No.1, (January 1985), pp. 169-175, ISSN 0019-9567

Page, R.C., Vandesteen, G.E., Ebersole, J.L., et al. (1985). Clinical and laboratory studies of a family with a high prevalence of juvenile periodontitis. *J Periodontol*. Vol.56, No.10, (October 1985), pp. 602-610, ISSN 0022-3492

Pontoriero, R., Wennström, J., Lindhe, J. (1999). The use of barrier membranes and enamel matrix proteins in the treatment of angular bone defects. A prospective controlled clinical study. *J Clin Periodontol*, Vol.26, No.12, (December 1999), pp. 833-840, ISSN 0303-6979

Rabie, A.B., Dan, Z., Samman, N. (1996). Ultrastructural identification of cells involved in the healing of intramembranous and endochondral bones. *Int J Oral Maxillofac Surg*, Vol.25, No.5, (October 1996), pp. 383-388, ISSN 0901-5027

Rescala, B., Rosalem, W. Jr., Teles, R.P., et al. (2010). Immunologic and microbiologic profiles of chronic and aggressive periodontitis subjects. *J Periodontol*, Vol.81, No.9, (2010), pp. 1308-1316, ISSN 1943-3670

Sarikaya, S., Haydar, B., Ciğer, S., et al. (2002). Changes in alveolar bone thickness due to retraction of anterior teeth. *Am J Orthod Dentofacial Orthop*, Vol.122, No.1, (July 2002), pp. 15-26, ISSN 0889-5406

Schätzle, M., Faddy, M.J., Cullinan, M.P., et al. (2009). The clinical course of chronic periodontitis: V. Predictive factors in periodontal disease. *J Clin Periodontol*, Vol.36, No.5, (2009), pp. 365-371, ISSN 1600-051X

Sculean, A., Windisch, P., Chiantella, G.C., et al. (2001). Treatment of intrabony defects with enamel matrix proteins and guided tissue regeneration. A prospective controlled clinical study. *J Clin Periodontol*, Vol.28, No.5, (May 2001), pp. 397-403, ISSN 0303-6979

Wachtel, H., Schenk, G., Böhm, S., et al. (2003). Microsurgical access flap and enamel matrix derivative for the treatment of periodontal intrabony defect: A controlled clinical study. *J Clin Periodontol*, Vol.30, No.6, (June 2003), pp. 496-504, ISSN 0303-6979

Vandevska-Radunovic, V., Kristiansen, A.B., Heyeraas, K.J., et al. (1994). Changes in blood circulation in teeth and supporting tissues incident to experimental tooth movement. *Eur J Orthod*, Vol.16, No.5, (October 1994), pp. 361-369, ISSN 0141-5387

9

Association Between Self-Efficacy and Oral Self-Care Behaviours in Patients with Chronic Periodontitis

Naoki Kakudate[1] and Manabu Morita[2]
[1]Department of Epidemiology and Healthcare Research,
Kyoto University School of Medicine and Public Health
[2]Department of Oral Health, Okayama University Graduate School of Medicine,
Dentistry and Pharmaceutical Sciences
Japan

1. Introduction

A number of major health behaviour theories have been academically established and include the Health Belief Model (HBM), Self-efficacy Theory, the Protection Motivation Theory (PMT), the Theory of Planned Behaviour (TPB), Locus of Control, Sense of Coherence, and the Transtheoretical Model. The HBM was originally developed to predict the likelihood of patients' participation in preventive health behaviours (Rosenstock, 1974). The HBM was later modified to incorporate the concept of self-efficacy, which is the strength of an individuals' belief that he or she can successfully enact behavioural change, improving the ability of this model to predict behavioural outcomes (Martin et al., 2010). Rogers (1975) expanded the HBM to include additional factors to improve the conceptual understanding of fear appeals. He further extended his proposed theory, the PMT, to a more general theory of persuasive communication that emphasized the cognitive processes underlying behavioural change (Rogers, 1983).

The TPB (Ajzen, 1991), which is an extension of the Theory of Reasoned Action (TRA) (Ajzen and Fishbein, 1980), targets situations in which individuals lack complete control over a particular behaviour. Similarly to the TRA, the central importance of this theory is not an individual's intention, but rather that behaviour is influenced by attitudes and subjective norms, in addition to perceived behavioural control, which closely resembles the concept of self-efficacy (Martin et al., 2010). Two additional constructs have been developed, the Health Locus of Control (Rotter, 1966) and the Sense of Coherence (Antonovsky, 1987), which evaluate an individual's psychological characteristics with respect to controlling health-related behaviours. Finally, the Transtheoretical Model of Behavioural Change is a model of intentional change that combines the Behaviour Modification Theory and an educational health programme (DiClemente et al., 1991). This model is comprised of five core constructs: stages of change, processes of change, decisional balance, temptation, and self-efficacy.

In this chapter, we describe the relationship between oral self-care and self-efficacy as it relates to chronic periodontitis patients. The self-efficacy theory has several important features that warrant its examination in this context. First, this theory has strong relationships with numerous health behavioural theories. Second, it has been demonstrated within a theoretical framework that enhancing self-efficacy leads to behaviour modification. Last, due to the simplicity of the self-efficacy theory, it can easily be applied in the daily clinical setting.

2. Self-efficacy theory

Bandura (1977) observed that the actions of individuals are associated with both outcome and efficacy expectations. The former is outcome expectancy related to achieving a desirable outcome by taking an action, whereas the latter is related to the confidence an individual has for performing an action necessary to produce the desired outcome and is termed self-efficacy (Bandura, 1977, 1997; Kakudate et al., 2010a). The existence of both types of expectations is needed for an individual to act (Figure 1). Thus, self-efficacy is an important factor for predicting individual action and controlling subsequent emotional responses.

Self-efficacy relates to the belief in one's general confidence to accomplish the actions necessary to reach a goal. When applied to the clinical setting, self-efficacy refers to a patient's perception of his or her ability to perform the actions needed to improve and maintain their health. Two levels of self-efficacy have been described: general self-efficacy, which reflects an individual's general and stable tendencies, and task-specific self-efficacy, which are beliefs related to a certain task (Sherer et al., 1982; Woodruff and Cashman, 1993; Stanley and Murphy, 1997).

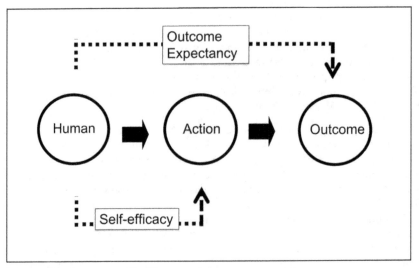

Fig. 1. Relationship between self-efficacy and outcome expectations

Self-efficacy is the belief in the capacity to perform a specific behaviour, whereas outcome expectations are the beliefs that carrying out a specific behaviour will lead to a desired outcome.

3. Self-efficacy in the clinical practice

In the clinical practice, the enhancement of self-efficacy has been shown to improve symptoms of chronic disease, such as diabetes, indicating that self-efficacy represents an antecedent to behaviour modification (Smarr et al., 1997; Wattana et al., 2007). For example, Smarr et al. (1997) examined the relationship between induced changes in self-efficacy following a stress management programme and outcome measures of depression, pain, health status, and disease status in rheumatoid arthritis patients, and found a significant association between self-efficacy modification and the clinically relevant outcome measures.

In the dental field, the relationship between self-efficacy and oral hygiene behaviour, such as toothbrushing or flossing, has been examined in several studies (McCaul et al., 1985; Tedesco et al., 1991, 1992; Stewart et al., 1997; Syrjälä et al., 1999, 2004). McCaul et al. (1985) analysed self-efficacy among college students with respect to brushing and flossing to predict task-related behaviours, and found that the retrospectively self-reported and prospective frequency of the two examined oral care factors were significantly associated with self-efficacy. Subsequently, Tedesco et al. (1991) reported that the addition of self-efficacy variables to the theory of reasoned action variables markedly increased the observed variance in brushing and flossing behaviours. Furthermore, it was demonstrated that cognitive behavioural intervention resulted in a delayed relapse in protective oral self-care behaviour and improved self-efficacy towards flossing (Tedesco et al., 1991). These researchers further analysed the associations between oral health behaviour and self-efficacy and the TRA, and found that linking the variables of the two theories significantly increased the variance in the brushing and flossing behaviours (Tedesco et al., 1992). Syrjälä et al. (2004) performed a comparative analysis to examine the relationships of psychological characteristics related to health behaviours, including intention, self-efficacy, locus of control, and self-esteem, and oral health-care habits, diabetes treatment adherence, number of dental caries and deepened periodontal pockets, and HbA1c (glycosylated haemoglobin) levels. Based on this analysis, only self-efficacy was found to be associated with both oral health-care habits and diabetes adherence.

Several cross-sectional studies have also examined self-efficacy and oral hygiene behaviour. For example, Stewart et al. (1997) measured self-efficacy with respect to toothbrushing and flossing using questionnaires, and demonstrated that self-efficacy scale scores are significantly associated with the frequency of brushing, flossing frequency, and dental visits, in addition to general dental knowledge. Notably, however, clinical periodontal parameters were not surveyed, nor is it clear whether the study participants suffered from periodontal disease. Syrjälä et al. (1999) conducted a cross-sectional survey for 149 insulin-dependent diabetic patients using a self-efficacy scale, which consisted of items related to the self-efficacies of toothbrushing, approximal tooth cleaning, and dental visits, and examined the associations of self-efficacy with oral health behaviour and dental plaque levels. The results of their analyses showed that the scores for all three examined items in the self-efficacy scale were related to self-reported oral health behaviours, and that visible plaque index values inversely correlated with the self-efficacies of toothbrushing and dental visits. However, again, it is unclear whether the study participants, who consisted of only diabetic patients, had periodontal disease.

4. Development of a self-efficacy scale for self-care (SESS) for patients with chronic periodontitis

In the context of periodontal disease, the efficacy of regular professional and patient self-care has been examined in detail (Kressin et al., 2003; Axelsson et al., 2004; Douglass, 2006). The adherence of periodontal disease patients to health-promoting behaviour is considered critical for the prevention and successful treatment of periodontal disease. In an effort to improve oral health-care behaviour, we previously conducted a cross-sectional study consisting of a questionnaire and a clinical assessment to develope a task-specific SESS for periodontal disease patients (Kakudate et al., 2007, 2008). The subjects of the study were 140 patients (64 females and 76 males, 19 to 86 years of age, mean age 51.7 ± 15.7) with mild to moderate chronic periodontitis.

The SESS consists of 15 items that are divided into three sub-scales: (i) self-efficacy for dentist consultations (SE-DC; five items), which relates to treatment adherence and regular dental check-ups (e.g., "I go to the dentist for treatment of periodontal disease"); (ii) self-efficacy for brushing of the teeth (SE-B; five items), which concerns the careful and thorough brushing of teeth (e.g., "I brush my teeth as instructed"); and (iii) self-efficacy for dietary habits (SE-DH; five items), which relates to adopting well-balanced eating and drinking habits (e.g., "I eat my meals at fixed times during the day"). All answers are scored using a five-point Likert scale (Tarini et al., 2007) ranging from 1 (not confident) to 5 (completely confident), and the scores for all 15 items are then summed to give total SESS scores ranging from 15 to 75 for each participant.

The reliability of the SESS was preliminarily verified using conventional methods (Carmines and Zeller, 1980; Syrjälä et al., 1999; Resnick et al., 2000; Travess et al., 2004; Champion et al., 2005; George et al., 2007; Rossen and Gruber, 2007) for both internal consistency (Cronbach's alpha = 0.86) and test-retest stability (Spearman's rank correlation coefficient = 0.73; $P < 0.001$). Based on Spearman's rank correlation coefficient analysis, the test-retest stability scores of the SE-DC, SE-B, and SE-DH components of the SESS were 0.57 ($P < 0.01$), 0.39 ($P < 0.05$), and 0.53 ($P < 0.01$), respectively. Construct validity of the scale was also demonstrated in a cross-sectional study that found periodontal patients with successful maintenance therapy had significantly higher SESS scores (mean value, 60.90 ± 6.64; n = 60) than those of initial-visit patients who had not received periodontal treatment (mean value, 56.86 ± 7.56; n = 129) ($P < 0.001$).

5. Predicting loss to follow-up in long-term periodontal treatment using the SESS

As described in Section 3, self-efficacy can be divided into general and task-specific self-efficacy. To compare these two types of efficacy with respect to oral care behaviour, we examined whether our developed SESS and a general self-efficacy scale (GSES) (Sakano and Tohjoh, 1986) could predict short-term compliance (within one year) for active periodontal treatment (Kakudate et al., 2008). The results of our pilot study revealed that only the SESS, particularly the SE-DC subscale, accurately predicted loss to follow-up from active periodontal treatment (Kakudate et al., 2008). As the continued maintenance of periodontal health care is considered critical for preventing relapse after active periodontal treatment, we further evaluated the hypothesis that SESS can predict loss to long-term follow-up during periodontal treatment by performing a 30-month longitudinal prospective cohort study for patients with mild to moderate chronic periodontitis. In our study, the odds ratios of the loss to follow-up for the middle- (54–59) and low-scoring (15–53) SESS groups were 1.05 (95% confidence interval: 0.36–3.07) and 4.56 (95% confidence interval: 1.11–18.74), respectively, compared to the high-scoring group (60–75) (Kakudate et al., 2010b). We therefore concluded that the assessment of self-efficacy specific to oral health care may allow prediction of loss to follow-up in long-term periodontal treatment. In addition, enhancing self-efficacy through psychoeducational intervention may reduce the number of patients lost to follow-up.

6. The four principal self-efficacy information sources

Self-efficacy beliefs are constructed from four principal sources of information: enactive mastery experience, vicarious experience, verbal persuasion, and physiological and affective states (Bandura, 1977, 1978, 1997). The first information source, enactive mastery experience, relates to an individual's accomplishments, with previous successes increasing expectations of mastery in subsequent tasks and repeated failures serving to lower them. The second source, vicarious experience, is obtained through the learning associated with observing a task or activity being successfully performed by others, and is often referred to as modelling. The third element, verbal persuasion, refers to the use of suggestive language to convince an individual that he or she can successfully perform a specific task. Common forms of verbal persuasion include coaching and evaluative feedback for performance, and help to support (persuade) an individual's belief that he or she possesses a certain capability. The fourth element, physiological and affective states, represents the physiological and emotional states, respectively, which influence an individual's assessment of self-efficacy. Through the effective exploitation of these four sources of information, it is therefore possible to enhance self-efficacy, which may have significant impacts with respect to oral health care in the field of dentistry. For example, Syrjälä et al. (2001) reported qualitative evidence that the sources of self-efficacy proposed by Bandura (1977), namely personal experience, emotional arousal, and modelling, are also supported in the context of oral health behaviour.

7. Enhancement of self-efficacy for self-care through six step method

The six-step method is a systematic approach that was designed to facilitate lifestyle changes in patients including principal self-efficacy information sources (Farquhar, 1987; Albright and Farquhar, 1992) and consists of the following six steps: (i) problem identification; (ii) instilling confidence and commitment; (iii) increasing behavioural awareness; (iv) developing and implementing an action plan; (v) plan evaluation; and (vi) maintaining the behavioural change and preventing relapse. Six-step method has been applied to periodontal dental practice as following steps (Kakudate et al., 2009).

Step 1. Identifying the problem

Knowledge, belief, and the barrier to periodontal self-care were clarified by person-to-person interviews. This information was obtained by asking the patient the following questions:

1. What do you do about self-care?
   a. How many times and how long do you brush?
   b. How many times do you perform inter-dental cleaning per week?
   c. When do you brush?
2. What do you know about self-care?
3. Have you tried to change your behavior in the past?
4. What inhibits the change in your belief? or What are your major barriers to change?

The patients are clearly told what the problems are, and the patients are told that their behaviors are harmful to their health and that modification of this behavior must be made.

Step 2. Creating confidence and commitment

There are many patients who have the conviction that changing their self-care behavior is not possible. Step 2 involves establishing commitment and confidence by conducting the clinical interview to incorporate counseling that assesses the patient's barrier to change his/her behavior. A story of a person who seems to be a model in a similar situation was introduced to raise the patient become aware of his/her assumption. In order to confirm intention and to promote motivation, the patient and the dentist signed a contract to begin working on a particular behavior change after face-to-face counseling.

Step 3. Increasing awareness of behavior

This step leads to increase in the patient's awareness of his or her behavior patterns through self-monitoring. The patients were asked to keep a diary of brushing and inter-dental cleaning every day until the next consultation and to describe their feelings at that time of brushing. The diary is used to determine the internal and external precursors to the behavior that often act as behavioral cues. The diary also helps to identify barriers to behavioral change in oral self-care.

Step 4. Developing and implementing the action plan

Based on the patient's behavior, description in the diary of oral hygiene measures, and oral hygiene states, a short-term action plan is set up by the principle of gradualism. The action plan was concrete, realistic, and achievable. For instance, the action plan includes "Brush twice a day", "Brush for more than three minutes", and "Use dental floss once a day at night" Then an incentive that a patient gives himself/herself when succeeding was decided. Small incentives such as beauty treatment, going to the movie, and shopping are selected. In the setting of the goal and the incentive, the dentist only supported the decision by the patient.

Step 5. Evaluating the plan

Whether or not the patient achieved the action plan is evaluated. Success is acknowledged and supported. When the plan succeeded, the success experience is acknowledged, and the subject is praised. If the patient fail, this is attributed to a failure of the plan, and a new plan that can be achieved is set up.

Step 6. Maintaining change and preventing relapse

Each patient has high-risk situations that might result in relapse. Unexpected long working hours, social events such as parties, and alcohol consumption often make it difficult to maintain newly acquired behaviors. Therefore, it is important for dentists and dental hygienists to help and encourage the patient to safeguard and reinforce the new behaviors. As in Step 4, incentives might be effective. Incentives can apply to a particular longer period of maintenance.

8. Evidence of behavioural approaches for self-care

According to a systematic review by the Cochrane Collaboration, several studies have suggested that psychological approaches to behavioral management can improve behaviours related to oral hygiene (Renz et al., 2007). This finding supports the use of psychological models in studies aimed at establishing intervention approaches for modifying oral health-related behaviour. In the review, four studies that applied psychological models were selected based on the Cochrane Oral Health Group methods (Renz et al., 2007). However, the reviewers concluded that overall quality of the included trials was low, thus limiting the conclusions that could be drawn, and in addition, the applied intervention was weakly designed and lacked key aspects of the major behavioural theories.

Since 2007, two randomized controlled trials (RCTs) have been conducted to evaluate intervention based on key aspects of the self-efficacy theory. Clarkson et al. (2009) conducted a RCT that was randomized by either patient (Patient) or dentist (Cluster) and included 87 dental practices and 778 adult patients (Patient RCT = 37 dentists / 300 patients; Cluster RCT = 50 dentists / 478 patients). The study patients were subjected to evidence-based intervention that targeted oral hygiene self-efficacy and action plans. After adjustment for baseline differences, patients who received the intervention exhibited improved behavioural (timing, duration, and method), cognitive (self-efficacy and planning), and clinical (plaque and gingival bleeding) outcomes. However, on comparison of the Patient and Cluster RCTs, the clinical outcomes were only significantly improved in the latter, suggesting that the trial design may have influenced the results.

In the second RCT, our group compared the efficacy of a six-step method to enhance self-efficacy with that of conventional oral hygiene instruction (Kakudate et al., 2009; Morita et al., 2010). Our RCT consisted of 38 patients with mild to moderate chronic periodontitis (Control group : Intervention group = 20 : 18) who were receiving periodontal treatment at a private dental clinic located in Sapporo, Japan. In both study groups, all examined variables, including Plaque Control Record (PCR) scores (O'Leary et al., 1972), tooth brushing duration, weekly frequency of interdental cleaning, and self-efficacy scores, significantly improved from the initial to the third clinic visit. Notably, we found that the intervention group, who received oral hygiene instruction using the six-step method, displayed higher self-efficacy than the control group, who were only provided with conventional oral hygiene instructions. In addition, PCR scores, toothbrushing duration, and weekly frequency of interdental cleaning also improved in the intervention group as compared with the control group.

In the two RCTs presented here, the enhancement of self-efficacy and ability to promote behavioural change through behavioural intervention was clearly observed; however, the methodology of intervention has yet to be fully established. Thus, further studies are needed to evaluate the suitability of these intervention methods with respect to oral health care in the clinical setting.

9. Conclusion

The assessment of self-efficacy towards oral health care is effective for the prediction of oral self-care behaviour in periodontal treatment. Therefore, by addressing low self-efficacy early and providing patient support to enhance self-efficacy in the clinical setting, loss to long-term follow-up during periodontal treatment can be minimized. Although behavioural approaches may enhance the self-efficacy for self-care habits and result in improved oral hygiene status, further research to evaluate the suitability of the specific intervention methodology is required. In addition, it is also important to determine whether applying methods developed based on past research results might provide any disadvantages to periodontal patients.

10. References

Ajzen I (1991). The theory of planned behaviour. *Organ Behav Hum Decis Process*, 50, 179–211, 0749-5978

Ajzen I, Fishbein M (1980). *Understanding attitudes and predicting social Behavior* (1 edition), Prentice Hall Inc, 0139364358, Enflewood cliffs

Albright CL, Farquhar JW (1992). Principles of behavioral change. In: *Introduction to clinical medicine*, Greene HM, pp. 596–601, BC Decker, Inc., 1556642334, Philadelphia

Antonovsky A (1987). *Unraveling the mystery of health: how people manage stress and stay well (1 edition)*, Jossey-Bass Publishers, 1555420281, San Francisco.

Axelsson P, Nystrom B, & Lindhe J (2004). The long-term effect of a plaque control program on tooth mortality, caries and periodontal disease in adults. Results after 30 years of maintenance. *J Clin Periodontol* 31: 749–757, 0303-6979

Bandura A (1977). Self-efficacy: toward a unifying theory of behavioral change. *Psychol Rev*, 84, 191–215, 0033-295X

Bandura A (1978). Reflections on self-efficacy. *Adv Behav Res Ther*, 1, 237–269, 0146-6402

Bandura A (1997). *Self-efficacy: the exercise of control*, W. H. Freeman and Company, 0716728508, New York City

Carmines EG, Zeller RA (1980). *Reliability and validity assessment*, SAGE Publications, 0803913710, London

Champion V, Skinner CS, & Menon U (2005). Development of a self-efficacy scale for mammography. *Res Nurs Health*, 28, 329–336, 0160-6891

Clarkson JE, Young L, Ramsay CR, Bonner BC, & Bonetti D (2009). How to influence patient oral hygiene behavior effectively. *J Dent Res*, 88, 933–937, 0022-0345

DiClemente CC, Prochaska JO, Fairhurst SK, Velicer WF, Velasquez MM, & Rossi JS (1991). The process of smoking cessation: an analysis of precontemplation contemplation, and preparation stage of change. *J Consult Clin Psychol*, 59, 295–304, 0022-006X

Douglass CW (2006). Risk assessment and management of periodontal disease. *J Am Dent Assoc*, 137, 27S–32S, 0002-8177

Farquhar JW (1987). *The American way of life need not be hazardous to your Health*, Da Capo Press, 0201121867, New York City

George S, Clark M, Crotty M (2007). Development of the Adelaide driving self-efficacy scale. *Clin Rehabil*, 21, 56–61, 0269-2155

Kakudate N, Morita M, Fujisawa M, Nagayama M, & Kawanami M (2007). Development of the Self-Efficacy Scale for Self-care (SESS) among periodontal disease patients (in Japanese). *J Jpn Soc Periodontol*, 49, 285–295, 0385-0110

Kakudate N, Morita M, & Kawanami M (2008). Oral health care-specific self-efficacy assessment predicts patient completion of periodontal treatment: a pilot cohort study. *J Periodontol*, 79, 1041–1047, 0022-3492

Kakudate N, Morita M, Sugai M, & Kawanami M (2009). Systematic cognitive behavioral approach for oral hygiene instruction: a short-term study. *Patient Educ Couns*, 74, 191–196, 0738-3991

Kakudate N, Morita M, Fukuhara S, Sugai M, Nagayama M, Isogai E, Kawanami M, & Chiba I (2010a). Development of the outcome expectancy scale for self-care (OESS) among periodontal disease patients. *J Eval Clin Pract* (in press), 1356-1294

Kakudate N, Morita M, Yamazaki S et al (2010b). Association between self-efficacy and loss to follow-up in long-term periodontal treatment. *J Clin Periodontol*, 37, 276–282, 0303-6979

Kressin NR, Boehmer U, Nunn ME, Spiro A 3rd (2003). Increased preventive practices lead to greater tooth retention. *J Dent Res*, 82, 223–227, 0022-0345

Martin LR, Haskard Zolnierek KB, DiMatteo MR (2010). *Health behavior change and treatment adherence: evidencebased guidelines for improving healthcare* (1 edition), Oxford University Press, 0195380401, New York City

McCaul KD, Glasgow RE, Gustafson C (1985). Predicting levels of preventive dental behaviors. *J Am Dent Assoc*, 111, 601–605, 0002-8177

Morita M, Kakudate N, Chiba I, Kawanami M (2010). *Assessment and enhancement of oral care self-efficacy*, Nova Science Publishers, 1608761135, New York City

O'Leary TJ, Drake RB, Naylor, J. E. (1972) The plaque control record. *J Periodontol*, 43, 38, 0022-3492

Renz A, Ide M, Newton T, Robinson PG, Smith D (2007). Psychological interventions to improve adherence to oral hygiene instructions in adults with periodontal diseases. *Cochrane Database Syst Rev*, 18, 1–17, 1469-493X

Resnick B, Zimmerman SI, Orwig D, Furstenberg AL, Magaziner J (2000). Outcome expectations for exercise scale: utility and psychometrics. *J Gerontol B Psychol Sci Soc Sci*, 55, S352–S356, 1079-5014

Rogers RW (1975). A protection motivation theory of fear appeals and attitude change. *J Psychology*, 91, 93–114, 0022-3980

Rogers R (1983). Cognitive and physiological processes in fear appeals and attitude change: a revised theory of protection motivation, In: *Social Psychophysiology*, J. Cacioppo & R. Petty, Guilford Press, 0898626269, New York City

Rosenstock IM (1974). Historical origins of the Health Belief Model. *Health Educ Monogr*, 2, 328–335, 0073-1455

Rossen EK, Gruber KJ (2007). Development and psychometric testing of the relocation self-efficacy scale. *Nurs Res*, 56, 244–251, 0029-6562

Rotter JB (1966). Generalized expectancies for internal versus external control of reinforcement. *Psychol monogr*, 80, 1–28, 0096-9753

Sakano Y, Tohjoh M (1986). The General Self-Efficacy Scale (GSES): scale development and validation (in Japanese). *Jap J Behav Ther*, 12, 73–82, 0910-6529

Sherer M, Maddux JE, Mercandante B, Prentice-Dunn S,Jacobs B, Rogers RW (1982). The Self-efficacy Scale: construction and validation. *Psychol Rep*, 51, 663–671, 0033-2941

Smarr KL, Parker JC, Wright GE et al (1997). The importance of enhancing self-efficacy in rheumatoid arthritis. *Arthritis Care Res*, 10, 18–26, 0893-7524

Stanley KD, Murphy MR (1997). A comparison of general self-efficacy with self-esteem. *Genet Soc Gen Psychol Monogr*, 123, 81–99, 8756-7547

Stewart JE, Strack S, Graves P (1997). Development of oral hygiene self-efficacy and outcome expectancy questionnaires. *Community Dent Oral Epidemiol*, 25, 337–342, 0301-5661

Syrjälä AM, Kneckt MC, Knuuttila ML (1999). Dental selfefficacy as a determinant to oral health behavior, oral hygiene and HbA1c level among diabetic patients. *J Clin Periodontol*, 26, 616–621, 0303-6979

Syrjälä AM, Knuuttila ML, Syrjälä LK (2001). Self-efficacy perceptions in oral health behavior. *Acta Odontol Scand*, 59, 1–6, 0001-6357

Syrjälä AM, Ylö stalo P, Niskanen MC, Knuuttila ML (2004). Relation of different measures of psychological characteristics to oral health habits, diabetes adherence and related clinical variables among diabetic patients. *Eur J Oral Sci*, 112, 109–114, 0909-8836

Tarini BA, Christakis DA, Lozano P (2007). Toward familycentered inpatient medical care: the role of parents as participants in medical decisions. *J Pediatr*, 151, 690–695, 0022-3476

Tedesco LA, Keffer MA, Fleck-Kandath C (1991). Selfefficacy, reasoned action, and oral health behavior reports: a social cognitive approach to compliance. *J Behav Med*, 14, 341–355, 0160-7715

Tedesco LA, Keffer MA, Davis EL (1992). Effect of a social cognitive intervention on oral health status, behavior reports, and cognitions. *J Periodontol*, 63, 567–575, 0022-3492

Travess HC, Newton JT, Sandy JR, Williams AC (2004). The development of a patient-centered measure of the process and outcome of combined orthodontic and orthognathic treatment. *J Orthod*, 31, 220–234, 1465-3125

Wattana C, Srisuphan W, Pothiban L, Upchurch SL (2007). Effects of a diabetes self-management program on glycemic control, coronary heart disease risk, and quality of life among Thai patients with type 2 diabetes. *Nurs Health Sci*, 9, 135–141, 1441-0745

Woodruff SL, Cashman JF (1993). Task, domain, and general efficacy: a reexamination of the Self-efficacy Scale. *Psychol Rep*, 72, 423–432, 0033-2941

10

Adjunctive Systemic Use of Beta-Glucan in the Nonsurgical Treatment of Chronic Periodontitis

Neslihan Nal Acar, Ülkü Noyan, Leyla Kuru, Tanju Kadir and Bahar Kuru
Department of Periodontology, Dental Faculty, Marmara University, İstanbul
Turkey

1. Introduction

Periodontal lesions in chronic periodontitis are associated with a subgingival microbiota predominated by gram-negative anaerobic rods, spirochetes and other motile microorganisms (Tanner et al., 1979). Chronic periodontitis is a complex process itself involving periodontal microorganisms, immune system and host factors. One reason for the augmented colonization of these periodontopathogens is believed to be related with a weak specific T helper 1-mediated immunity (Bartova et al., 2000; Breivik & Thrane, 2001; Wassenar et al., 1998) and, the immune response in patients with periodontal lesions may be inclined towards a strong T helper 2-mediated immunity. Immune functions can be enhanced by activating macrophages and establishing Th1 dominance (Inoue et al., 2002; Lee et al., 2002). The use of certain immunomodulating agents may stimulate immune response and activate macrophages and neutrophils. Beta-glucan (β-glucan), a polysaccharide extracted from cell walls of *Saccharomyces cerevisiae*, has been found to have immunomodulatory effects in animals and humans (Babineau et al., 1994; Bleicher & Mackin, 1995; Chan et al., 2009; Engstad, 1994; Engstad et al., 2002). It increases resistance to bacterial infections and cancer cells while stimulating wound healing (Brown & Gordon, 2001; Chan et al., 2009; Yun et al., 2003). Numerous studies have shown that β-glucan is a stimulator activating phagocytosis, respiratory burst, and the production of cytokines and chemokines in macrophages (Kankkunen et al., 2010; Sherwood et al., 1987, Williams & Di Luzio, 1980). Recently, the possibility of subcutaneous injections of β-glucan being able to modulate allergic sensitisation has been demonstrated in children (Sarinho et al., 2009). The authors proposed a new therapeutic strategy in allergic diseases as β-glucan possesses a beneficial action in restoring T helper 2 function (Sarinho et al., 2009). Furthermore, besides its antibacterial effects, antiviral and antifungal properties of β-glucan have been put forward (Bedirli et al., 2003; Di Luzio et al., 1980; Jung et al., 2004; Kenyon, 1983; Kernodle et al., 1998; Leblanc et al., 2006; Nicoletti et al., 1992; Tzianabos, 2000). The protective effect of β-glucan has been established to *Staphylococcus aureus* (Di Luzio & Williams, 1978), *Escherichia coli, Listeria monocytogenes, Mycobacterium leprae, Candida albicans* (Williams et al., 1978), *Pneumocytis carinii, Leishmania donovani* and *Influenza virus* (Jung et al., 2004).

Transforming growth factor-beta1 (TGF-β1) plays a part in many different clinical processes, such as embryonal development, cellular proliferation and differentiation, wound healing, and angiogenesis via supression of collagenase production by fibroblasts and macrophages

(Edwards et al., 1987; Page, 1991) and inhibition of the release of procollagenase. Moreover, it increases the synthesis of extracellular matrix molecules by stimulating numerous cell types including fibroblasts and osteoblasts (Chen et al., 1987; Hakkinen et al., 1996; Matsuda et al., 1992). Expression and production of this growth factor both at periodontally healthy and diseased sites suggest that it contributes to maintenance of tissue integrity (Buduneli et al., 2001; Kuru et al., 2004a; Kuru et al., 2004b; Steinsvoll et al., 1999; Wright et al., 2003). Thus, these properties of TGF-β1 show its important role in the pathogenesis of periodontal disease and wound healing.

Since β-glucan affects immune function with quickened macrophage activation and establishment of T helper 1 dominance, the tissue destruction seen in periodontal disease may be inhibited by the usage of this immunomodulating agent. Chaple et al. (1998) have reported that there was a failure of the recruitment and activation of macrophages in the gingival samples obtained from untreated advanced periodontitis patients, compared with those of patients with gingivitis. Thus, the ability of β-glucan to stimulate macrophages seems to be very crucial. Breivik et al. (2005) evaluated the effect of β-1,3/1,6 glucan on the progression of ligature-induced periodontal disease in animals. Their findings showed that orally administrated β-glucan significantly reduced periodontal bone loss as measured on digital x-rays. Stashenko et al. (1995) tested the effect of this biological response modifier on infection-stimulated alveolar bone resorption in an *in vivo* model. Their findings supported the concept that β-glucan can decrease hard and soft tissue destruction in animals. Although β-glucan has been suggested to enhance endogenous antibacterial mechanisms in neutrophils and to increase the healing potential of damaged tissues (Bedirli et al., 2003; Browder et al., 1988, Browder et al., 1990, Stashenko et al., 1995), so far, its effect on periodontal tissue healing as an adjunct to nonsurgical periodontal therapy (NPT) has never been investigated in humans.

The aim of this chapter is to present the results of a controlled study investigating the effects of NPT with an adjunctive use of systemic β-glucan on clinical, microbiological parameters and gingival crevicular fluid (GCF) TGF-β1 levels in chronic periodontitis patients over a 3-month period.

2. Materials and methods

2.1 Study population

Twenty subjects between 30-56 years of age were selected among chronic periodontitis patients who applied to the clinics of Department of Periodontology, Dental Faculty, Marmara University, Istanbul, Turkey. Medical and dental histories were obtained and intraoral examinations were carried out at pre-screening visit. Patients were diagnosed to have chronic periodontitis according to the clinical and radiographic findings (Armitage 1999). Inclusion criteria were as follows: to be systemically healthy, have at least two sites with a probing depth ≥ 5 mm in each quadrant and radiographic evidence of moderate to advanced chronic periodontitis. None of the patients had received antibiotics or periodontal treatment within the 6 months preceeding the study. Women who were pregnant, breast-feeding or using oral contraceptives were excluded. In addition, 10 systemically and periodontally healthy subjects were selected as the healthy control group. None of these subjects had bleeding on probing or a history of medication in the past 6 months. All patients were non-smokers. The protocol of the study was approved by the Ethics Commitee of Marmara University (Number: B.30.2.MAR.0.01.00.02/AEK-232). Patients who fulfilled the inclusion criteria provided written informed consent and participated in the study.

2.2 Study design

This study was a randomized, controlled, parallel group clinical trial of 3-month duration. With the purpose of evaluating the adjunctive effect of β-glucan, 20 chronic periodontitis patients were randomly divided into 2 groups: group 1 (n=10) received NPT only, group 2 received NPT and adjunctive β-glucan (n=10). A total of two sessions of NPT were applied to all patients and group 2 patients used systemic β-glucan (10 mg, 1x1) for 40 days (Fig. 1).

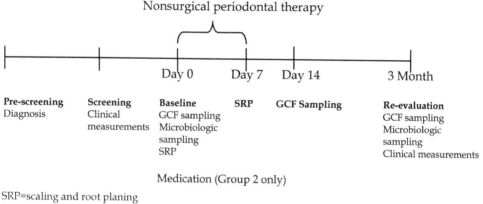

SRP=scaling and root planing
GCF= gingival crevicular fluid

Fig. 1. Study design.

As shown in Fig. 1, this study was consisted of four main stages including pre-screening, screening, baseline (Day 0) and re-evaluation (3 month - day 91). Screening examination was conducted to assess the patient's eligibility for participation. The periodontal status of each patient was assessed by a single blinded examiner (N.N.A.). The periodontal clinical measurements included gingival index (Löe & Sillness, 1963), plaque index (Sillness & Löe, 1964) and bleeding on probing. Additionally, probing depth and relative attachment level were measured to the nearest mm with a periodontal probe using an individual occlusal stent as a reference point for probe placement. Sampling was performed from sites with a probing depth ≥ 5 mm and subgingival microbiological and GCF samples were collected from different periodontal sites.

Patients who were eligible for the study, returned to our clinic at baseline visit for sampling and application of NPT. At baseline, oral hygiene instructions including brushing and flossing were given. Then, full mouth scaling and root planing (SRP) was performed in all patients using an ultrasonic scaler (Cavitron® EMZ, Switzerland) and Gracey curettes (Hu-Friedy Ins. Co, USA) until smooth root surfaces were achieved. The group 2 patients were further instructed to take one capsule of β-glucan (10 mg, 1x1) in the morning for 40 days.

At day 7, full mouth SRP was applied again in all patients. GCF samples were obtained at day 14. Clinical measurements and sampling procedures were repeated at 3-month re-evaluation stage.

2.3 Collection of GCF samples

GCF samples were obtained at days 0 and 14, and 3 months after therapy. Two GCF samples from each chronic periodontitis patient were collected from mesio- and disto-buccal aspects of single rooted teeth exhibiting probing depth ≥ 5 mm. In the healthy control group, two GCF samples were collected from mesio- or disto-buccal aspect of single rooted matching teeth exhibiting probing depth ≤ 3 mm without any clinical sign of gingival inflammation and alveolar bone loss.

Prior to GCF sampling, the selected sites were isolated with cotton rolls, saliva was removed using a high-power suction tip and supragingival plaque was removed using a periodontal probe to prevent saliva and/or plaque contamination (Griffiths et al., 1992). Paper strips (Periopaper; ProFlow, Inc., Amityville, NY, USA) were placed at the entrance of the crevice until mild resistance was felt and left in position for 30 seconds (Lamster et al., 1985). Strips contaminated with blood or saliva were discarded. The volumes of GCF collected were measured by weighing the papers, before and after sample collection, using a micro balance (AND 200-HM, Japan) (Kuru et al., 2004b). The weight of the fluid was converted to volume by assuming that the density of GCF was 1.0 (Cimasoni & Giannopoulou, 1988). The GCF samples were stored at -80°C until the day of laboratory analysis.

2.4 TGF-β1 analysis in GCF

The paper strips were allowed to thaw at room temperature for 30 minutes. GCF samples were eluted from the strips by placing them in 100 μl of phosphate-buffered saline (PBS) and stored at 4°C for up to 24 h prior to the laboratory procedures (Kuru et al., 2004a).

GCF TGF-β1 levels were analysed by enzyme linked immunosorbent assay, using a commercially available Colorimetric Sandwich enzyme linked immunosorbent assay Kit (Quantikine DB100, R&D Systems, Minneapolis, MN, USA). In order to measure biological active TGF-β1, GCF samples were acidified using 20 μl 1 N HCL at room temperature for 10 minutes. Then, the samples were neutralized by adding 20 μl 1.2 NaOH/0.5 M HEPES. The activated GCF samples were further analysed as described previously (Kuru et al., 2004a). Briefly, an aliquot of 200 μl of known concentrations (0, 31.2, 62.5, 125, 250, 500, 1000 and 2000 pg/ml) of the activated recombinant human TGF-β1 standard and of the activated samples of GCF were added to the plate, which had been pre-coated with a recombinant human soluble receptor II which specifically binds human TGF-β1. The plate was covered with an adhesive strip and incubated at room temperature for 3 hours. Each well was aspirated and washed 3 times with 400 μl of the wash buffer provided, after which 200 μl of the detecting antibody (horseradish peroxidase-conjugated polyclonal antibody against TGF-β1) was added. The plate was again covered with an adhesive strip and incubated at room temperature for 1.5 hour. After washing 3 times, 200 μl of the substrate solution (tetramethylbenzidine containing H_2O_2) was added to each well and incubated at room temperature for 20 minutes. Following the addition of 50 μl of 2 M H_2SO_4 to stop the reaction, the absorbance at 450 nm was measured using a spectrophotometer. The absorbance was also measured at 570 nm to determine any optical imperfections between the wells, and this value was subtracted from the absorbance at 450. A standard curve was prepared for each experiment and concentrations of TGF-β1 in samples were then calculated from this curve. The minimum detection limit of the assay kit was 4.61 pg/ml.

2.5 Subgingival microbiological sampling

Subgingival microbiological samples were collected at baseline and 3 months after therapy. The mesio- or disto-buccal site of a single-rooted tooth in the upper right quadrant exhibiting probing depth ≥ 5 mm was selected as the microbiological sampling site. Supragingival plaque was removed from the sampling site with a sterile curette followed by isolation using a cotton roll. Subgingival plaque sample was collected with a standardized 30# sterile paper point by inserting it into the crevice, and leaving in place for 10 seconds. Paper points contaminated with saliva or blood were discarded.

2.6 Microbiological analysis

The proportion of anaerobic microorganisms in the total flora was determined by microbiological culture method as described previously (Kuru et al., 1999; Noyan et al., 1997; Yilmaz et al., 2002). Immediately after obtaining subgingival plaque, each sample was aseptically transferred into 4.5 ml of PBS and dispersed using a vortex mixer at maximal setting for 60 s. The dispersed samples were serially diluted and 0.2 ml portion of 10^{-1}, 10^{-2},....10^{-5} dilutions were spread on a solid agar medium using sterile bent glass rods. Trypticase soy agar plate (Oxoid, Oxoid Ltd., England) enriched with 0.0005 % hemin (Sigma, Sigma Chemical Co., USA), 0.00005 % menadione (Sigma), and 5 % defibrinated sheep blood, was inoculated for non-selective bacterial growth (Wolff et al., 1985). Furthermore, trypticase soy agar plate enriched with 5 % defibrinated sheep blood was used for cultivation for facultative anaerobic microorganisms.

After 7 days of incubation of the supplemented trypticase soy agar plates in Gas Pak jars (Gas generating kit, Oxoid) in an atmosphere of 95 % H_2 and 5 % CO_2 at 37ºC, the total viable count was determined from the dilution giving 30-300 colonies. After 5 days of incubation of trypticase soy agar plate in air and 10 % CO_2 at 37ºC, the total number of facultative anaerobes was determined.

All the microbiological data were expressed as colony forming units/ml (CFU/ml). Obligate anaerobic bacteria was calculated as the total counts of anaerobically cultivable bacteria minus the total counts of facultatively anaerobic bacteria and expressed as a percentage of total viable count.

2.7 Statistical analysis

SPSS for Windows (Release 10.0, SPSS Inc., USA) was used for statistical analyses. The mean values for each periodontal measurement was calculated as the mean of whole mouth for each patient. The mean for each periodontal parameter was also calculated separately for periodontal sites selected for microbial sampling with initial probing depth ≥5 mm for each patient. Comparisons between the groups were carried out using the Mann-Whitney U test, and multiple comparisons within each group were performed using the Friedman test followed by the Wilcoxon Sign test for comparisons of values between different time points. *P* values <0.05 were considered statistically significant. Lack of significance is indicated by not significant (NS).

3. Results

All of patients enrolled in this study completed the study protocol. None of the patients in group 2 complained of any adverse effects due to the systemic usage of β-glucan. Patient demographics are outlined in Table 1.

	Group 1	Group 2
n	10	10
Age (mean years ± SD)	44.5 ± 9.4	42.4 ± 7.7
Age range	30-56	33-52
Gender (male:female)	8:2	4:6

Table 1. Demographic characteristics of patients participated in the study.

3.1 Clinical findings

The self-performed plaque control program resulted in improved oral hygiene in all patients supported by the finding of significant reductions in full mouth plaque index scores in both groups (p<0.01) (Table 2). No significant difference was found between the groups regarding the plaque index values (p>0.05). Significant reductions were detected in full mouth gingival index and bleeding on probing parameters after therapy in both groups (p<0.01). However, the changes in mean gingival index and bleeding on probing values of the group 1 were not different than those of the group 2 (p>0.05). Probing depth measurements at sampling sites demonstrated significant reductions from baseline to 3 month in both groups (p<0.01). When the probing depth reduction between the groups was compared, there was no significant difference (p>0.05). Significant attachment gain at sampling sites was achieved in both groups (p<0.01) (Table 2), but intergroup comparison yielded no significant difference between the groups (p>0.05) (data not shown).

	Group 1		Group 2	
Parameter	Baseline	3 Months	Baseline	3 Months
PI(Full mouth)	2.17 ± 0.38	0.36 ± 0.23*	2.28 ± 0.31	0.44 ± 0.31*
GI(Full mouth)	2.36 ± 0.37	0.33 ± 0.21*	2.16 ± 0.47	0.45 ± 0.42*
BOP(%)(Full mouth)	88 ± 11	9 ± 4*	84 ± 14	10 ± 6*
PD (mm)(Sampling sites)	5.28 ± 0.16	3.35 ± 0.33*	5.38 ± 0.14	3.49 ± 0.15*
RAL (mm)(Sampling sites)	9.40 ± 1.14	8.18 ± 1.23*	9.56 ± 0.80	8.44 ± 0.72*

All values are expressed as mean ± standard deviation.
* (p<0.01), Wilcoxon Sign test
PI=Plaque index, GI= gingival index, BOP= bleeding on probing, PD= probing depth,
RAL= relative attachment level

Table 2. Clinical parameters of the study groups at baseline and 3 months after treatment.

3.2 Biochemical findings

GCF volume of the groups 1 and 2 showed significant decreases during the experimental period (p<0.05) and intragroup comparisons revealed that the decreases between days 0-14, 14-91 and 0-91 were significant in both groups (p<0.05) (Fig. 2). However, there were no significant differences in the changes of GCF volume between the groups (p>0.05).

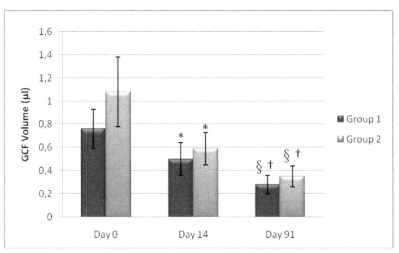

* p<0.05, between days 0-14, Wilcoxon Sign test, § p<0.05, between days 0-91, Wilcoxon Sign test.
† p<0.05, between days 14-91, Wilcoxon Sign test.

Fig. 2. Mean GCF volume of sampling sites in study groups.

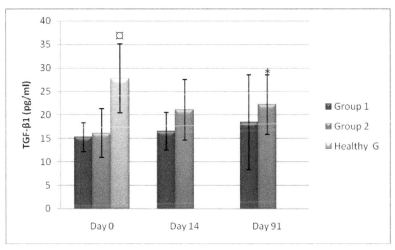

¤ p<0.01, compared to groups 1 and 2, Mann-Whitney U test
* p<0.05, respective baseline value, Wilcoxon Sign test.

Fig. 3. GCF TGF-β1 levels (pg/ml) of sampling sites in study groups at baseline and after therapy.

When baseline GCF TGF-β1 concentrations of the groups 1 and 2 and the healthy group were compared, healthy group showed a significantly higher level of TGF-β1 than that of the groups 1 and 2 ($p < 0.01$) (Fig. 3). At day 91, TGF-β1 concentration in GCF increased in the groups 1 and 2 when compared to their respective baseline values, but only the increase in the group 2 was found to be significant ($p < 0.05$) (Fig. 3). However, no significant difference was found between the groups in the GCF TGF-β1 concentration level.

3.3 Microbiological findings

Total anaerobically grown microorganisms expressed as total viable counts in subgingival plaque samples before and 3 month after different treatment modalities, are given in Table 3. NPT applied to the group 1 resulted in a decrease in total viable counts. A similar decrease was also noted when the group 2 patients received adjunctive β-glucan. However, these reductions were not significant ($p > 0.05$). Furthermore, intergroup comparisons revealed no significant differences between the two groups ($p > 0.05$). Fig. 4 demonstrates the proportions of obligate and facultative anaerobes of the study groups. Significant reductions were detected in the percentage of obligate anaerobic bacteria along with significant increases in the percentage of facultative anaerobic bacteria in both groups after therapy ($p < 0.01$). However, no differences were found between the groups ($p > 0.05$).

		Group 1	Group 2	p[¥]
Baseline	mean	49	88	NS
	range	0.51-178	0.43-260	
3 Month	mean	2	14	NS
	range	0.05-6	0.06-130	
	p[Ω]	NS	NS	

[¥] Mann-Whitney U test, [Ω]Wilcoxon Sign test, NS=not significant

Table 3. Total viable counts (x10^4 CFU/ml) of subgingival samples at baseline and after 3 months.

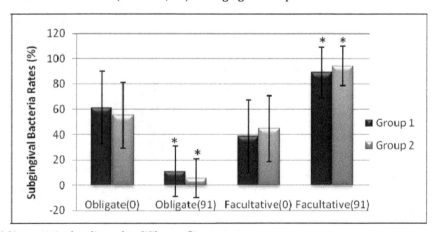

* $p < 0.01$, respective baseline value, Wilcoxon Sign test.

Fig. 4. Proportions of obligate and facultative anaerobes in subgingival plaque samples of the groups 1 and 2.

4. Discussion

This chapter presented a randomized, controlled, parallel group clinical study which was designed to evaluate the effects of NPT with or without adjunctive use of systemic β-glucan on clinical, microbiological and biochemical parameters in chronic periodontitis patients over a 3-month period. NPT is the first stage of periodontal therapy that aims to reduce the number of pathogen microorganisms in periodontal pocket leading to the resolution of inflammatory response and arresting the progression of disease, resulting in probing depth reduction and attachment gain (Greenstein, 1992; Cobb, 1996; Noyan et al., 1997, Yilmaz et al., 2002). It is well known that the efficacy of nonsurgical therapy is related to the baseline probing depth, and inflammatory changes are more pronounced in deeper pockets. Therefore, the effectiveness of NPT and adjunctive β-glucan in this study was evaluated for only periodontal sites with baseline probing depth ≥5 mm. Significant improvements in all measured clinical parameters (plaque index, gingival index, bleeding on probing, probing depth, relative attachment level) were observed 3 months following SRP procedure, as expected. Moreover, SRP supplemented with β-glucan resulted in significant clinical outcome. However, β-glucan appears to have no additional effect on clinical parameters recorded in the present study, as evidenced by insignificant difference between the groups.

β-glucan acts as an immunostimulant agent enhancing host-mediated immune responses to pathogens, especially by activating macrophages (Brown & Gordon 2001, Suzuki et al., 2001). β-glucan stimulates macrophage phagocytosis (Lee et al., 2002) and changes the balance from immunglobulin G1 antibodies (T helper 2 dependent antibody subclasses) towards a T helper 1 dependent immunglobulin G2a response (Suzuki et al., 2001). It also stimulates the production of T helper 1-stimulating cytokine interferon-γ but suppresses interleukin-4 which induces T helper 2 responses (Inoue et al., 2002). Therefore, β-glucan skew the T helper 1/T helper 2 balance towards a T helper 1-dominated response (Suzuki et al., 2001). The presence of a T helper 2-biased response to the periodontopathogens is supported by the observation that peripheral blood cells of patients release more T helper 2 cytokines in response to periodontopathogens *in vitro* (Bartova et al., 2000, Wassenaar et al., 1998). In the present study, concentration of GCF TGF-β1 increased following both therapies but the increase was significant only in the group 2 which received β-glucan. As TGF-β1 is a T helper 1 stimulating cytokine, the increase of this cytokine can be explained by this mechanism.

In the present study, the level of TGF-β1 in GCF samples obtained from chronic periodontitis patients was investigated and compared with periodontally healthy individuals. TGF-β1 has a very important role in the pathogenesis of periodontal diseases and also in wound healing. To the best of our knowledge, no data is available on periodontal treatment with adjunctive use of β-glucan. Hence this is the first study to explore any effect of this immunomodulator agent on the treatment of chronic periodontitis patients.

In the present study we have demonstrated that the healthy group had higher GCF TGF-β1 concentration than the groups 1 and 2. This finding is in agreement with previous reports which found lower GCF TGF-β1 concentrations at inflamed sites when compared with healthy sites (Buduneli et al., 2001, Gürkan et al., 2005; Kuru et al., 2004a). Expression of

GCF constituents as concentration could result in higher levels at healthy sites where GCF volume is very low (Curtis et al., 1988, Emingil et al., 2000). Therefore, in healthy sites, high levels of TGF-β1 in GCF may be related to low GCF volume.

TGF-β1 is a key mediator in resolution of inflammation (Sodek & Overall, 1992, Steinsvoll et al., 1999). This multifunctional growth factor has both pro-inflammatory and anti-inflammatory properties (Wahl et al., 1993). Its effects on cell proliferation and differentiation suggest a key role for this cytokine in wound healing, tissue remodeling and regeneration (Sporn & Roberts, 1993). Thus, these properties of TGF-β1 indicate its important role in inflammatory wound healing. In the present study, concentration of GCF TGF-β1 increased following both therapies. After the elimination of microbial factors, as shown by decrease in the preposition of anaerobic species, there will be a rapid restoration of the periodontium; this might be the reason why the cytokine levels increased in our study. This increase was significant only in β-glucan group between day 0 and day 91. Since systemic β-glucan usage activates macrophages and neutrophils which produce TGF-β1 when activated (Igarasi et al., 1993), the significant increase in group 2 might have occurred due the effect of β-glucan. In the study of Gürkan et al. (2005), only GCF TGF-β1 levels of subantimicrobial dose doxycycline group was significantly higher than baseline and placebo group at 3 months. On the other hand, the GCF TGF-β1 concentration in the subantimicrobial dose doxycycline group decreased while it increased in the placebo group at the end of 6-month period. The authors concluded that the drug efficacy at the biochemical level may continue as long as the agent is used. In accordance with our results, Gürkan et al. (2005), have demonstrated that the level of this growth factor increased after resolution of inflammation. Thus, it could be hypothesized that antiinflammatory role of TGF-β1 may be more potent than its proinflammatory properties during healing after NPT. However, the levels of this cytokine at different stages of healing process needs to be clarified with further studies.

The demonstration of bacterial specificity in periodontal disease allows the clinician to direct therapy toward the elimination or suppression of the periodontopathogens in terms of antimicrobial treatment. As antibiotics have important disadvantages including side effects, drug resistance etc., recent researches have focused on new therapeutic agents alternative to antibiotics. Since β-glucan has been suggested to possess antimicrobial activity (Bedirli et al., 2003, Di Luzio et al., 1980, Nicoletti et al., 1992), we evaluated the microbiological effect of β-glucan as an adjunct to NPT. In this study, a reduction in the proportion of obligate anaerobic bacteria occurred in both groups. A decrease in the number of anaerobic bacteria is synonimous with a successful treatment of periodontal infections and reflects the antimicrobial effect following NPT, as expected (Greenstein, 1992; Noyan et al., 1997; Yilmaz et al., 2002). But as there are no significant differences between the two groups, we can assume that β-glucan has no additional antimicrobial effect when used systemically as an adjunct to NPT in patients with chronic periodontitis.

Regarding the duration of systemic β-glucan usage, no data is available so far on its systemic usage in the periodontal diseases. Treatment duration with β-glucan varies from 39 days to 90 days in animal and human studies according to the type and severity of the problem (Breivik et al.,2005; Kabasakal et al., 2011; Lin et al., 2011; Sarinho et al., 2009; Turunen et al., 2011). Biagini et al. (1988) documented soft tissue healing after NPT and found precisely oriented collagen bundle fibres by 30 days to 60 days. Furthermore, Magnusson et al. (1984) reported that repopulation of subgingival microbiota occurred between 30 to 60 days. Therefore, our patients in this study were put on β-glucan medication for 40 days according to the combination of the aforementioned data.

5. Conclusion

This is the first preliminary report investigating the effects of NPT plus β-glucan on clinical parameters, subgingival microflora and GCF TGF-β1 level in patients with chronic periodontitis. Within its limits, systemic β-glucan used as an adjunct to NPT did not provide additional clinical and microbiological effects. However, β-glucan might increase the concentration of TGF-β1 thereby augmenting periodontal healing potential. As β-glucans are inexpensive and have a good margin of safety (Chan et al., 2009), their potential therapeutic value deserves further detailed investigations for clarifying the paucity of information in the literature in order to design a strategy for their possible use in clinical periodontal practice.

6. Aknowledgements

This study was supported by a grant from Marmara University Scientific Research Project Commission with the number SAĞ-BGS-081004-0100.

7. References

Armitage G.C. (1999). Development of a classification system for periodontal diseases and conditions. *Ann Periodontol*, Vol:4, pp.1-7, ISSN:1553-0841.

Babineau T.J., Marcello P., Swails W., Kenler A., Bistrian B., & Forse R.A. (1994). Randomized phase I/II trial of a macrophage-specific immunomodulator (PGG-glucan) in high-risk surgical patients. *Ann Surg*, Vol:220, pp.601-609, ISSN:0003-4932.

Bartova J., Kratka O.Z., Prochazkova J., Krejsa O., Duskova J., Mrklas L., Tlaskalova H.,& Cukrowska B. (2000). Th1 and Th2 cytokine profile in patients with early onset periodontitis and their healthy siblings. *Mediators of Inflammation*, Vol:9, pp.115-120, ISSN:0962-9351.

Bedirli A., Gokahmetoglu S., Sakrak O., Ersoz N., Ayangil D., & Esin H. (2003). Prevention of intraperitoneal adhesion formation using beta-glucan after ileocolic anastomosis in a rat bacterial peritonitis model. *Am J Surg*, Vol:185, No:4, pp.339-343, ISSN:0002-9610.

Biagini G., Checchi L., Miccoli M.C., Vasi V., & Castaldini C. (1988). Root curettage and gingival repair in periodontics. *J Periodontol*, Vol:59, pp.124-129, ISSN: 0022-3492.Bleicher P., & Mackin W. (1995). Betafectin PGG glucan: A novel carbohydrate immunomodulator with antiinfective properties. *Annu Rev Pharmacol Toxicol*, Vol:37, pp.143-166, ISSN:0362-1642.

Breivik T., & Thrane P.S. (2001). Psychoneuroimmune interactions in periodontal disease. Chapter 63, In *Psychneuroimmunology*, Ader R., Felten L., & Cohen N. (eds)., 3rd edition, pp. 627-644. Academic Press, ISBN:0-12-088576-x, San Diego.

Breivik T., Opstad P.K., Engstad R., Gundersen G., Gjermo P., & Preus H. (2005). Soluble β-1,3/1,6-glucan from yeast inhibits experimental periodontal disease in Wistar rats. *J Clin Periodontol*, Vol:32, pp.347-352, ISSN:0303-6979.

Browder W., Williams D., Lucore P., Pretus H., Jones E., & McNamee R. (1988). Effect of enhanced macrophage function on early wound healing. *Surgery*, Vol:104, No:2, pp.224-230, ISSN:0039-6060.

Browder W., Williams D., Pretus H., Olivero G., Enrichens F., Mao P., & Franchello A. (1990) Beneficial effect of enhanced macrophage function in the travma patient. *Ann Surg*, Vol:211, pp.605-611, ISSN:0003-4932.

Brown G.D., & Gordon S. (2001). Immune recognition. A new receptor for beta-glucans. *Nature*, Vol:6, No:413, pp.36-37, ISSN:0028-0836.

Buduneli N., Kütükçüler N., Aksu G. & Atilla G. (2001). Evaluation of transforming growth factor-β1 level in crevicular fluid of cyclosporin A-treated patients. *J Periodontol*, Vol:72, pp. 526-531, ISSN:0022-3492.

Chan G.C., Chan W.K., & Sze D.M. (2009). The effects of β-glucan on human immune and cancer cells. *J Hematol Oncol*, Vol:2, pp.25-36, ISSN:1756-8722.

Chaple C.C., Srivastrava M., & Hunter N. (1998). Failure of macrophage activation in destructive periodontal disease. *J Pathol*, Vol:186, pp.281-286, ISSN: 1096-9896.

Chen J.K., Hoshi H., & McKeehan W.L. (1987). Transforming growth factor type β specifically stimulates synthesis of proteoglycan in human adult arterial smooth muscle cells. *Proc Natl Acad Sci USA*, Vol:84, pp.5287-5291, ISSN:1091-6490.

Cimasoni G., & Giannopoulou C. (1988). Can crevicular fluid component analysis asist in diagnosis and monitoring periodontal breakdown? In: *Periodontology Today*, ed. Guggenheim, B., pp. 260-270. Karger, ISBN:978-3-8055-4843-4, Basel.

Cobb C.M. (1996). Nonsurgical pocket therapy: Mechanical. *Ann Periodontol*, Vol:1, pp.443-490, ISSN:1553-0841.

Curtis M.A., Griffiths G.S., Price S.J., Culthurst S.K., & Johnson N.W. (1988). The total protein concentration of gingival crevicular fluid. Variation with sampling time anf gingival inflammation. *J Clin Periodontol*, Vol:15, pp.628-632, ISSN:0303-6979.

Di Luzio N.R., Williams D.L., McNamee R.B., & Malshet V.G. (1980). Comparative evaluation of the tumor inhibitory and antibacterial activity of solubilized and particulate glucan. *Recent Results Cancer Res*, Vol:75, pp.165-172, ISSN:0080-0015.

Di Luzio N.R., & Williams D.L. (1978). Protective effect of glucan against systemic Staphylococcus aureus septicemia in normal and leukemic mice. *Infect Immun*, Vol:20, pp.804-810, ISSN:0019-9567.

Edwards D.R., Murphy G., Reynolds J.J., Whitham S.E., Docherty A.J., Angel P., & Heath J.K. (1987). Transforming growth factor beta modulates the expression of collagenase and metalloproteinase inhibitor. *J Bone Miner Res*, Vol:6, pp.1899-1904, ISSN:0884-0431.

Emingil G., Çoker I., Atilla G., & Hüseyinov A. (2000). Levels of leukotriene B$_4$ and platelet activating factor in gingival crevicular fluid in renal transplant patients receiving cyclosporine-A. *J Periodontol*, Vol:71, pp.50-57, ISSN:0022-3492.

Engstad C.S., Engstad R.E., Olsen J.O., & Osterud B. (2002). The effect of soluble beta 1,3-glucan and lipopolysaccharide on cytokine production and coagulation activation in whole blood. *International Immunopharmacology*, Vol:2, pp.1585-1597, ISSN:1567-5769.

Engstad R.E. (1994). Yeast β-glucan as an immunostimulant in Atlantic salmon (Salmo salar L.): Biological effects, recognition and structural aspects. Tromsø: University of Tromsø.

Greenstein G. (1992). Periodontal response to mechanical non surgical therapy: A review. *J Periodontol*, Vol:63, pp.118-130, ISSN:0022-3492.

Griffiths G.S., Wilton J.M., & Curtis M.A. (1992). Contamination of human gingival crevicular fluid by plaque and saliva. *Arch Oral Biol*, Vol:37, pp.559-564, ISSN:0003-9969.

Gürkan A., Çınarcık S., & Hüseyinov A. (2005). Adjunctive subantimicrobial dose doxycycline: effect on clinical parameters and gingival crevicular fluid transforming growth factor-β1 levels in severe, generalized chronic periodontitis. *J Clin Periodontol*, Vol:32, pp.244-253, ISSN:0303-6979.

Hakkinen L., Westermarck J., Kahari V.M., & Larjava H. (1996). Human granulation-tissue fibroblasts show enhanced proteoglycan gene expression and altered response to TGF-β1. *J Dent Res*, Vol:75, pp.1767-1778, ISSN:0022-0345.

Igarasi A., Okochi H., Bradham D.M., & Grotendorst G.R. (1993). Regulation of connective tissue growth factor gene expression in human skin fibroblasts and during wound repair. *Mol Biol Cell*, Vol:4, pp.637-645, ISSN:0898-7750.

Inoue A., Kodama N., & Nanba H. (2002). Effect of maitake (Grifola frondosa) D-fraction on the control of the T lymph node Th-1/Th-2 proportion. *Biol Pharm Bull*, Vol:25, pp.536-540, ISSN:0918-6158.

Jung K., Ha Y., Ha S., Han D.U., Kim D., & Moon W.K. (2004). Antiviral effect of Saccharomyces cerevisae β-glucan to Swine Influenza virus by increased production of interferon-γ and nitric oxide. *J Vet Med B Infect Dis Vet Public Health*, Vol:51, pp.72-76, ISSN:0931-1793.

Kabasakal L, Sener G, Balkan J, Doğru-Abbasoğlu S, Keyer-Uysal M, & Uysal M. (2011). Melatonin and beta-glucan alone or in combination inhibit the growth of dunning prostatic adenocarcinoma. *Oncol Res*, Vol:19, pp.259-263, ISSN: 0965-0407.

Kankkunen P., Teirila L., Rintahakka J., Alenius A., Wolff H., & Matikainen S. (2010). (1,3)-β-glucans activate both dectin-1 and NLRP3 inflammasome in human macrophages. *J Immunol*, Vol:184, pp.6335-6342, ISSN:0022-1767.

Kenyon A.J. (1983). Delayed wound healing in mice associated with viral alteration of macrophages. *Am J Vet Res*, Vol:44, No:4, pp.652-656, ISSN:0002-9645.

Kernodle D.S., Gates H., & Kaiser A.B. (1998). Prophylactic anti-infective activity of poly-(1-6)-β-D-glucopyranosyl-(1-3)-β-D-glucopyranose glucan in a guinea pig model of staphylococcal wound infection. *Antimicrob Agents Chemother*, Vol:42, No:3, pp.545-549, ISSN:0066-4804.

Kuru B., Yilmaz S., Noyan Ü., Acar O, & Kadir T. (1999). Microbiological features and crevicular fluid aspartate aminotransferase enzyme activity in early onset periodontitis patients. *J Clin Periodontol*, Vol:26, pp.19-25, ISSN:1600-051x.

Kuru L., Griffiths G.S., Petrie A., & Olsen I. (2004a). Changes in transforming growth factor-beta1 in gingival crevicular fluid following periodontal surgery. *J Clin Periodontol*, Vol:31, No:7, pp.527-533, ISSN:0303-6979.

Kuru L., Yılmaz S., Kuru B., Köse K.N., & Noyan U. (2004b). Expression of growth factors in the gingival crevice fluid of patients with phenytoin-induced gingival enlargement. *Arch Oral Biol*, Vol:49, pp.945-950, ISSN:0003-9969.

Lamster I.B., Hartley L.J., & Oshrain R.L. (1985). Evaluation and modification of spectrophotometric procedures for analysis of lactat dehydrogenase, beta-glucoronidase and arylsulphatase in human gingival crevicular fluid collected with fitler-paper strips. *Arch Oral Biol*, Vol:30, pp.235-242, ISSN:0003-9969.

Leblanc B.W., Albina J.E., Reichner J.S. (2006). The effect of PGG-(beta)-glucan on neutrophil chemotaxis in vivo. *J Leukoc Biol*, Vol:79, pp.667-675, ISSN:0741-5400.

Lee D.Y., Ji I.H., Chang H.I., & Kim C.W. (2002). High-level TNF-alpha secretion and macrophage activity with soluble beta-glucans from Saccharomyces cerevisiae. *Biosci Biotechnol Biochem*, Vol:66, pp.233-238, ISSN:0916-8451.

Lin S, Pan Y, Luo L, & Luo L. (2011). Effects of dietary β-1,3-glucan, chitosan or raffinose on the growth, innate immunity and resistance of koi (Cyprinus carpio koi). *Fish Shellfish Immunol*, doi:10.1016/j.fsi.2011.07.013, ISSN 1050-4648.

Löe H., & Sillness J. (1963). Periodontal disease in pregnancy (I). Prevalence and severity. *Acta Odontologica Scandinavica*, Vol:21, pp.533-551, ISSN:0001-6357.

Magnusson I., Checchi L., Miccoli M.C., Vasi V., & Castaldini C. (1988). Root curettage and gingival repair in periodontics. *J Periodontol*, Vol:59, pp.124-129, ISSN:0022-3492.

Matsuda N., Lin W.L., Kumar N.M., Cho M.I., & Genco R.J. (1992). Mitogenic, chemotactic and synthetic responses of rat periodontal ligament cells to polypeptide growth factors in vitro. *J Periodontol*, Vol:63, pp.515-525, ISSN:0022-3492.

Nicoletti A., Nicolette G., Ferraro G., Palmieri G., Mattaboni P., & Germogli R. (1992). Preliminary evaluation of immunoadjuvant activity of an orally administered glucan extracted from Candida albicans. *Arzneimittelforschung*, Vol:42, pp.1246-1250, ISSN:0004-4172.

Noyan Ü., Yilmaz S., Kuru B., Kadit T., Acar O., & Büget E. (1997). A clinical and microbiological evaluation of systemic and local metronidazole delivery in adult periodontitis patients. *J Clin Periodontol*, Vol:24, pp.158-165, ISSN:1600-051x.

Page R. (1991). The role of inflammatory mediators in the pathogenesis of periodontal disease. *J Periodontal Res*, Vol:26, pp.230-242, ISSN:0022-3484.

Sarinho E., Medeiros D., Schor D., Silva A.R., Sales V., Motta M.E., Costa A., Azoubel A., & Rizzo J.A. (2009). Production of interleukin-10 in asthmatic children after beta-1-3-glucan. *Allergol Immunopathol (Madr.)*, Vol:37, pp.188-192, ISSN:0301-0546.

Sherwood E.R., Williams D.L., Mcnamee R.B., Jones E.L., Browder I.W., & DiLuzio N.R. (1987). *In vitro* tumoricidal activity of resting and glucan-activated Kupffer cells. *J Leukocyte Biol*, Vol:42, pp.69-75, ISSN:0741-5400.

Sillness J., & Löe H. (1964). Periodontal disease in pregnancy II. Correlation between oral hygiene and periodontal condition. *Acta Odontologica Scandinavica*, Vol:22, pp.121-135, ISSN:0001-6357.

Sodek J., & Overall C.M. (1992). Matrix metalloproteinases in periodontal tissue remodeling. *Matrix Suppl.*, Vol:1, pp.352-362, ISSN:0940-1199.

Sporn M.B., & Roberts A.B. (1993). A major advantage in the use of growth factors to enhance wound healing. *J Clin Invest*, Vol:92, pp.2565-2566, ISSN:0021-9738.

Stashenko P., Wang C.Y., Riley E., Wu Y., Ostroff G., & Niederman R. (1995). Reduction of infection-stimulated periapical bone resorption by the biological response modifier PGG Glucan. *J Dent Res*, Vol:74, No:1, pp.323-330, ISSN:0022-0345.

Steinsvoll S., Halstensen T.S., & Schenck K. (1999). Extensive expression of TGF-β1 in chronically-inflamed periodontal tissue. *J Clin Periodontol*, Vol:26, pp.366-373, ISSN:0303-6979.

Suzuki Y., Adachi Y., Naohito O., & Yadomae T. (2001). Th1/Th2-balancing immunomodulating activity of gel-forming (1-3)-β-glucans from fungi. *Biol Pharm Bull*, Vol:24, pp.811-819, ISSN:0918-6158.

Tanner A.C.R., Haffer C., Brathall G.T., Visconti R.A., & Socransky S.S. (1979). A study of bacteria associated with advancing periodontitis in man. *J Clin Periodontol*, Vol:6, pp.278-307, ISSN:0303-6979.

Turunen K, Tsouvelakidou E, Nomikos T, Mountzouris KC, Karamanolis D, Triantafillidis J, Kyriacou A. (2011). Impact of beta-glucan on the faecal microbiota of polypectomized patients: A pilot study. *Anaerobe*, doi: 10.1016/j.anaerobe.2011.03.025.

Tzianabos A.O. (2000). Polysaccharide immunomodulators as therapeutic agents: Structural aspects and biologic function. *Clin Microbiol Rev*, Vol:13, pp.523-533, ISSN:0938-8512.

Wahl S.M., Costa G.L., Mizel D.E., Allen J.B., Skaleric U., & Mangan D.F. (1993). Role of transforming growth factor beta in pathophysiology of chronic inflammation. *J Periodontol*, Vol:64, pp.450-455, ISSN:0022-3492.

Wassenaar A., Reinhardus C., Abraham I.L., Snijders A., & Kievits F. (1998). Characteristics of Prevotella intermedia-specific CD4+ T cell clones from peripheral blood of a chronic adult periodontitis patient. *Clin Exp Immunol*, Vol:113, pp.105-110, ISSN:0009-9104.

Williams D.L., Cook J.A., Hoffmann E.O., & Di Luzio N.R. (1978). Protective effect of glucan in experimentally induced candidiasis. *J Reticuloendothel Soc*, Vol:23, pp.479-490, ISSN:0033-6890.

Williams D.L., DiLuzio N.R. (1980). Glucan-induced modification of murine viral hepatitis. *Science*, Vol:208, pp.67-69, ISSN:0036-8075.

Wolff L.F., Liljemark W.F., Bloomquist C.G., Philström B.L., Schaffer E.M., & Bandt C.L. (1985). The distribution of Actinobacillus actinomyecetemcomitans in human plaque. *J Periodontal Res*, Vol:20, pp.237-250, ISSN:0022-3484.

Wright H.J., Chapple I.L.C., & Matthews J.B. (2003). Levels of TGF-β1 in gingival crevicular fluid during a 21-day experimental model of gingivitis. *Oral Dis*, Vol:9, pp.88-94, ISSN:1354-523x.

Yilmaz S., Kuru B., Kuru L., Noyan Ü., Argun D., & Kadir T. (2002). Effect of galium arsenide diode laser on human periodontal disease: a microbiological and clinical study. *Lasers Surg Med*, Vol:30, pp.60-66, ISSN:1096-9101.

Yun C.H., Estrada A., Van Kessel A., Park B.C., & Laarveld B. (2003). Beta-glucan, extracted from oat, enhances disease resistance against bacterial and parasitic infections. *FEMS Immunol Med Microbiol*, Vol:21, No:1, pp.67-75, ISSN:0928-8244.

11

Japanese Apricot (*Ume*): A Novel Therapeutic Approach for the Treatment of Periodontitis

Yoko Morimoto-Yamashita[1], Masayuki Tokuda[1],
Takashi Ito[1], Kiyoshi Kikuchi[2], Ikuro Maruyama[1],
Mitsuo Torii[1] and Ko-ichi Kawahara[1,3]
[1]*Kagoshima University Graduate School of Medical and Dental Sciences*
[2]*Yame Public General Hospital*
[3]*Osaka Institute of Technology*
Japan

1. Introduction

A lot of fruits contain nutrient substances that can prevent, cure or suppress various diseases. They are nature's true medicines, and diets rich in fruits are consistently associated with a decreased risk of cancer and other chronic diseases. Apricot "*Prunus armeniaca*" is the fruit of a rosaceous tree (*rosaceae*), which is produced in most parts of the world (Gur, 1985). The name *Prunus armeniaca* is thought to be a misnomer based upon the long-held view that apricots initially originated in Armenia. It is known that apricots originated in the Far East, most likely in the Himalayas, the Northern and Western regions of China from where they spread to Armenia and Russia (Gu, 1979; Gulcan, 1988). Apricot is found semi-wild and wild in the northern hills of China and in a broad belt across the hills, mountains, and plateaus of Central Asia as far as the Caucasus Mountains. The first record of the domestication of apricots is an account of their cultivation in China, about 4000 years ago. It is likely that tribe people of Central Asia established traditional rights to harvest their parts of the apricot forests for millennia before this time.

The apricot variety found in Japan is "*Prunus mume Sieb. et Zucc*" widely known as *Ume* (Figure 1). The Japanese people started to grow *Ume* trees more than 2000 years ago, most likely imported from China. Soon they discovered the health enhancing effects of apricot fruits, and over many centuries, through cultivation, they have improved their apricot tree variety to produce healthier fruits. Accordingly, there is a long-standing view that the Japanese apricot juice can suppress cancer in tumour bearing hosts and inhibit the growth of bacteria.

This article reviews the current knowledge on *Ume*, including its correlation with some diseases and periodontitis.

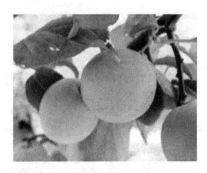
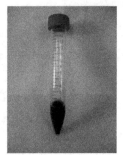

Japanese apricot fruits   MK615

Fig. 1. MK615 is made from Japanese apricot (*Ume*).

2. Anti-cancer effects of an extract from *Ume*

MK615 is an extract mixture containing hydrophobic substances from *Ume* (AdaBio, Gunma, Japan) (Figure 1). It contains several triterpenoids and has been shown to exert an anti-neoplastic effect against human cancers, such as breast cancer, stomach cancer, hepatocellular carcinoma, colon cancer and malignant melanoma. The mechanisms responsible for the anti-neoplastic effects of MK615 include induction of apoptosis and autophagy, and suppression of Aurora A kinase in cancer cells (Nakagawa et al., 2007; Adachi et al., 2007; Okada et al., 2007; Mori et al., 2007; Matsushita et al., 2010).

3. Inhibitory effects of an extract from *Ume* on *Helicobacter pylori*

Helicobacter pylori infection is an important factor in human gastric disorders, including chronic active gastritis, peptic ulcers, intestinal metaplasia and cancer.

In the *in vitro* study, *Ume* extract had an immediate bactericidal effects on *H. pylori* (Miyazawa et al., 2006; Enomoto et al., 2010). In the *in vivo* study, *Ume* extract suppress chronic active gastritis in the glandular stomachs of *H. pylori*-infected Mongolian gerbils (Otsuka et al., 2005). *H. pylori*-inoculated gerbils were given *Ume* extract in their drinking water for 10 weeks. The microscopic scores for gastritis and mucosal hyperplasia in the *Ume* extract groups were significantly lower than in the *H. pylori*-inoculated control group, with dose-dependence. Additionally, it was reported that *Ume* extract showed the antibacterial effect on *H. pylori* in the human stomach in vivo pilot study (Nakajima et al., 2006). Therefore, *Ume* extract may have potential as a safe and inexpensive agent to control *H. pylori*-associated gastric disorders, including gastric neoplasia.

4. Anti-inflammatory effects of an extract from *Ume*

The high mobility group box 1 protein (HMGB1), a nuclear protein, has two distinct functions in cellular systems. In the nucleus, HMGB1 acts as an intracellular regulator of the transcription process with a crucial role in the maintenance of DNA functions (Lu et al., 1996). In the extracellular space, HMGB1 is released by all eukaryotic cells upon necrosis or by various cells in response to inflammatory stimuli such as endotoxins, tumor necrosis factor (TNF)- α, and C-reactive protein (Wang et al., 1999; Taniguchi et al., 2003; Kawahara et al., 2008). Extracellular HMGB1 can act as a potent inducer of proinflammatory cytokines including TNF- α, interleukin (IL)-6, and IL-1s from a wide variety of cells, thus playing a major role in various inflammatory diseases such as sepsis, rheumatoid arthritis, disseminated intravascular coagulation, periodontitis, xenotransplantation and atherosclerosis (Wang et al., 1999; Taniguchi et al., 2003; Kawahara et al., 2008; Ito et al., 2007; Morimoto et al., 2008; Kawahara et al., 2007; Porto et al., 2006). Therefore, agents capable of inhibiting HMGB1 can be considered to possess therapeutic potential.

It was reported that an extract of *Ume*, an abundant source of triterpenoids, strongly inhibited HMGB1 release from lipopolysaccharide (LPS)-stimulated macrophage-like RAW264.7 cells (Kawahara et al., 2009). The inhibitory effect on HMGB1 release was enhanced by authentic oleanolic acid (OA), a naturally occurring triterpenoid. Similarly, the HMGB1 release inhibitor in *Ume* extract was found to be OA. Regarding the mechanisms of the inhibition of HMGB1 release, the OA or *Ume* extract was found to activate the transcription factor Nrf2, which binds to the antioxidative responsive element, and subsequently the heme oxygenase (HO)-1 protein was induced, indicating that the inhibition of HMGB1 release from LPS-stimulated RAW264.7 cells was mediated via the Nrf2/HO-1 system; an essentially antioxidant effect. These results suggested that natural sources of triterpenoids warrant further evaluation as 'rescue' therapeutics for sepsis and other potentially fatal systemic inflammatory disorders.

5. Periodontal disease

5.1 Symptoms

Periodontal disease, which includes gingivitis and periodontitis, is the most common chronic disorder of infectious origin known in humans, with a prevalence of 10–60% in adults depending on the diagnostic criteria used (Papapanou, 1996). Periodontitis is a chronic inflammatory disease of which the primary etiological factor is microbial dental plaque which causes an inflammatory response (Loe et al., 1965). Periodontitis destroys the periodontal tissue and eventually causes loss of teeth . Chronic and progressive bacterial infection leads to gingival connective tissue destruction and irreversible alveolar bone resorption (Ranny, 1993). Periodontal disease has various states and stages, ranging from easily treatable gingivitis to irreversible severe periodontitis and is increased by several risk factors such as systemic disease, medications (hypotensors, anti-epilepsy drugs and anti-cancer drugs), cigarette smoking, ill-fitting bridges, and trauma caused by occlusion (Papapanou, 1996; Slavin & Taylor, 1987; Grossi et al., 1997; Bjorn et al., 1969; Glickman, 1965). In addition to these variables, medical conditions that trigger host antibacterial defense mechanisms, such as neutrophil disorders and human immunodeficiency virus (HIV) infection, are likely to promote periodontal disease (Clark et al., 1977; Mealey, 1996).

The most prevalent form of periodontal disease is a mild form called gingivitis. Gingivitis is characterized by inflammation of the gums, redness, swelling, and frequent bleeding on probing (Greenstein, 1984). More advanced forms of periodontitis are also prevalent. The symptoms are similar to those of gingivitis, but are more severe due to the stronger inflammatory responses. Periodontitis is characterized by loss of gingival connective tissue attachments and alveolar bone resorption.

For diagnosing the extent of periodontal disease, probing depth is a good indicator of how far the disease has advanced (Greenstein, 1997). In clinically healthy periodontium, there is no apical migration of epithelial attachment or pocket formation and the probing depth is 1-3 mm . Patients with probing depths of 4 mm or more are diagnosed with periodontitis. Patients with probing depths of 6 mm or more are diagnosed with advanced, or severe periodontitis. Due to mild nature of symptoms, such as gingival bleeding and attachment loss many individuals neglect to treat their disease which, if left untreated, may progress to irreversible periodontitis and eventually tooth loss.

5.2 Pathogenesis of periodontal disease

The presence of large numbers of oral bacteria can induce tissue destruction indirectly by activating host defense cells, which in turn, release mediators that stimulate the effectors of connective tissue destruction. The components of microbial plaques have the capacity to induce an initial infiltrate of inflammatory cells that includes lymphocytes, macrophages, and polymorphonuclear leukocytes (PMNs) (Kowashi et al., 1980; Zappa et al., 1991). Microbial components, especially LPS, activate macrophages, which synthesize and secrete a variety of proinflammatory mediators including IL-1, IL-6, IL-8, TNF-α, prostaglandin E_2 (PGE$_2$) and hydrolytic enzymes (Birkedal-Hansen, 1993). Similarly, bacterial substances induce T lymphocytes to produce IL-1 and lymphotoxin (LT), a molecule with similar properties to TNF-α. These cytokines play a key role in periodontal tissue destruction through the induction of collagenolytic enzymes such as matrix metalloproteinases (MMPs) (Sorsa et al., 1992). These latent collagenolytic enzymes are activated by reactive oxygen species in the inflammatory environment, leading to elevated levels of interstitial collagenase in inflamed gingival tissue.

5.3 Periodontal disease and systemic disease

In the last decade, many studies have been published indicating a positive relationship between periodontal disease and various systemic diseases. Significant associations between periodontal disease and cardiovascular disease, diabetes mellitus, preterm low birth weight and osteoporosis have been reported (Jemin, & Salomon, 2006), bridging the once wide gap between medicine and dentistry. Researchers have hypothesized the etiologic role of periodontitis in the pathogenesis of these systemic diseases. Therefore, patients diagnosed with periodontal disease may be at a higher risk due to a compromised immune system as infectious and opportunistic microbes responsible for periodontal infection may prove a burden to the rest of the body. Furthermore, these microbes can release products that elicit an inflammatory response. Periodontal lesions are recognized as continually renewing reservoirs for the systemic spread of bacterial antigens, Gram-negative bacteria, cytokines and other proinflammatory mediators. Therefore,   development of new treatment modalities for periodontitis may contribute to the effective inhibition of systemic inflammatory diseases.

5.4 Treatment of periodontal disease

Once diagnosed, most periodontal diseases can be treated successfully. Therapeutic goals are to eliminate bacteria and other contributing risk factors, thereby preventing progression of the disease and maintaining healthy state of periodontal tissues. The recurrence of periodontitis must also be prevented. In severe cases, regeneration of the periodontal attachment must be attempted. The nonsurgical step involves a special cleaning technique called scaling and root planing. Supplemental treatment tools may include an antiseptic mouth rinse and other medications, either to aid the healing process, to suppress inflammation, or to further control the bacterial infection. Often, antibiotics are administered. Tetracyclines, or a combination of amoxicillin and metronidazole, may be used to kill a broad range of bacteria in microbial dental plaque(Hayes et al., 1992; Van Winkelhoff et al., 1992). However, if overused, these agents may become uneffective. Another drawback to antibiotic therapy lies in the difficulty of identifying and targeting a specific pathogen due to the numerous species residing in the plaque.

6. Possible new treatments for periodontitis

6.1 Anti-inflammatory effects of an extract from *Ume*

Natural compounds such as catechins in green tea, naringenin, a major flavanone, in grapefruits, and polyphenols in cranberries may be useful for the prevention and treatment of inflammatory periodontal diseases (Makimura et al., 1993; Bodet et al., 2008; Bodet et al., 2008). Consequently, natural compounds with the capacity to modulate host inflammatory responses have received considerable attention, with the suggestion that they may be potential new therapeutic agents for the treatment of periodontal disease (Paquette & Williams, 2000). Some studies indicate that MK615 extracted from *Ume* may have not only anti-cancer effects, but also strong anti-inflammatory effects. MK615 contains several triterpenoids, including oleanolic acid and ursolic acid, and may have anti-inflammatory effects. Recent studies have suggested that triterpenoids have both anti-tumor and anti-inflammatory effects (Nakagawa et al., 2007; Adachi et al., 2007; Okada et al., 2007; Okada et al., 2008; Kawahara et al., 2009). MK615 inhibits the release of HMGB1, a novel inflammatory mediator, by LPS-stimulated RAW264.7 cells (Kawahara et al., 2009). The inhibitory mechanism is mediated via the antioxidant compounds heme oxygenase-1, NQO-1 and glutathione-s transferase, which are induced by oleanolic acid. This strongly suggests that MK615 may suppress inflammation.

In the periodontal field, MK615 inhibits cytokine release, including that of TNF-α and IL-6, by *P. gingivalis* LPS-stimulated cells in dose-dependent manners (Morimoto et al., 2009). It is clearly indicating that MK615 contains an inhibitor of cytokine release. The continuous high secretion of various cytokines including TNF-α and IL-6 by host cells following stimulation with periodontal pathogens and their products is a critical determinant of periodontal tissue destruction. Therefore, blockade of TNF-α and IL-6 secreted by periodontal pathogens or other cytokines may suppress pro-inflammatory responses, and inhibit the development and progression of periodontal disease. It has been reported that LPS possibly induces TNF-α and IL-6 expressions through transient phosphorylation of ERK1/2, JNK, and p38MAPK (Matsuzaki et al., 2004; Kim et al., 2007; Son et al., 2008; Neuder et al., 2009; Xiao et al., 2007). Additionally, it has been also reported that the production of inflammatory cytokines requires nuclear factor kappaB (NF-κB) activation (D'Acquisto et al., 1997). The inhibitory mechanism of MK615 is mediated by the attenuation of MAPK phosphorylation (Figure 2) and subsequent inactivation of NF-κB to suppress LPS-induced translocation and phosphorylation of the p65 subunit (Figure 3 &4). These results support the notion that MK615 has anti-inflammatory effects, and MK615 may represent a key molecule with therapeutic potential for periodontitis. Therapeutic approaches that inhibit cytokine production are receiving increasing attention as options for managing chronic periodontitis.

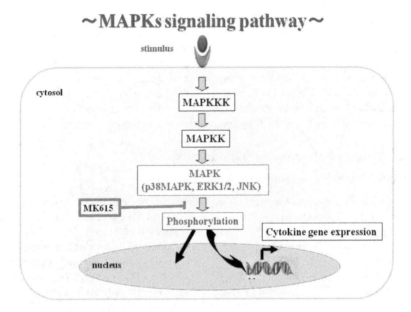

Fig. 2. MK615 inhibits phosphorylation of MAPKs.

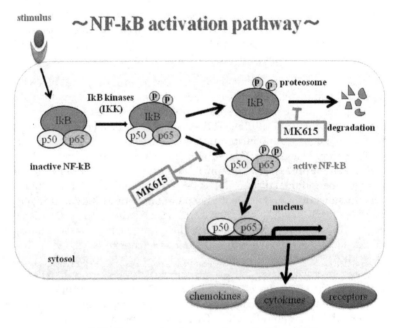

Fig. 3. MK615 suppresses NF-κB activation but not degradation of IκB.

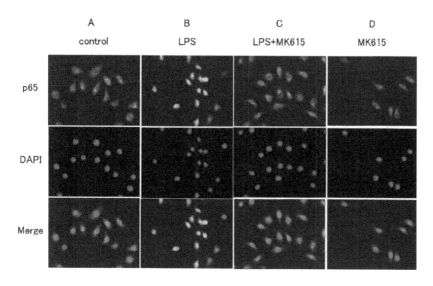

Figure 4 Morimoto et.al

Fig. 4. MK615 suppresses *P. gingivalis* LPS-induced nuclear translocation of NF-κB p65 in RAW264.7 cells. Cells were left untreated or pretreated with MK615 and stimulated with LPS. (A) In untreated cells, NF-κB p65 is limited to the cytoplasm. (B) LPS-stimulated cells show NF-κB p65 (green) translocation into the nucleus. (C) LPS-stimulated cells pretreated with MK615 show a significant reduction in p65 nuclear translocation. (D) Cells treated with MK615 alone show no effect. Cells stained with DAPI were used to verify the nuclear localization (blue). Original magnification: ×400.

6.2 Anti-microbial effects of an extract from *Ume*

Periodontitis and dental caries are major oral diseases. The formation of dental plaque, which plays an important role in the development of periodontal disease and caries in humans, can be initiated by several strains of oral streptococci (Freedman & Tanzer, 1974; Tanzer et al., 1974). *Streptococcus mutans* is the main pathogen for dental caries, although other acidogenic microorganisms can also be involved (Murata, 2008). *S. mutans* produces three types of glucosyltransferase (GTFB, GTFC and GTFD), and synthesizes an adherent and water-insoluble glucan from sucrose that allows adherence of *S. mutans* to the tooth surface and dental plaque formation (Edwardsson, 1968; Hamilton-Miller, 2001).

There is great interest in the use of antimicrobial agents for the prevention and treatment of periodontitis and caries. The prevention of periodontal disease and dental caries requires control of the pathogens that exist in the oral dental plaque biofilm. Chlorhexidine is a potent antiplaque chemical agent. However, it has some side effects, such as altered taste sensation, desquamation and soreness of the oral mucosa (Makimura et al., 1993). Thus, it is important to develop alternative antiplaque agents from natural sources that have no side effects.

It is reported that MK615 has not only anti-inflammatory effects for periodontal tissues but also antimicrobial activity against periodontal bacteria, such as *A. actinomycetemcomitans* and *P. gingivalis* (Table 1). In addition, MK615 exerted antibacterial activity against cariogenic bacteria, such as *S. mutans*, *S. gordonii* and *S. sanguinis*, with an expected anti-caries effect (Table 1). Moreover, it was found that MK615 exhibited an inhibitory effect on *S. mutans* biofilm formation. The most effective treatment against dental caries and periodontitis would be one that prevents early biofilm formation (Wei et al., 2006). MK615 is known to contain active components with anti-inflammatory and anti-oxidative properties, such as oleanolic acid (Kawahara et al., 2009). A previous study suggested that oleanolic acid has antimicrobial actions against *S. mutans* (Kozai et al., 1999), while another study showed that oleanolic acid markedly inhibits water-insoluble glucan synthesis from sucrose by the crude glucosyltransferase of *S. mutans* (Kozai et al., 1987). Therefore, MK615 has potential as a therapeutic agent for treating and preventing oral diseases such as periodontitis and dental caries. Further studies will focus on the active antimicrobial components in MK615, which should be identified and investigated for their mechanisms of action. Additionally, further studies are required to investigate the effects of local application of MK615 as an adjunctive treatment to conventional therapy for patients with periodontitis. Such studies may lead to the development of novel periodontal therapies and improved strategies for public oral health.

MICs of MK615 against oral
microorganisms.

Species	(mg/ml)
A. actinomycetemcomitans 57	6.5
A. actinomycetemcomitans IDH	6.5
P. gingivalis	1.6
S. mutans UA159	13
S. mutans MT403R	13
S. mutans RIMD	13
S. gordonii	13
S. salivarius	(-)
S. sanguinis	13

Table 1.

7. Conclusion

With the growing recognition of their benefits for public health in recent years, natural foods are now being highlighted with special reference to their effects on human health in addition to their pharmacological actions. Japanese *Ume* has been used as a herbal medicine with several biological activities, including anticancer, antioxidant and anti-inflammation effects (Nakagawa et al., 2007; Adachi et al., 2007; Okada et al., 2007; Mori et al.,2007; Kawahara et al., 2009).

MK615, an extract of compounds from Japanese *Ume*, has not only anti-inflammatory effects for periodontal tissues but also antimicrobial activity against periodontal bacteria, such as *A. actinomycetemcomitans* and *P. gingivalis*. In addition, MK615 exerted antibacterial activity against cariogenic bacteria, such as *S. mutans, S. gordonii* and *S. sanguinis*, with an expected anti-caries effect. Moreover, it was found that MK615 exhibited an inhibitory effect on *S. mutans* biofilm formation. MK615 has potential as a therapeutic agent for treating and preventing oral diseases such as periodontitis and dental caries. Further studies will focus on the active anti-inflammatory and antimicrobial components in MK615, which should be identified and investigated for their mechanisms.

MK615 is safe in food for providing health benefits, and this remains unquestioned even when it is prescribed for oral therapy. Moreover, it is also used as a treatment for patients with liver cancer. In the future, it may be added to toothpastes, mouth rinses and other oral products that can be used easily by the majority of the populationranging from youngsters to the elderly. In addition, MK615 may be applicable to the total body through examining its possible effects on not only oral bacteria but also *Staphylococcus aureus* and *Candida albicans*.

8. References

Adachi, M. Suzuki, Y. Mizuta, T. Osawa, T. Adachi, T. Osaka, K. Suzuki, K. Shiojima, K. Arai, Y. Masuda, K. Uchiyama, M. Oyamada, T. & Clerici, M. (2007). The " *Prunus mume Sieb. et Zucc*" (Ume) is a rich natural source of novel anti-cancer substance, *International Journal of Food Properties Int. J. Food. Prop.* Vol. 10: 375-384.

Birkedal-Hansen, H. (1993). Role of cytokines and inflammatory mediators in tissue destruction, *J. Periodont. Res.* Vol. 28: 500–510.

Bjorn, AL. Bjorn, H. & Grcovic, B. (1969). Marginal fit of restorations and its relation to periodontal bone level, *Odont Revy.* Vol. 20: 311-321.

Bodet, C. Grenier, D. Chandad, F. Ofek, I. Steinberg, D. & Weiss, EI. (2008). Potential oral health benefits of cranberry, *Crit. Rev. Food. Sci. Nutr.* Vol. 48: 672-680.

Bodet, C. La, VD. Epifano, F. & Grenier, D. (2008). Naringenin has anti-inflammatory properties in macrophage and *ex vivo* human whole-blood models, *J. Periodontal. Res.* Vol. 43: 400-407.

Clark, RA. Page, RC. & Wilde, G. (1977). Defective neutrophil chemotaxis in juvenile periodontitis, *Infect. Immun.* Vol. 18 (3): 694-700.

D'Acquisto, F. Cicatiello, L. Iuvone, T. Ialenti, A. Ianaro, A. Esumi, H. Weisz, A. & Carnuccio, R. (1997). Inhibition of inducible nitric oxide synthase gene expression by glucocorticoid-induced protein(s) in lipopolysaccharide-stimulated J774 cells, *Eur. J. Pharmacol.* Vol. 339: 87–95.

Edwardsson, S. (1968). Characteristics of caries-inducing human streptococci resembling Streptococcus mutans, *Arch Oral Biol.* Vol. 13: 637-646.

Enomoto, S. Yanaoka, K. Utsunomiya, H. Niwa, T. Inada, K. & Ichinose, M. (2010). Inhibitory effects of Japanese apricot (Prunus mume Siebold et Zucc.; Ume) on Helicobacter pylori-related chronic gastritis, *Eur J Clin Nutr.* Vol. 64: 714-719.

Freedman, ML. & Tanzer, JM. (1974). Dissociation of plaque formation from glucan induced agglutination in mutants of Streptococcus mutans, *Infect Immun.* Vol. 10: 189-196.

Glickman, I. (1965). Clinical significance of trauma from occlusion, *J. Am. Dent. Assoc.* Vol. 70: 607-618.

Greenstein, G. (1984). The role of bleeding upon probing in the diagnosis of periodontal disease. A literature review, *J. Periodontol.* Vol. 55 (12): 684-688.

Greenstein, G. (1997). Contemporary interpretation of probing depth assessments: diagnostic and therapeutic implications. A literature review, *J. Periodontol.* Vol. 68 (12): 1194-1205.

Grossi, SG. Zambon, J. Machtei, EE. Schifferle, R. Andreana, S. Genco, RJ. Cummins, D. & Harrap, G. (1997). Effects of smoking and smoking cessation on healing after mechanical periodontal therapy, *J. Am. Dent. Assoc.* Vol. 128 (5): 599-607.

Gu, M. (1979). Apricot Cultivars in China, *Acta Horticulturae* Vol. 209: 63-67.

Gulcan, R. (1988). Apricot Cultivars in Near East, *Acta Horticulturae* Vol. 209: 49-54.

Gur, AR. (1985). Deciduous Fruit Trees. *In Handbook of Flowering*, CRC Press, pp. 355-389.

Hamilton-Miller, JM. (2001). Anti-cariogenic properties of tea (Camellia sinensis), *J Med Microbiol.* Vol. 50: 299-302.

Hayes, C. Antezak-Bouckoms, A. & Burdick, E. (1992). Quality assessment and meta-analysis of systemic tetracycline use in chronic adult periodontitis, *J Clin Periodontol.* Vol. 9: 164–168.

Ito, T. Kawahara K. Nakamura, T. Yamada, S. Nakamura, T. Abeyama, K. Hashiguchi, T. & Maruyama, I. (2007). High-mobility group box 1 protein promotes development of microvascular thrombosis in rats, *J. Thromb. Haemost.* Vol. 5: 109-116.

Jemin, Kim. & Salomon, Amar. (2006). Periodontal disease and systemic conditions: a bidirectional relationship, *Odontology* Vol. 94: 10-21.

Kawahara, K. Biswas, KK. Unoshima, M. Ito, T. Kikuchi, K. Morimoto, Y. Iwata, M. Tancharoen, S. Oyama, Y. Takenouchi, K. Nawa, Y. Arimura, N. Jie, MX. Shrestha, B. Miura, N. Shimizu, T. Mera, K. Arimura, S. Taniguchi, N. Iwasaka, H. Takao, S. Hashiguchi, T. & Maruyama, I. (2008). C-reactive protein induces high mobility group box-1 protein release through a p38MAPK in the macrophage cell line RAW264.7 cells, *Cardiovasc. Pathol.* Vol. 17: 129-138.

Kawahara, K. Hashiguchi, T. Masuda, K. Saniabadi, AR. Kikuchi, K. Tancharoen, S. Ito, T. Miura, N. Morimoto, Y. Biswas, KK. Nawa, Y. Meng, X. Oyama, Y. Takenouchi, K. Shrestha, B. Sameshima, H. Shimizu, T. Adachi, T. Adachi, M. & Maruyama, I. (2009). Mechanism of HMGB1 release inhibition from RAW264.7 cells by oleanolic acid in Prunus mume Sieb. et Zucc, *Int. J. Mol. Med.* Vol. 23: 615-620.

Kawahara, K. Setoyama, K. Kikuchi, K. Biswas, KK. Kamimura, R. Iwata, M. Ito, T. Morimoto, Y. Hashiguchi, T. Takao, S. & Maruyama, I. (2007). HMGB1 release in co-cultures of porcine endothelial and human T cells, *Xenotransplantation* Vol. 14: 636-641.

Kim, Do Y. Jun, JH. Lee, HL. Woo, KM. Ryoo, HM. Kim, GS. Baek, JH. & Han, SB. (2007). N-acetylcysteine prevents LPS-induced pro-inflammatory cytokines and MMP2 production in gingival fibroblasts, *Arch. Pharm. Res.* Vol. 30: 1283-1292.

Kowashi, Y. Jaccardand, F. & Cimasoni, G. (1980). Sulcular polymorphonuclear leucocytes and gingival exudate during experimental gingivitis in man, *J. Periodont. Res.* Vol. 15: 151-158.

Kozai, K. Miyake, Y. Kohda, H. Kametaka, S. Yamasaki, K. & Nagasaka, N. (1987) Inhibition of Glucosyltransferase from Streptococcus mutans by Oleanolic acid and Ursolic Acid, *Caries. Res.* Vol 21: 104-108.

Kozai, K. Suzuki, J. Okada, M. & Nagasaka, N. (1999). Effect of oleanolic acid-cyclodextrin inclusion compounds on dental caries by in vitro experiment and rat-caries model, *Microbios* Vol. 97: 179-188.

L. Manogue, KR. Faist, E. Abraham, E. Andersson, J. Andersson, U. Molina, PE. Abumrad, NN. Sama, A. & Tracey, KJ. (1999). HMG-1 as a late mediator of endotoxin lethality in mice, *Science* Vol. 285: 248-251.

Loe, H. Theilade, E. & Jensen SB. (1965). Experimental gingivitis in man, *J. Periodontol.* Vol. 36: 177-187.

Lu, J. Kobayashi, R. & Brill, SJ. (1996). Characterization of a high mobility group 1/2 homolog in yeast, *J. Biol. Chem.* Vol. 271: 33678-33685.

Makimura, M. Hirasawa, M. Kobayashi, K. Indo, J. Sakanaka, S. Taguchi, T. & Otake, S. (1993). Inhibitory effect of tea catechins on collagenase activity, *J. Periodontol.* Vol. 64: 630-636.

Matsushita, S. Tada, KI. Kawahara, KI. Kawai, K. Hashiguchi, T. Maruyama, I. & Kanekura, T. (2010). Advanced malignant melanoma responds to *Prunus mume Sieb. et Zucc* (Ume) extract: Case report and *in vitro* study, *Experimental and Therapeutic Medicine* Vol. 1: 569-574.

Matsuzaki, H. Kobayashi, H. & Yagyu, T. (2004). Bikunin inhibits lipopolysaccharide-induced tumor necrosis factor-alpha induction in macrophages, *Clin. Diag. Lab. Immunol.* Vol. 11: 1140–1147.

Mealey, BL. (1996). Periodontal implications: medically compromised patients, *Ann Periodontol.*, Vol. 1: 256-321.

Miyazawa, M. Utsunomiya, H. Inada, K. Yamada, T. Okuno, Y. & Tatematsu, M. (2006). Inhibition of *Helicobacter pylori* Motility by (+)-Syringaresinol from Unripe Japanese Apricot, *Biol Pharm Bull.* Vol. 29: 172-173.

Mori, S. Sawada, T. Okada, T. Ohsawa, T. Adachi, M. & Keiichi K. (2007). New anti-proliferative agent, MK615, from Japanese apricot 'Prunus mume' induces striking autophagy in colon cancer cells in vitro, *World J. Gastroenterol.* Vol. 13: 6512-6517.

Morimoto, Y. Kawahara, KI. Kikuchi, K. Ito, T. Tokuda, M. Matsuyama,T. Noma, S. Hashiguchi, T. Torii, M. & Maruyama, I. (2009). MK615 attenuates *Porphyromonas gingivalis* lipopolysaccharide-induced pro-inflammatory cytokine release via MAPK inactivation in murine macrophage-like RAW264.7 cell, *Biochemical and Biophysical Research Communications* Vol. 389: 90-94.

Morimoto, Y. Kawahara, KI. Tancharoen, S. Kikuchi, K. Matsuyama, T. Hashiguchi, T. Izumi, Y. & Maruyama, I. (2008). Tumor necrosis factor-alpha stimulates gingival epithelial cells to release high mobility-group box 1, *J. Periodontal. Res.* Vol. 43: 76-83.

Murata, RM. Branco de Almeida, LS. Yatsuda, R. Dos Santos, MH. Nagem, TJ. & Koo H. (2008). Inhibitory effects of 7-epiclusianone on glucan synthesis, acidogenicity and biofilm formation by Streptococcus mutans, *FEMS Microbiol Lett.* Vol. 282: 174-181.

Nakagawa, A. Sawada, T. Okada, T. Ohsawa, T. Adachi, M. & Kubota K. (2007). New antineoplastic agent, MK615, from UME (a variety of) Japanese apricot inhibits growth of breast cancer cells in vitro, *The Breast Journal Breast. J.* Vol. 13: 44-49.

Nakajima, S. Fujita, K. Inoue, Y. Nishino, M. Seto, Y. (2006). Effect of the folk remedy, Bainiku-ekisu, a concentrate of Prunus mume juice, on Helicobacter pylori infection in humans, *Helicobacter* Vol. 11(6): 589-591.

Neuder, LE. Keener, JM. Eckert, RE. Trujillo, JC. & Jones SL. (2009). Role of p38 MAPK in LPS induced pro-inflammatory cytokine and chemokine gene expression in equine leukocytes, Vet. Immunol. Immunopathol. Vol. 129: 192-199.

Okada, T. Sawada, T. Osawa, T. Adachi, M. & Kubota K. (2008). MK615 inhibits pancreatic cancer cell growth by dual inhibition of Aurora A and B kinases, *World J. Gastroenterol.* Vol. 14: 1378-1382.

Okada, T. Sawada, T. Osawa, T. Adachi, M. & Kubota, K. (2007). A novel anti-cancer substance, MK615, from Ume, a variety of Japanese apricot, inhibits growth of hepatocellular carcinoma cells by suppressing Aurora A kinase activity, *Hepatogastroenterology* Vol. 54: 1770-1774.

Otsuka, T. Tsukamoto, T. Tanaka, H. Inada, K. Utsunomiya, H. Mizoshita, T. Kumagai, T. Katsuyama, T. Miki, K. Tatematsu, M. (2005). Suppressive effects of fruit-juice concentrate of Prunus mume Sieb. et Zucc. (Japanese apricot, Ume) on Helicobacter pylori-induced glandular stomach lesions in Mongolian gerbils, *Asian. Pac. J. Cancer. Prev.* Vol. 6(3): 337-341.

Papapanou, PN. (1996). Periodontal diseases: Epidemiology, *Ann. Periodontal.* Vol. 1 (1): 1-36.

Paquette, DW. & Williams, RC. (2000). Modulation of host inflammatory mediators as a treatment strategy for periodontal diseases, *Periodontol. 2000.* Vol. 24: 239-252.

Porto, A. Palumbo, R. Pieroni, M. Aprigliano, G. Chiesa, R. Sanvito, F. Maseri, A. & Bianchi, ME. (2006). Smooth muscle cells in human atherosclerotic plaques secrete and proliferate in response to high mobility group box 1 protein, *FASEB J.* Vol. 20: 2565-2566.

Ranny, R. (1993). Classification of periodontal disease, *Periodontol. 2000.* Vol. 2: 13-25.

Slavin, J. & Taylor, J. (1987). Cyclosporine, nifedipine and gingival hyperplasia, *Lancet* Vol. 2: 739.

Son, YH. Jeong, YT. Lee, KA. Choi, KH. Kim, SM. Rhim, BY. & Kim, K. (2008). Roles of MAPK and NF-kappaB in interleukin-6 induction by lipopolysaccharide in vascular smooth muscle cells, J. Cardiovasc. Pharmacol. Vol. 51: 71-77.

Sorsa, T. Ingman, T. Suomalainen, K. Haapasalo, M. Konttinen, YT. Lindy, O. Saari, H. & Uitto, VJ. (1992). Identification of proteases from periodontopathogenic bacteria as activators of latent human neutrophil and fibroblast-type interstitial collagenases, *Infect Immun.* Vol. 60: 4491-4495.

Taniguchi, N. Kawahara, K. Yone, K. Hashiguchi, T. Yamakuchi, M. Goto, M. Inoue, K. Yamada, S. Ijiri, K. Matsunaga, S. Nakajima, T. Komiya, S. & Maruyama, I. (2003). High mobility group box chromosomal protein 1 plays a role in the pathogenesis of rheumatoid arthritis as a novel cytokine, *Arthritis. Rheum.* Vol. 48: 971-981.

Tanzer, JM. Freedman, ML. Fitzgerald, RJ. & Larson RH. (1974). Diminished virulence of glucan synthesis defective mutants of Streptococcus mutans, *Infect Immun.* Vol. 10: 197-203.

Van Winkelhoff, AJ. Tijhof, CJ. & de Graaff, J. (1992). Microbiological and clinical results of metronidazole plus amoxicillin therapy in *Actinobacillus actinomycetemcomitans*-associated periodontitis, J. Periodontol. Vol. 63: 52-57.

Wang, H. Bloom, O. Zhang, M. Vishnubhakat, JM. Ombrellino, M. Che, J. Frazier, A. Yang, H. Ivanova, S. Borovikova,

Wei, G. Campagna, NA. & Bobek, AL. (2006). Effect of MUC7 peptides on the growth of bacteria and on Streptococcus mutans biofilm, J. Antimicrob. Chemother. Vol. 57: 1100-1009.

Xiao, ZY. Zhou, WX. Zhang, YX. Cheng, JP. He, JF. Yang, RF. & Yun, LH. (2007). Inhibitory effect of linomide on lipopolysaccharide-induced proinflammatory cytokine tumor necrosis factor-alpha production in RAW264.7 macrophages through suppression of NF-κB, p38, and JNK activation, Immunol. Lett. Vol. 114: 81-85.

Zappa, U. Reinking-Zappa, M. Grafand, H. & Espel, M. (1991). Cell populations and episodic periodontal attachment loss in humans, J. Clin. Periodontol. Vol. 18: 508-515.

12

Alternative Treatment Approaches in Chronic Periodontitis: Laser Applications

Livia Nastri and Ugo Caruso

Seconda Università degli Studi di Napoli - Dept. of Stomatologic,
Orthodontic and Surgical Sciences, Naples,
Italy

1. Introduction

Periodontal disease is initiated by pathogenic plaque biofilm and characterized by bacteria-induced inflammatory destruction of tooth-supporting structures and alveolar bone (Lui & Corbet, 2011). With a constant bacterial challenge, the periodontal tissues are continuously exposed to specific bacterial components that have the ability to alter many local functions. The role of the inflammatory process is to protect the host and limit the pathogenic effect of biofilm, thus determining some tissue destruction as a collateral effect of the defence. The extent and severity of damage vary among individuals and over time (Offenbacher, 1996;Kinane et al., 2005; Karlsson et al., 2008), mainly influenced by individual's immune and inflammatory responses to microbial challenge. In some patients gingivitis progresses to periodontitis, with a slower or faster progression, that is characterized by the destruction of the supporting structures of the teeth, including periodontal ligament and bone, and cementum alterations, that may in turn ultimately cause tooth loss (Kinane, 2001). Unfortunately, little and still uncertain is the possibility to interfere with individual response, to redirect inflammatory and immune defences or, as it is commonly defined, to perform a "host modulation". The rationale behind this approach is to aid the host in its fight against infectious agents by supplementing the natural defence mechanism or to modify its responses by changing the course of inflammatory systems. Therefore, pharmaceutical inhibition of host response with an anti-inflammatory mechanism may prove to be an effective strategy for treating periodontal diseases. Current research has focused on the use of subantimicrobial dose of doxycycline (SDD) as a treatment modality, and SDD is the only systemically used host modulatory drug approved by the United States Food and Drug Administration. (Deo et al., 2010) (Figure 1).

At present state, an effective and widely accepted treatment approach for periodontal disease is the mechanical removal of the bacterial biofilm and their toxins from the tooth surface by scaling and root planing, making it compatible with biologic reattachment that is the basis of any eventual adjunctive therapy (Sigusch et al., 2010). Traditionally, scaling and root planing procedures can be performed by hand and/or powered instruments. However, complete removal of bacterial deposits within the periodontal pockets is not necessarily achieved with conventional mechanical therapy. In addition, access to areas such as furcations, concavities, grooves, and distal sites of molars is limited (Aoki et al., 2004).

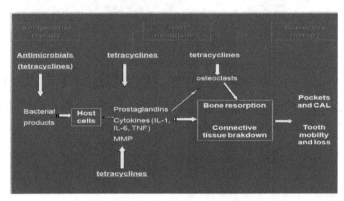

Fig. 1. Scheme of pathogenesis of periodontal disease; role of tetracycline in different phases.

Currently, efficient anti-infective treatments with reduced side effects are being searched for. Local and systemic antibiotics may lead to bacterial resistance, allergies, gastrointestinal disorders and others, reducing patient compliance or advising against the prescription (Quirynen et al., 2003; Rodrigues et al., 2004).

Therefore, development of novel systems for scaling and root planing, as well as further improvement of currently used mechanical instruments, is required.

For its various characteristics, such as ablation or vaporization, haemostasis and sterilization effect, the use of laser may serve as an adjunct or alternative treatment to conventional periodontal therapy (Aoki et al., 2004).

2. Characteristics of lasers

The word LASER is the acronym for Light Amplification by Stimulated Emission of Radiation. A laser is a device that emits light through a process called stimulated emission, featuring collimated (parallel) and coherent (temporally and spatially constant) electromagnetic radiation of a single wavelength. Laser light is produced by pumping (energizing) a certain substance, or gain medium, within a resonating chamber (Figure 2).

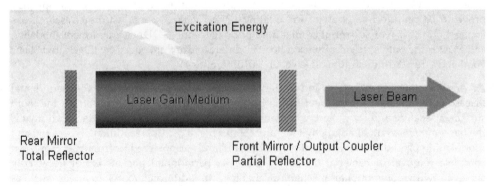

Fig. 2. Schematic drawing of the main component of a laser system.

The process of lasing occurs when an exited atom is stimulated to emit a photon before the process occurs spontaneously. Spontaneous emission of a photon by one atom stimulates the release of a subsequent photon and so on. This stimulated emission generates a very coherent and synchronous wave, of a single wavelength and in a collimated form (parallel rays) of light that is found nowhere else in nature. The various laser systems are usually named after the ingredients of the gain medium, but three factors are important to the final characteristics of the laser light: as said before, gain medium, source of pump energy, design of resonating chamber. Clinically, that is for medical applications, both the laser-delivery system (e.g. optical fiber or articulated arm with mirrors) and the application tip are of paramount importance, as they may condition the ease of use, range of applications and energy efficiency of a laser system. The most common classifications of lasers are those related to the type of gain medium and characteristics of the laser light.

The characteristics of lasers depend on their wavelength (table 1 and figure 3).

Laser type		Wavelength	Color
Excimer lasers	Argon Fluoride (ArF)	193 nm	Ultraviolet
	Xenon Chloride (XeCl)	308 nm	Ultraviolet
Gas lasers	Argon	488 nm	Blue
		514 nm	Blue-green
	Helium Neon (HeNe)	637 nm	Red
	Carbon Dioxide (CO_2)	10,600 nm	Infrared
Diode lasers	Indium Gallium Arsenide Phosphorus (InGaAsP)	655 nm	Red
	Gallium Aluminum Arsenide (GaAlAs)	670–830 nm	Red-infrared
	Gallium Arsenide (GaAs)	840 nm	Infrared
	Indium Gallium Arsenide (InGaAs)	980 nm	Infrared
Solid state lasers	Frequency-doubled Alexandrite	337 nm	Ultraviolet
	Potassium Titanyl Phosphate (KTP)	532 nm	Green
	Neodymium:YAG (Nd:YAG)	1,064 nm	Infrared
	Holmium:YAG (Ho:YAG)	2,100 nm	Infrared
	Erbium, chromium:YSGG (Er,Cr:YSGG)	2,780 nm	Infrared
	Erbium:YSGG (Er:YSGG)	2,790 nm	Infrared
	Erbium:YAG (Er:YAG)	2,940 nm	Infrared

Table 1. Type and wavelength of lasers (from Aoki et al. 2004)

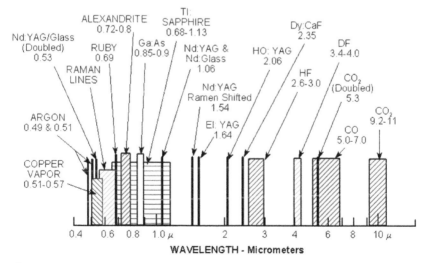

Fig. 3. Electromagnetic spectrum and wavelengths of lasers.

The term "waveform" describes the way of laser delivery over time, either as a continuous or as a pulsed beam emission (table 2). A continuous wave laser beam emits an uninterrupted beam at the output power set for as long as the switch is turned on. The pulsed beam may be delivered in two different modalities: a free-running pulse, in which pulsation is stored for a certain time and the emission has a peak power greater than the power selected on the panel, or gated pulse, in which a continuous wave beam is interrupted at various rates by a shutter, having the laser the same power set.

Criteria	Types	Examples
Output Energy	Low-output, soft, or therapeutic	Low-output diodes
	High-output, hard, or surgical	Diodes, CO_2, Nd:YAG, Er:YAG, Er,Cr:YSGG
State of the gain medium	Solid-state	Nd:YAG, Er:YAG, Er,Cr:YSGG, KTP
	Gas	HeNe, Argon, CO_2
	Excimer	F_2,ArF, KrCl, XeCl
	Diode	GaAlAs, InGaAs
Oscillation mode	Continous-wave	CO_2, Diodes
	Pulsed- wave	CO_2, Diodes, Nd:YAG, Er:YAG, Er,Cr:YSGG, KTP

Table 2. Mode of irradiation and laser denomination.

The first prototype of laser was developed by Maiman in 1960, using a crystal medium of ruby that emitted a coherent radiant light from the crystal when stimulated by energy. The first application of laser in dental field was reported by Goldman et al. (1964), describing the effect of the ruby laser on enamel and dentin while attempting to remove caries in vitro using the ruby laser. Since then, many researchers investigated the effects of various laser types on dental hard tissue and caries. However, previous laser systems where basically not indicated for hard tissue procedures due to major thermal damage (Frentzen et al., 2002).

The effect of the laser on a tissue depends on its behaviour within it. It can reflect, scatter, be absorbed or transmitted to surrounding tissues (Figure 4).

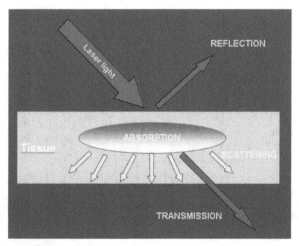

Fig. 4. Possible effects of laser irradiation on tissue.

Basically, as the absorption increases, the reflection, scattering and transmission decrease. For most biological tissues, higher absorption occurs in wavelengths with greater absorbance in water. The more absorbance occurs, the less the laser light penetrates the surrounding tissues with a shallower layer of laser-affected tissue (Ishikawa et al. 2009).

Since the periodontium is composed of gingiva, periodontal ligament, cementum and alveolar bone, both soft and hard tissues are involved in a lasering process. The high power carbon dioxide (CO_2) and neodymium-doped yttrium aluminium garnet (Nd:YAG) lasers are capable of excellent soft tissue ablation with a good haemostatic effect. As such, these lasers have been generally proposed for periodontal surgery and oral surgery (Aoki et al. 2004). However, these lasers are not suitable for treatment of root surface or alveolar bone, due to carbonization of these tissues and major thermal side-effects on the target and surrounding tissues, with a limitation of employment indications to gingivectomy and frenectomy.

In the late eighties Keller and Hibst (1989) and Kayano et al. (1991) reported the possibility of dental hard tissue ablation by erbium yttrium aluminium garnet (Er:YAG) laser irradiation, which is highly absorbed by water, without producing major thermal side-effects. Er:YAG laser was then proved for periodontal hard tissue procedures such as dental calculus removal and decontamination of the diseased root surface.

Diode and Nd:YAG lasers are also currently under investigation and used by clinicians because of their flexible fiber delivery system, which is suitable for pocket insertion. Nd.YAG, CO2, Diodes, Er:YAG, erbium chromium-doped yttrium scandium gallium and garnet (Er,Cr:YSGG), Argon, excimer and alexandrite lasers are being studied in vitro or are in clinical use (table 3).

Laser type		Current/Potential dental application
Excimer lasers	Argon Fluoride (ArF) Xenon Chloride (XeCl)	Hard tissue ablation, Dental calculus removal
Gas lasers	Argon (Ar)	Curing of composite materials, Tooth whitening, Intraoral soft tissue surgery, Sulcular debridement (subgingival curettage in periodontitis and peri-implantitis)
	Helium Neon (HeNe)	Analgesia, Treatment of dentin hypersensitivity, Aphthous ulcer treatment
	Carbon Dioxide (CO₂)	Intraoral and implant soft tissue surgery, Aphthous ulcer treatment, Removal of gingival melanin pigmentation, Treatment of dentin hypersensitivity, Analgesia
Diode lasers	Indium Gallium Arsenide Phosphorus (InGaAsP)	Caries and calculus detection
	Galium Aluminum Arsenide (GaAlAs) and Gallium Arsenide (GaAs)	Intraoral general and implant soft tissue surgery, Sulcular debridement (subgingival curettage in periodontitis and peri-implantitis), Analgesia, Treatment of dentin hypersensitivity, Pulpotomy, Root canal disinfection, Aphthous ulcer treatment, Removal of gingival melanin pigmentation
Solid state lasers	Frequency-doubled Alexandrite	Selective ablation of dental plaque and calculus
	Neodymium:YAG (Nd:YAG)	Intraoral soft tissue surgery, Sulcular debridement (subgingival curettage in periodontitis), Analgesia, Treatment of dentin hypersensitivity, Pulpotomy, Root canal disinfection, Removal of enamel caries, Aphthous ulcer treatment, Removal of gingival melanin pigmentation
	Erbium group Erbium:YAG (Er:YAG), Erbium:YSGG (Er:YSGG), Erbium.chromium:YSGG (Er.Cr:YSGG)	Caries removal and cavity preparation, Modification of enamel and dentin surfaces, Intraoral general and implant soft tissue surgery, Sulcular debridement (subgingival curettage in periodontitis and peri-implantitis), Scaling of root surfaces, Osseous surgery, Treatment of dentin hypersensitivity, Analgesia, Pulpotomy, Root canal treatment and disinfection, Aphthous ulcer treatment, Removal of gingival melanin/metal-tattoo pigmentation

Table 3. Characteristics and actual or potential clinical use of different laser lights (from Aoki et al. 2004)

Characteristics, possible development and actual studies will be analyzed for different laser types.

2.1 CO₂ laser

The CO_2 laser has a wavelength of 10.600 nm and can be used in either pulsed-wave or continuous-wave modes. Because of an excellent capacity for soft tissue ablation, CO_2 lasers have been successfully used as an adjunctive tool to de-epithelialize the mucoperiosteal flap during traditional flap surgery (Centty et al. 1997). The scattering of laser energy within the surrounding tissues is low and the layer of heat-altered tissue that remains after vaporization is relatively shallow; however the vaporization temperature is high and the irradiated surface is easily carbonized. With the CO2 laser, the performance advantages are the rapid and simple vaporization of soft tissues with strong haemostasis, which produces a clear operating field and requires no suturing (Pick et al., 1995). Gingival hyperplasia is a typical indication for CO2 laser treatment. Inorganic components of hard tissues, like bone and cementum (and also dental calculus), can reach very high temperatures, due to their content in apatite, especially phosphate ions ($-PO_4$), that absorb CO_2 laser wavelength much more than water (Featherston, 2000).

2.1.1 Periodontal applications of CO₂ laser

Several studies reported major thermal side effects, such as melting, cracking or carbonization when CO_2 lasers were used directly on root surface (Aoki et al. 2004). However, these negative effects were avoided when irradiation was performed in a pulsed mode with a de-focused beam (Barone et al., 2002). The defocused mode of the CO2 laser has root conditioning effects, such as smear layer removal, decontamination and the preparation of a surface favourable to fibroblast attachment (Crespi et al., 2002).

Transmission of the CO2 laser through optical fibers was very difficult and therefore the system previously employed mirror systems using articulated arms for laser beam delivery. In the case of the CO2 laser, because of the lack of an appropriate flexible delivery system with suitable contact tips for periodontal pocket therapy, only a few clinical studies have been reported on the effects of this laser in the non surgical treatment of periodontitis (Miyazaki et al., 2003; Mullins et al., 2007). Also, CO2 irradiation of the periodontal pocket using a special tip failed to result in a reduction of bacterial counts, and potentially damaged the soft tissue surrounding the periodontal pocket itself with cases of residual melted calculus being reported.

2.2 Nd:YAG laser

The Nd:YAG laser has a wavelength of 1.064 nm and operates in a free running pulsed mode. It is commonly used in periodontal therapy to incise and excise soft tissues as well for the curettage and disinfection of periodontal pockets. The Nd:YAG laser has low absorption in water, and the energy scatters or penetrates into the biological tissues. In water, the Nd:YAG laser will theoretically penetrate to a depth of 60mm before it is attenuated to 10% of its original strength (AAP, 2002). In soft tissue treatments, this laser is very effective at producing coagulation and haemostasis, in a relatively thick layer of soft tissues. Hence, the Nd:YAG laser is basically effective for ablation of potentially hemorrhagic soft tissue, being the width of coagulation from 0.3 to 0.8 mm at 3-10 W of laser power. However these effects are primarily caused by tissue heating and therefore irradiated surfaces usually exhibit a thick layer of coagulated tissue. Because of its high penetrability, the possible thermal effects on tissues laying below the irradiated are, such as dental pulp or bone tissue, is occasionally a matter of concern during periodontal treatment (Schwarz et al., 2009).

In dentistry, soft tissue surgery using the Nd:YAG laser has been widely accepted. In 1990, the FDA approved soft tissue removal by means of a pulsed Nd:YAG laser for intraoral soft tissue application without anaesthesia, with a minimal bleeding compared to scalpel surgery. The delivery system of the laser is flexible and suitable for periodontal employment, being a flexible optical fiber with a contact tip of 400 μm. In 1997 the FDA approved the use of Nd:YAG laser in sulcular debridement (Aoki et al., 2004).

2.2.1 Periodontal applications of Nd:YAG laser

The first in vitro studies on the use of Nd:YAG laser for calculus removal showed that its ability to remove calculus at a level equivalent to mechanical treatment is not easily clinically expectable. Different studies with different irradiation power and mode gave different degrees of calculus removal from the root and different effects on the root itself. Tseng & Liew (1990) demonstrated that partial removal and detachment of the calculus from the root surface was achieved by 2.0 to 2.75 W of power at 20 Hz pulse. However, melting of calculus and thermal damage was noted in localized areas of cementum and even dentin.

Morlock et al. (1992) showed that the Nd:YAG laser at 1.25-1.50 W, pulse 20 Hz, produced surface pitting and crater formation with charring, carbonization, melting, even when irradiation was performed parallel to root surface. Other authors demonstrated how the root surface was modified by Nd:YAG irradiation in a way that affected fibroblast recolonization and reattachment.

Also the removal of smear layer from the root surface is obtained only at powers that are not suitable for clinical use, either for a root alteration or for significant intrapulpal temperature rise.

Other authors demonstrated the possibility of calculus removal from the root with more or less extent of root damages. As subgingival calculus is often dark coloured, the Nd:YAG laser has the advantage of being absorbed by deposits. However the energy capable of detaching the calculus may be inappropriate for clinical usage due to increased thermal side-effects. Clinically an application of a low power Nd:YAG laser can result in an ineffective and patchy removal of calculus from the root surface. However, it would result in an alteration of calculus that should followed by facilitation of mechanical debridement.

Nd:YAG laser was the first to be approved by FDA for applying in periodontal pockets . It has been widely used by general practioners because of its ease of use. However, in spite of its long time use, there is still very insufficient proof of a positive effect from scientific studies.

Nd:YAG laser cannot achieve root surface debridement to a satisfactory degree, due to insufficient ability to remove calculus and to distinguish calculus from the root. If utilized, Nd:YAG laser should employed as an adjunct to conventional mechanical treatment to exploit the ability of curettage of the soft wall of pocket, to remove infected granulation tissue and epithelium, as for its ability of detoxification at a relatively low energy level.

Nonetheless, it has to be kept in mind that Nd:YAG laser has the capability of a deep penetration in oral tissue and the risk of a pulpal or alveolar bone temperature rise is high.

2.3 Nd:YAP laser

The Nd:YAP laser has a wavelength of 1.340 nm and it is mainly absorbed by black-pigmented tissues. Its employment in periodontal pocket treatment is still under investigation at first stages, however the concern related to a potential increase in temperature of the target is similar to that of Nd:YAG laser (Lee et al., 2005).

2.4 Er:YAG laser

The Er:YAG laser has a wavelength of 2.940 nm. It has a great absorption in water, theoretically 10.000 -20.000 times higher than that of CO2 and Nd:YAG lasers. Its light is well absorbed by all biological tissue that contain water molecules, so that Er:YAG laser is indicated not only for soft tissues but also for ablation of hard tissues (Aoki et al., 2004). In dental hard tissues the Er:YAG laser is absorbed by intrinsic water in apatite crystals and by OH group of the mineral apatite. So, Er:YAG laser has been used in a free-running pulse mode for caries removal and cavity preparation (Cozean et al., 1997).

Er:YAG laser was first approved for cavity preparation, and in 1999 it was accepted for soft tissue surgery, sulcular debridement and finally for osseous surgery. The huge absorption by water minimize, in fact, the thermal effect on surrounding tissues during irradiation, with a very thin penetration in soft tissues (10-50 μm) and only some degrees of heating in hard tissue. Because of the very low water content of hard tissues, since the Er:YAG laser emits in the infrared spectrum, some water coolant is advisable to reduce heat generation and absorb excessive laser energy (Burkes et al., 1992).

During Er:YAG laser irradiation, the laser energy is absorbed selectively by water molecules and hydrous organic components of biological tissues, causing evaporation of water by a "photothermal evaporation". Moreover, in hard tissue procedures, the water vapour production induces an increase of internal pressure within the tissue, resulting in an explosive expansion called "microexplosion" (Aiko et al., 2004) principle because of hard tissue ablation. The absorption of the Er:YAG laser by inorganic components (Hydroxyapatite) is however much lower than that of the CO2 laser, so that the absorption in water and in organic compounds with a water content is fast and occurs before heat accumulation into inorganic compounds. For these characteristics, Er:YAG laser received much attention by researcher both for soft tissue and for hard tissue applications.

2.4.1 Periodontal applications of Er:YAG laser

The ability of Er:YAG laser to remove subgingival dental calculus has already been shown in in vitro studies (Aoki et al., 1994; Aoki et al. ,2000; Folcwaczny et al.,2000; Frentzen et al., 2002). In 1994 Aoki et al. first documented the capacity of Er:YAG laser to remove dental calculus in an in vitro study, using a pulsed mode under irrigation. The laser was set at 30 mJ/pulse (energy density of single pulse at the tip:10.6 J/cm^2 per pulse) and 10 Hz, in the contact mode, directed perpendicular to the root surface using a conventional 600μm tip. The ablation of cementum was of little substance and the rise in pulpal temperature moderate. Stock et al. (1996) introduced a new tip, a chisel tip, suitable for root surface treatment within periodontal pockets. The authors utilized the tip with a power of 120 mJ/pulse (8 J/cm^2 per pulse) and 15 Hz with water spray and an angulation of the tip of 20° to the root surface, reporting that only smooth ablation traces were visible in the cementum. The calculus was completely removed without thermal change of the root surface. Aoki et al. (1994) evaluated the effectiveness of Er:YAG laser compared to conventional ultrasonic scaling. The panel set was 40 mJ/pulse (14.2 J/cm^2 per pulse) and 10 Hz with water spray using a conventional tip at 30° to the root surface. The level of calculus removal by laser was similar to that with ultrasonic scaling, although the laser was slightly less efficient. The depth of cementum removal varies between 15 and 150 μm depending on the output power. At a power up to 100 mJ/pulse (12.2 J/cm^2 per pulse) the root substance removal is similar to that with curettes and a selective calculus removal can be feasible using lower radiation energies (Aoki et al. 2000).

Thus, the Er:YAG laser does not accomplish selective ablation of dental calculus in vitro, as the tissue underlying dental calculus is also removed. However, for a safe but effective clinical use, a combination of a higher pulse repetition rate and a lower energy output is recommended to obtain a smooth root surface with less tissue removal.

On the contrary, supragingival scaling on enamel is contraindicated, since complete calculus removal occurs with a certain removal of enamel too, and this fact has no positive relevance compared to the removal of a thin layer of contaminated cementum.

Er:YAG laser does not cause carbonization of the irradiated root surface, that becomes chalky due to the mechanical ablation. In particular the layer just beneath the ablated cementum reveals more structural changes and damages, with microstructural degradation and thermal denaturation. The use of a water coolant results in less damage and a cleaner surface (Aoki et al. 2004). On periodontal diseased root, the Er:YAG laser treatment shows a better attachment and a better condition for fibroblast adherence compared to a diseased root treated only by mechanical means. These better results may be due to detoxification and disinfection obtained by laser and to the absence of a smear layer on the surface.

In animal studies Er:YAG laser showed no major thermal side-effects on pulp, when used under irrigation. It may be presumed that Er:YAG laser subgingival scaling at low level energy, especially with the contact tip directed obliquely or parallel to the root surface, does not produce any major deleterious outcomes in the pulp tissue.

The Er:YAG laser offers several antimicrobial advantages over conventional mechanical scaling, due to its bactericidal effect, degradation and removal of bacterial endotoxins, ablation effects without producing a smear layer (Aiko et al. 2004). Ando et al. (1996) observed a bactericidal effect against *P. gingivalis* and *A. actinomycetemcomitans* even at low energy level (Ando et al. 1996). Moreover, the wavelength of Er:YAG laser correspond to the peak of absorbance of bacterial lipopolysaccharide, so that the Er:YAG laser can effectively and rapidly remove most of the lipopolysaccharide that coat the teeth (Yamaguchi et al.,1997).

Based on the results of several in vitro studies, a clinical phase of controlling the effects of Er:YAG laser started in 1996 by Watanabe et al. (1996). The laser scaling was performed with a panel set of 40 mJ/pulse (11.3 J/cm^2 per pulse) at 10 Hz using a straight contact tip of 600 μm. According to authors 95% of calculus was removed, with only some irregularity left on tooth surface. More recently, Schwarz et al. (2001) reported a split mouth study comparing the effects of conventional scaling and root planing with two different laser tips. Periodontal pockets were treated under anaesthesia with hand instruments or one of the two tips, in an angulation of 15-20° to the root surface. Laser setting was 160 mJ/pulse with an energy density of 18.8 J/cm^2 or 14.5 J/cm^2 according to the tip. Laser treatment required less time than scaling and root planing, with similar or better results in terms of periodontal parameters (reduction of pockets, reduction of bleeding on probing, gain of attachment level). Laser advantage was higher in deep pockets and the clinical attachment gain obtained by laser was stable for 2 years.

Schwarz et al. (2001) showed that the clinical use of Er:YAG laser resulted in a smooth root surface, favourable for new attachment. However, histological studies have not been performed yet.

For clinical application the Er:YAG laser has some limitations that have to be taken into account. When used subgingivally, with a water coolant, it causes a splash of water and blood from pockets as the result of explosive ablation and so it requires an extraoral apparatus for high speed evacuation. Moreover, in periodontal pockets, the operator cannot see the calculus and the irradiated surface. Recently as a novel application of laser, the use of diode fluorescence spectroscopy for detection of dental calculus has been suggested by Hibst et al. (2001) and Keller et al. (2001).

In summary, in vitro and in vivo researches indicated the safety and effectiveness of clinical application of the Er:YAG laser for periodontal pocket treatment. However, the energy set, the energy output, the energy at the tip, the shape of the tip, the contact mode are key factors to obtain a satisfying clinical result. More studies are needed to design protocols of employment, however Er:YAG laser can be considered a promising adjunctive or alternative method for non surgical periodontal therapy.

2.5 Diode lasers

These lasers are a group of laser operating by a solid-state semiconductor, among which the most commonly used are the Gallium-aluminium-arsenide (GaAlAs) laser with a wavelength of 810 nm, and the indium-gallium-arsenide-phosphide (InGaAsP) laser at 980 nm of wavelength. The laser is emitted in continuous-wave mode and gated-pulsed mode using a flexible fiber optic delivery system (Figure 5).

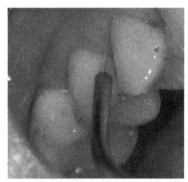

Fig. 5. The diode laser fiber in clinical use in a pocket of a patient with chronic periodontitis.

Laser light at 800-980 nm is very poorly absorbed by water and by hard tissues, being highly absorbed by haemoglobin and pigments. The diode laser is indicated for soft tissue surgery and for curettage. The diode laser exhibits a great thermal effect at the tip, caused by heat accumulation and produces a very good haemostasis, with an effect similar to electrocauterization (ALD, 2000).

The very user-friendly hand-piece and the low cost of the unit, would make it suitable for periodontal pocket therapy, however the features of the laser light are more indicated for sulcular debridement.

2.5.1 Periodontal applications of diode lasers

The diode laser used on the root surface after scaling and root planing with curettes, showed no alteration on the root microstructure and the periodontal ligament cells attached on the treated roots as on the control roots which were unirradiated (Kreisler et al., 2001). However if the root was covered by blood, the roots were altered by laser irradiation with severe damages till carbonization. Temperature elevation was time and energy-dependant. The diode laser irradiation may jeopardize pulp vitality during root surface instrumentation.

Schwarz et al. (2003) performed in vivo on hopeless roots, a GaAlAs diode laser treatment (810 nm wavelength). They reported that diode laser was ineffective in removing calculus and altered the root in an unfavourable way. However, given the recommended parameters, the possibility of inducing root surface damages is virtually absent (Cobb et al. 2010).

Some studies demonstrated that diode laser is effective in bacterial elimination, resulting in a better healing. Moritz et al. (1997) showed a significant reduction of bacteria, as *A. actynomicetemcomitans*, with a parallel improvement of periodontal parameters. Caruso et al. (2008) compared the effectiveness of a diode laser (980 nm wavelength) used as an adjunct to SRP to SRP alone, with a power output of 2.5 W in a pulse mode (30 Hz) and a tip (400 µm) angulated at 20°. Findings indicated a slightly better periodontal healing, in terms of clinical parameters at 4, 8 and 12 weeks. However, the microbiological parameters revealed no differences between groups, showing no additional benefit of diode laser on the treated pockets.

Most recently, 655 nm InGaAsP (indium gallium arsenide phosphate) diode laser radiation has been included in an Er:YAG laser device to induce fluorescence in subgingival calculus (Folwaczny et al. 2002, Krause et al. 2003). Preliminary clinical and histological results have shown that fluorescence- controlled (feedback system) Er:YAG laser radiation enabled an effective removal of subgingival calculus and a predictable root surface preservation in comparison with hand instruments (Schwarz et al. 2006, Krause et al. 2007).

In recent years, it has also been suggested that GaAlAs radiation within the milliwatt range, referred to as "low-level laser therapy", may have a positive influence on the proliferation of gingival fibroblasts or periodontal ligament fibroblasts, thus supporting periodontal wound healing (Khadra et al. 2005)

2.6 Argon laser

The argon laser operates at a wavelength of 488 nm (blue) and 514 nm (blue-green). It is poorly absorbed by water so that it is not indicated for hard tissue treatments. It is well absorbed in pigmented tissues, including haemoglobin and melanin, and in pigmented bacteria. Thanks to this characteristic the argon laser was clinically studied to test its effect on pigmented bacteria in periodontal pockets in combination with mechanical root planing (Finkbeiner 1995). The author reported a significant pocket reduction. Considering the advantages of eradication of pigmented bacteria, this laser may be useful for the treatment of periodontal pockets, requiring, however, further studies.

2.7 Alexandrite laser

In 1995 Rechmann & Henning assumed that the wavelength of alexandrite laser (337nm) may be favourable for selective calculus ablation, basing the theory on the difference in spectral region of fluorescence emission from dentin and that from subgingival calculus. Their study revealed that the alexandrite laser at the power of 1 J/cm^2 of pulse and pulse repetition of 55Hz under water cooling, could selectively ablate dental calculus, supra and sub-gingivally, as well as dental plaque. The laser has a wavelength in the spectrum of ultraviolet and does not produce any damage or effect on enamel or cementum. The development of this laser is widely expected in relation to its capability of being selective, however, there is a main concern regarding the use of ultraviolet light and further studies are needed to demonstrate the safety and effectiveness of this laser.

3. Photodynamic laser therapy

Photodynamic therapy (PDT) is a minimally invasive process that utilizes photosensitizing drugs (photosensitizers), which, when administered systemically or locally to a patient, may be selectively retained by diseased tissues preferentially over normal healthy tissues. These drugs can be activated by intense and wavelength-specific light to achieve selective photochemical destruction of diseased cells, by the generation of a reaction that produces singlet oxygen and free radicals with a subsequent cytotoxic and vasculotoxic effect. Due to the highly reactive nature of radicals formed trough the process, activity is confined to their immediate environment. Thus activity is selective and dependent on the delivery of the photosensitizer to the target (Nastri et al., 2010). Theoretically, neither the photosensitizer nor light alone can induce an efficient cytotoxic effect on the cells. The light that activates the photosensitizer must be of a specific wavelength with a relatively high intensity. With the discovery of lasers that are collimated, coherent and monochromatic, the process became more specific and it was possible to use intensive light with low-level energy.

Depending on the type of drug, photosensitizer may be injected intravenously, ingested orally, or applied topically. Currently, PDT has been approved in many countries for clinical uses, mostly for the treatment of cancer (Meisel & Kocher, 2005).

Several studies have shown that PDT has also antimicrobial properties (Photodynamic Antimicrobial Therapy).

The human tissue efficiently transmits the red light and a wider wavelength activation photosensitising results in a deeper penetration of light. Most of the photosensitizers are activated by red light between 630 nm and 700 nm, corresponding to a depth of penetration of light by 0.5 cm (630 nm) to 1.5 cm (about 700 nm). This limits the degree of necrosis or apoptosis, and defines the therapeutic effect. While not every district in the human body is accessible to light, the periodontal pockets are easily exposed by using particular hand piece and the PDT could be effective.

Various photoactive compounds, natural and synthetic, have a photosensitising potential; they include degradation products of chlorophyll polyacetilen, thiophene (Meisel & Kocher, 2005).

In antimicrobial photodynamic therapy, the particular photosensitizers are toluidine blue O, methylene blue, erithrosine, povidone-iodine, which have been shown to be safe when employed in the medical field and are effective in both gram+ and gram- bacteria. As a light source, the diode lasers are the light source predominantly applied.

Nastri et al.(2010) presented a research with the aim of evaluating the bactericidal *in vitro* effect of laser diodes 830 nm (as the light source) after photosensitization with Toluidine Blue (TBO), on periopathogenic bacteria as *Aggregatibacter actinomycetemcomitans, Porphyromonas gingivalis, Fusobacterium nucleatum* and *Prevotella intermedia*. After evaluating the effect on the single bacterial strain, authors also evaluated the ability of Diode Laser to disrupt the structure of biofilms produced by *A. actinomycetemcomitans* after photosensitization with TBO.

The study suggested that the association of TBO and diode laser light 830 nm was effective for the killing of both the main periopathogenic species alone (*Aggregatibacter actinomycetemcomitans, Prevotella intermedia, Porphyromonas gingivalis, Fusobacterium nucleatum*) and biofilms.

In a recent split-mouth study, it was demonstrated that non surgical periodontal treatment performed on patients with aggressive periodontitis, by applying photodynamic therapy alone, showed clinical improvements similar to that of conventional scaling and root planing (De oliveira et al., 2007). Also, it has been demonstrated that scaling and root planing combined with photo disinfection, or the application of photodynamic therapy alone, leads to reduction of pocket depth and clinical attachment gain (Andersen et al., 2007).

Braun et al. (2008) evaluated the effect of adjunctive antimicrobial photodynamic therapy (methylene blue + 100 mW diode laser) in chronic periodontitis using a split mouth design. After 3 months of healing, the adjunctive use of photodynamic therapy resulted in a significant higher change in mean relative attachment level, probing pocket depth, sulcus fluid flow rate and bleeding on probing at the sites receiving PDT than the control sites.

Taken together, the few data available from controlled studies suggest that in patients with chronic periodontitis, the adjunctive use of PDT to scaling and root planing may result in higher reductions in bleeding on probing, probing depth and higher CAL gain on a short term basis (3 to 6 months).

Therefore, photodynamic therapy as a low-level therapy, using a diode laser with short irradiation time, is considered not to produce side effects, like thermal changes, injuries to gingival or pulp tissues and to the intact periodontal apparatus at the basis of the pocket. Nevertheless, it is important to remind that the dye itself can be cytotoxic and that it remains in the pocket, potentially interfering with periodontal reattachment and compromise patients aesthetics by producing temporary pigmentation of the periodontal tissue (Takasaki et al., 2009). In addition it has to be clarified if selective killing of periodontopathogens by antimicrobial photodynamic therapy really occurs without affecting the normal oral microflora. However, it is still not known how many applications of PDT are necessary to completely eliminate bacteria and to prevent recolonization.

New basic and controlled clinical studies are needed to clarify the advantages or the limits of PDT, if it has to become widely applied in clinical practice. However, there can be several indications for PDT, as an adjunctive therapy to mechanical periodontal treatment, during surgical therapy or during maintenance.

4. Advantages of lasers

Irradiation shows a great power of ablation, haemostasis, detoxification and bactericidal effects. These features could potentially be a tool for periodontal therapy, especially for cutting of soft tissues as in the debridement of diseased tissue, in this sense being the laser an adjunctive therapy to mechanical approaches. However, laser showed strong thermal effects, causing melting, carbonization and cracking of hard tissues, such as root and bone (Ishikawa et al. 2009).

The recently developed Er:YAG and Er,Cr:YSGG lasers, can ablate both soft and hard tissues and are applicable with water irrigation to a safe periodontal therapy such as scaling and root planing, even in an alternative, unique treatment. These lasers may be capable of effective removing not only dental plaque but also calculus from the root surface, with extremely low mechanical stress and no formation of smear layer on the treated root surface.

Furthermore, potential biostimulation effects of scattering and penetrating lasers on the cells surrounding the irradiated tissues may be helpful for reduction of inflammation and healing of periodontal tissues.

Moreover, considering that most periodontopathogens have the capability of soft tissue invasion, not only debridement of the root surface but also removal of the epithelium lining and granulation tissue of the gingival wall within the pocket, could be important factors in the treatment of moderate to deep pockets in order to promote reattachment (Aoki et al. 2004). This may be particularly important for non healed pockets or for recurrent acute phase in residual pockets.

5. Disadvantages of lasers

Although the use of lasers for subgingival curettage and calculus removal in the treatment of periodontal pockets has been increasing among practioners, the scientific studies indicating positive results of laser are still insufficient. The use of lasers in a safe mode during routine clinic is still far to become a reality. The clinician should have a precise knowledge of characteristics and effects, of risks and disadvantages of each type of laser before using one of them for a certain clinical procedure. It has also to be reminded that different lasers have different characteristics and are not useful for everything. Due to the high cost of each apparatus, it is very difficult to have all the different lasers indicated for different procedures in a private practice

Improper irradiation of teeth and periodontal pockets by lasers can damage the tooth and root surface as well as the attachment at the base of the pockets. Possible damages to underlying bone and pulp are also to be considered. The risk of thermal injuries has always to be considered, as explained before, and the set of the laser power always accurately chosen in order to provide the less risk of damage to bone, root, pulp and surrounding tissues.

Lasers are completely different from conventional mechanical therapy because they exert their effects not only in a contact mode but also at distance. Inadvertent irradiation of patient's eyes or tissue outside the target must be strictly prevented. It is necessary that patient, operator and assistant wear special glasses to protect for the wavelength of the laser that has to be used. Use of wet gauze packs may be occasionally useful for protection of the surrounding tissues from accidental beam impact.

Furthermore, high speed evacuation systems are required to capture the water and blood vaporization produced by laser light and development of new apparatus with little hand pieces and thin tips, useful in periodontal pockets, is still at work.

6. Conclusions

Laser periodontal treatment for periodontitis is being receiving much attention both from researchers and clinicians. At the present state, there is a great need to develop an evidence-based approach to the study of lasers. The different studies and clinical application, even if performed with the same wavelength, may be different in several other set parameters, making it very difficult to compare the lasers and the gold standard of periodontal therapy: mechanical scaling and root planing. If CAL gain is the main parameter of success in periodontal non surgical therapy, there is scarce evidence that laser therapy can be superior to conventional treatment. Moreover, the evidence of some additional benefits coming from laser therapy as an adjunctive treatment to conventional mechanical treatment is minimal.

In conclusion, the use of lasers still requires many studies to become a routine therapy with the same advantages and low risks of conventional periodontal therapy. The most promising one is Er:YAG laser for its ability of calculus removing and with a relatively safe modality of use under water cooling. However, the high cost and the little demonstration of real superiority to conventional therapy is still a refrain. The perfect wavelength, power set and tip have not been studied yet. A reliable procedure for laser application in non surgical periodontal therapy should be established by further studies, and clinicians should have the precise knowledge of the potential benefits or damages before using this relatively new instruments, which are still under debate.

In summary, the use of lasers to debride root surface is in its infancy. They showed several positive effects, due to their characteristics of working in a noncontact mode, useful for very deep pockets and furcations, of bacterial detoxification and decontamination, to be more patient –tolerated etc. However, lasers show a history of significant side-effects, that should at least induce caution for their safe use.

7. References

AAP (The American Academy of Periodontology). (2002)The Research, Science and Therapy Committee of the American Academy of Periodontology, Cohen RE, Ammons WF. Revised by Rossman JA. Lasers in Periodontics (Academy report). J Periodontol: 73: 1231–1239.

Adriaens PA, Edwards CA, De Boever JA, Loesche WJ. (1988) Ultrastructural observations on bacterial invasion in cementum and radicular dentin of periodontally diseased human teeth. J Periodontol: 59: 493–503.

ALD (The Academy of Laser Dentistry). (2000) Featured wavelength: diode – the diode laser in dentistry (Academy report) Wavelengths: 8: 13

Andersen R, Loebel N, Hammond D, Wilson M. (2007) Treatment of periodontal disease by photodisinfection compared to scaling and root planing. J Clin Dent: 18: 34–38

Ando Y, Aoki A, Watanabe H, Ishikawa I (1996). Bactericidal effect of erbium YAG laser on periodontopathic bacteria. Lasers Surg Med: 19: 190–200.

Aoki A, Ando Y, Watanabe H, Ishikawa I. (1994) In vitro studies on laser scaling of subgingival calculus with an erbium: YAG laser. J Periodontol: 65: 1097-1106

Aoki A, Miura M, Akiyama F, Nakagawa N, Tanaka J, Oda S, Watanabe H, Ishikawa I. (2000) In vitro evaluation of Er:YAG laser scaling of subgingival calculus in comparison with ultrasonic scaling. J Periodontal Res: 35: 266-277.

Aoki A, Sasaki KM, Watanabe H, Ishikawa I. (2004) Lasers in nonsurgical periodontal therapy. Periodontol 2000: 36: 59-97.

Barone A, Covani U, Crespi R, Romanos GE. (2002) Root surface morphological changes after focused versus defocused CO2 laser irradiation: a scanning electron microscopy analysis. J Periodontol: 73: 370-373.

Braun A, Dehn C, Krause F, Jepsen S. (2008) Short-term clinical effects of adjunctive antimicrobial photodynamic therapy in periodontal treatment: a randomized clinical trial. J Clin Periodontol: 35: 877-884.

Burkes EJ Jr, Hoke J, Gomes E, Wolbarsht M. (1992) Wet versus dry enamel ablation by Er:YAG laser. J Prosthet Dent. 67: 847-851

Caruso U, Nastri L, Piccolomini R, d'Ercole S, Mazza C, Guida L. (2008) Use of diode laser 980 nm as adjunctive therapy in the treatment of chronic periodontitis. A randomized controlled clinical trial. New Microbiol. Oct;31(4):513-8.

Centty IG, Blank LW, Levy BA, Romberg E, Barnes DM. (1997)Carbon dioxide laser for de-epithelialization of periodontal flaps. J Periodontol: 68: 763-769.

Cobb CM, Low SB, Coluzzi DJ. (2010) Lasers and the treatment of chronic periodontitis. Dent Clin North Am. Jan;54(1):35-53

Cozean C, Arcoria CJ, Pelagalli J, Powell GL. (1997) Dentistry for the 21st century? Erbium:YAG laser for teeth. J Am Dent Assoc: 128: 1080-1087.

Crespi R, Barone A, Covani U, Ciaglia RN, Romanos GE. (2002) Effects of CO2 laser treatment on fibroblast attachment to root surfaces. A scanning electron microscopy analysis. J Periodontol: 73: 1308-1312.

de Oliveira RR, Schwartz-Filho HO, Novaes AB Jr, Taba M Jr. (2007) Antimicrobial photodynamic therapy in the non-surgical treatment of aggressive periodontitis: a preliminary randomized controlled clinical study. J Periodontol: 78: 965-973.

Deo V, Bhongade ML (2010) Pathogenesis of periodontitis: role of cytokines in host response Dent Today. Sep;29(9):60-2, 64-6

Featherstone JDB. (2000) Caries detection and prevention with laser energy. Dent Clin North Am: 44: 955-969.

Finkbeiner RL. (1995) The results of 1328 periodontal pockets treated with the argon laser: selective pocket thermolysis. J Clin Laser Med Surg: 13: 273-281

Folwaczny M, Mehl A, Haffner C, Benz C, Hickel R. (2000) Root substance removal with Er:YAG laser radiation at different parameters using a new delivery system. J Periodontol: 71: 147-155.

Folwaczny, M., Heym, R., Mehl, A. & Hickel, R. (2002) Subgingival calculus detection with fluorescence induced by 655nm InGaAsP diode laser radiation. Journal of Periodontology 73, 597-601.

Frentzen M, Braun A, Aniol D. (2002)Er:YAG laser scaling of diseased root surfaces. J Periodontol: 73: 524-530.

Goldman L, Hornby P, Meyer R, Goldman B. (1964) Impact of the laser on dental caries. Nature: 25: 417.

Hibst R, Paulus R, Lussi A. (2001) Detection of occlusal caries by laser fluorescence: basic and clinical investigations. Med Laser Appl: 16: 205-213.

Ishikawa I, Aoki A, Takasaki AA, Mizutani K, Sasaki KM, Izumi Y. (2009) Application of lasers in periodontics – True Innovation or Myth? Periodontol 2000: 50: 90–126.

Karlsson MR, Diogo Löfgren CI, Jansson HM. (2008) The effect of laser therapy as an adjunct to non-surgical periodontal treatment in subjects with chronic periodontitis: a systematic review. J Periodontol. Nov;79(11):2021-8

Kayano T, Ochiai S, Kiyono K, Yamamoto H, Nakajima S, Mochizuki T. (1991) Effect of Er:YAG laser irradiation on human extracted teeth. J Clin Laser Med Surg: 9: 147–150.

Keller U, Hibst R. (1989) Experimental studies of the application of the Er:YAG laser on dental hard substances. II. Light microscopic and SEM investigations. Lasers Surg Med: 9: 345–351.

Keller U, Hibst R. (1991) Tooth pulp reaction following Er:YAG laser application. Proc SPIE: 1424: 127–133

Khadra M, Kasem N, Lyngstadaas SP, Haanaes HR, Mustafa K. (2005) Laser therapy accelerates initial attachment and subsequent behaviour of human oral fibroblasts cultured on titanium implant material. A scanning electron microscope and histomorphometric analysis. Clin Oral Implants Res: 16: 168–175.

Kinane DF. (2001) Causation and pathogenesis of periodontal disease. Periodontol 2000.;25:8-20

Kinane DF, Attstrom R, European Workshop in Periodontology group B. (2005) Advances in the pathogenesis of periodontitis. Group B consensus report of the fifth European Workshop in Periodontology. J Clin Periodontol; 32(Suppl. 6):130-131.

Krause, F., Braun, A. & Frentzen, M. (2003) The possibility of detecting subgingival calculus by laser-fluorescence in vitro. Lasers in Medical Science 18, 32–35.

Krause, F., Braun, A., Brede, O., Eberhard, J., Frentzen, M. & Jepsen, S. (2007) Evaluation of selective calculus removal by a fluorescence feedback-controlled Er:YAG laser in vitro. Journal of Clinical Periodontology 34, 66–71.

Kreisler M, Meyer C, Stender E, Daubla¨nder M, Willershausen Zo¨nnchen B, d'Hoedt B. (2001) Effect of diode laser irradiation on the attachment rate of periodontal ligament cells: an in vitro study. J Periodontol: 72: 1312–1317

Lee BS, Chang CW, Chen WP, Lan WH, Lin CP. (2005) In vitro study of dentin hypersensitivity treated by Nd:YAP laser and bioglass. Dent Mater: 21: 511–519.

Lui J, Corbet EF, Jin L. (2011) Combined photodynamic and low-level laser therapies as an adjunct to nonsurgical treatment of chronic periodontitis. J Periodontal Res. Feb;46(1):89-96

Maiman TH. (1960) Stimulated optical radiation in ruby. Nature: 187: 493–494.

Meisel P, Kocher T. (2005) Photodynamic therapy for periodontal diseases: state of the art. J Photochem Photobiol B. May 13;79(2):159-70

Miyazaki A, Yamaguchi T, Nishikata J, Okuda K, Suda S, Orima K, Kobayashi T, Yamazaki K, Yoshikawa E, Yoshie H. (2003)Effects of Nd:YAG and CO2 laser treatment and ultrasonic scaling on periodontal pockets of chronic periodontitis patients. J Periodontol: 74: 175–180.

Moritz A, Gutknecht N, Doertbudak O, Goharkhay K, Schoop U, Schauer P, Sperr W. (1997) Bacterial reduction in periodontal pockets through irradiation with a diode laser: a pilot study. J Clin Laser Med Surg: 15: 33–37

Morlock BJ, Pippin DJ, Cobb CM, Killoy WJ, Rapley JW. (1992)The effect of Nd:YAG laser exposure on root surfaces when used as an adjunct to root planing: an in vitro study. J Periodontol: 63: 637–641

Mullins SL, MacNeill SR, Rapley JW, Williams KB, Eick JD, Cobb CM. (2007) Subgingival microbiologic effects of one-time irradiation by CO2 laser: a pilot study. J Periodontol: 78: 2331-2337.

Nastri L, Donnarumma G, Porzio C, De Gregorio V, Tufano MA, Caruso F, Mazza C, Serpico R. (2010) Effects of toluidine blue-mediated photodynamic therapy on periopathogens and periodontal biofilm: in vitro evaluation. Int J Immunopathol Pharmacol. Oct-Dec;23(4):1125-32

Offenbacher S. (1996) Periodontal diseases: Pathogenesis.Ann Periodontol;1:821-878

Pick RM, Pecaro BC, Silberman CJ. (1985)The laser gingivectomy. The use of the CO2 laser for the removal of phenytoin hyperplasia. J Periodontol: 56: 492-496.

Quirynen M, Teughels W, van Steenberghe D. (2003) Microbial shifts after subgingival debridement and formation of bacterial resistance when combined with local or systemic antimicrobials. Oral Dis.;9 Suppl 1:30-7

Rechmann P, Henning T. (1995) Selective ablation of sub- and supragingival calculus with a frequency-doubled Alexandrite laser. Proc SPIE: 2394: 203-210

Rodrigues RM, Gonçalves C, Souto R, Feres-Filho EJ, Uzeda M, Colombo AP. (2004) Antibiotic resistance profile of the subgingival microbiota following systemic or local tetracycline therapy. J Clin Periodontol. Jun;31(6):420-7

Schwarz F, Putz N, Georg T, Reich E. (2001) Effect of an Er:YAG laser on periodontally involved root surfaces: an in vivo and in vitro SEM comparison. Lasers Surg Med: 29: 328-335.

Schwarz F, Sculean A, Berakdar M, Georg T, Becker J. (2003) In vivo and in vitro effects of an Er:YAG laser, a GaAlAs diode laser and scaling and root planing on periodontally diseased root surfaces. A comparative histologic study. Lasers Surg Med: 32: 359-366.

Schwarz F, Sculean A, Georg T, Reich E. (2001) Periodontal treatment with an Er:YAG laser compared to scaling and root planing. A controlled clinical study. J Periodontol: 72: 361-367.

Schwarz, F., Bieling, K., Venghaus, S., Sculean, A., Jepsen, S. & Becker, J. (2006) Influence of fluorescence-controlled Er:YAG laser radiation, the Vector system and hand instruments on periodontally diseased root surfaces in vivo. Journal of Clinical Periodontology 33, 200-208.

Sigusch BW, Engelbrecht M, Völpel A, Holletschke A, Pfister W, Schütze J. (2010) Full-mouth antimicrobial photodynamic therapy in Fusobacterium nucleatum-infected periodontitis patients. J Periodontol. Jul;81(7):975-81

Stock K, Hibst R, Keller U. (1996)Er:YAG removal of subgingival calculi: efficiency, temperature and surface quality. Proc SPIE: 2922: 98-106.

Takasaki AA, Aoki A, Mizutani K, Schwarz F, Sculean A, Wang CY, Koshy G, Romanos G, Ishikawa I, Izumi Y. (2009) Application of antimicrobial photodynamic therapy in periodontal and peri-implant diseases. Periodontol 2000.;51:109-40

Tseng P, Liew V. (1990)The potential applications of a Nd:YAG dental laser in periodontal treatment. Periodontology (Australia): 11: 20-22.

Watanabe H, Ishikawa I, Suzuki M, Hasegawa K. (1996) Clinical assessments of the erbium:YAG laser for soft tissue surgery and scaling. J Clin Laser Med Surg: 14: 67-75

Yamaguchi H, Kobayashi K, Osada R, Sakuraba E, Nomura T, Arai T, Nakamura J. (1997) Effects of irradiation of an erbium:YAG laser on root surfaces. J Periodontol: 68: 1151- 1155

Permissions

The contributors of this book come from diverse backgrounds, making this book a truly international effort. This book will bring forth new frontiers with its revolutionizing research information and detailed analysis of the nascent developments around the world.

We would like to thank Dr. Nurcan Buduneli, for lending her expertise to make the book truly unique. She has played a crucial role in the development of this book. Without her invaluable contribution this book wouldn't have been possible. She has made vital efforts to compile up to date information on the varied aspects of this subject to make this book a valuable addition to the collection of many professionals and students.

This book was conceptualized with the vision of imparting up-to-date information and advanced data in this field. To ensure the same, a matchless editorial board was set up. Every individual on the board went through rigorous rounds of assessment to prove their worth. After which they invested a large part of their time researching and compiling the most relevant data for our readers. Conferences and sessions were held from time to time between the editorial board and the contributing authors to present the data in the most comprehensible form. The editorial team has worked tirelessly to provide valuable and valid information to help people across the globe.

Every chapter published in this book has been scrutinized by our experts. Their significance has been extensively debated. The topics covered herein carry significant findings which will fuel the growth of the discipline. They may even be implemented as practical applications or may be referred to as a beginning point for another development. Chapters in this book were first published by InTech; hereby published with permission under the Creative Commons Attribution License or equivalent.

The editorial board has been involved in producing this book since its inception. They have spent rigorous hours researching and exploring the diverse topics which have resulted in the successful publishing of this book. They have passed on their knowledge of decades through this book. To expedite this challenging task, the publisher supported the team at every step. A small team of assistant editors was also appointed to further simplify the editing procedure and attain best results for the readers.

Our editorial team has been hand-picked from every corner of the world. Their multi-ethnicity adds dynamic inputs to the discussions which result in innovative outcomes. These outcomes are then further discussed with the researchers and contributors who give their valuable feedback and opinion regarding the same. The feedback is then collaborated with the researches and they are edited in a comprehensive manner to aid the understanding of the subject.

Apart from the editorial board, the designing team has also invested a significant amount of their time in understanding the subject and creating the most relevant covers. They scrutinized every image to scout for the most suitable representation of the subject and create an appropriate cover for the book.

The publishing team has been involved in this book since its early stages. They were actively engaged in every process, be it collecting the data, connecting with the contributors or procuring relevant information. The team has been an ardent support to the editorial, designing and production team. Their endless efforts to recruit the best for this project, has resulted in the accomplishment of this book. They are a veteran in the field of academics and their pool of knowledge is as vast as their experience in printing. Their expertise and guidance has proved useful at every step. Their uncompromising quality standards have made this book an exceptional effort. Their encouragement from time to time has been an inspiration for everyone.

The publisher and the editorial board hope that this book will prove to be a valuable piece of knowledge for researchers, students, practitioners and scholars across the globe.

List of Contributors

Timo Sorsa and Taina Tervahartiala
Department of Oral and Maxillofacial Diseases, Helsinki University Central Hospital, Finland
Institute of Dentistry, University of Helsinki, Helsinki, Finland

Jorge Gamonal and Rolando Vernal
Laboratory of Periodontal Biology, Faculty of Dentistry, University of Chile, Chile

Päivi Mäntylä
Institute of Dentistry, University of Helsinki, Helsinki, Finland

Marcela Hernández
Laboratory of Periodontal Biology, Faculty of Dentistry, University of Chile, Chile
Department of Pathology, Faculty of Dentistry, University of Chile, Chile

Shigenobu Kimura, Yu Shimoyama, Taichi Ishikawa and Minoru Sasaki
Iwate Medical University, Japan

Yuko Ohara-Nemoto
Nagasaki University Graduate School of Biomedical Sciences, Japan

Takeshi Yamanaka, Kazuyoshi Yamane, Chiho Mashimo, Takayuki Nambu, Hugo Maruyama and Hisanori Fukushima
Osaka Dental University, Japan

Kai-Poon Leung
US Army Dental and Trauma Research Detachment, Institute of Surgical Research, USA

Catalina Pisoschi, Camelia Stanciulescu and Monica Banita
University of Medicine and Pharmacy, Craiova, Romania

Nurcan Buduneli
Department of Periodontology, School of Dentistry, Ege University, İzmir, Turkey

Maria Grazia Cifone, Annalisa Monaco, Davide Pietropaoli, Rita Del Pinto and Mario Giannoni
University of L'Aquila – Department of Health Sciences, San Salvatore Hospital Building Delta 6 – 67100 - L'Aquila, Italy

Jae Hyun Park, Kiyoshi Tai, John Morris and Dorotea Modrin
Arizona School of Dentistry & Oral Health, A. T. Still University, U.S.A.

Tetsutaro Yamaguchi, Yoko Tomoyasu, and Koutaro Maki
Department of Orthodontics, Showa University School of Dentistry, Tokyo, Japan

Kazushige Suzuki and Matsuo Yamamoto
Department of Periodontology, Showa University School of Dentistry, Tokyo, Japan

Naoki Kakudate
Department of Epidemiology and Healthcare Research, Kyoto University School of Medicine and Public Health, Japan

Manabu Morita
Department of Oral Health, Okayama University Graduate School of Medicine, Dentistry and Pharmaceutical Sciences, Japan

Neslihan Nal Acar, Ülkü Noyan, Leyla Kuru, Tanju Kadir and Bahar Kuru
Department of Periodontology, Dental Faculty, Marmara University, İstanbul, Turkey

Ko-ichi Kawahara
Kagoshima University Graduate School of Medical and Dental Sciences, Japan
Osaka Institute of Technology, Japan

Kiyoshi Kikuchi
Yame Public General Hospital, Japan

Yoko Morimoto-Yamashita, Masayuki Tokuda, Takashi Ito, Ikuro Maruyama and Mitsuo Torii
Kagoshima University Graduate School of Medical and Dental Sciences, Japan

Livia Nastri and Ugo Caruso
Seconda Università degli Studi di Napoli - Dept. of Stomatologic, Orthodontic and Surgical Sciences, Naples, Italy

9 781632 413192